Pharmacy Practice Research Methods

D1743702

Zaheer-Ud-Din Babar

Editor

Pharmacy Practice Research Methods

Second Edition

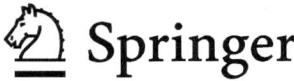 Springer

Editor
Zaheer-Ud-Din Babar
Department of Pharmacy, School of Applied Sciences
University of Huddersfield
Huddersfield
UK

ISBN 978-981-15-2995-5   ISBN 978-981-15-2993-1   (eBook)
https://doi.org/10.1007/978-981-15-2993-1

This Springer imprint is published by the registered company Springer Nature Singapore Pte Ltd.
The registered company address is: 152 Beach Road, #21-01/04 Gateway East, Singapore 189721, Singapore

To Danyal

Preface

Globally, pharmacists and pharmacies have played a central role to promote the safe and effective use of medicines. In the last 30 years or so, the "practice of pharmacy" has changed significantly, and it has also impacted and changed the way the consumers use medicines. According to an estimate, only about one-fourth of the dispensed medicines are used properly. In this context, it is vital to "understand and to perform research on the factors, behaviours, practices, and experiences of patients and consumers on the issues which influence their decisions influencing the 'use of medicines'. The data and literature suggest that valid research techniques and methods could lead to reliable findings, in turn helping to "*improve the use of medicines*".

Pharmacy practice research studies are not simple observations, and it is said that with the sound methodologies and techniques, one can come up with reliable and valid results which could significantly add to improve the "quality use of medicines". *Pharmacy Practice Research Methods* comes into play in this context, and the first edition of the book was written to highlight and showcase methodologies used in the field. There were other books on pharmacy practice research; however, the emphasis was on how to conduct a pharmacy practice research project.

Nevertheless, in this book *Pharmacy Practice Research Methods*, the focus was on techniques, the strength, and weaknesses and how these methodologies provide richness to pharmacy practice literature. This was coupled with the case studies and examples and about generating evidence and impact. In the first edition, the chapters include "evidence and impact in pharmacy practice research", "quantitative and qualitative techniques used in pharmacy practice research", "action research in pharmacy practice", "the role of pharmacoeconomics and pharmacoepidemiology", "mixed methods research", and the "future of pharmacy practice".

The current second edition updates the field with the seven new chapters including "quality improvement methods in pharmacy practice research", "covert and overt observations", "grounded theory in pharmacy practice research", "realist research", "information sources used for pharmacy practice research", "systematic reviews and meta-analysis", and "randomized controlled trials and pharmacy practice". The chapters on evidence and impact, pharmacoepidemiology, mixed methods research, action research, qualitative and quantitative techniques are written from a fresh perspective.

The book aims to strengthen this rapidly evolving field, and I hope it would be useful for students, researchers, and academics around the globe.

Brighouse, UK   Zaheer-Ud-Din Babar
19 March 2020

Contents

About the Editor

Zaheer-Ud-Din Babar is the Professor in Medicines and Healthcare and the Director of the Centre for Pharmaceutical Policy and Practice Research at the University of Huddersfield, United Kingdom. A pharmacist by training, Prof. Babar is the recipient of the prestigious "Research Excellence Award" from the University of Auckland. He understands the health and pharmacy systems and is known for his work in pharmaceutical policy and practice, including quality use of medicines, access to medicines, medicine prices and issues related to pharmacoeconomics. He has published in high impact journals such as *PLoS Medicine* and *The Lancet* and has acted as a consultant for the World Health Organization, Royal Pharmaceutical Society, Health Action International, International Union Against Tuberculosis and Lung Disease, World Bank, International Pharmaceutical Federation (FIP) and for the Pharmaceutical Management Agency of New Zealand. His edited work includes *Economic Evaluation of Pharmacy Services*, *Pharmacy Practice Research Methods*, *Global Pharmaceutical Policy Pharmaceutical Prices in the 21st Century*, *Pharmaceutical Policies in Countries with Developing Healthcare Systems*, *Equitable access to high cost medicines* and the *Encyclopedia of Pharmacy Practice and Clinical Pharmacy*. Published by Elsevier and Adis/Springer, the books are used in curriculum design, policy development and as a reference resource all around the globe. Professor Babar is the Editor-in-Chief of the BMC *Journal of Pharmaceutical Policy and Practice*.

Chapter 1
Pharmacy Practice Research: Evidence, Impact and Synthesis

Christine Bond

Abstract This chapter summarises the current challenges which exist in matching increasing demand for healthcare services to available capacity and funding. This has led to a drive to implement new services and redesign existing services in line with evidence of their clinical effectiveness and cost-effectiveness. These principles are then translated into the context of pharmacy with consideration of the quality of the evidence available for pharmacy and related medicine services. There is an examination of the interplay between practice, policy and research, and examples are given on different ways in which research can inform policy. The chapter concludes with a summary of the remaining challenges that need to be addressed to ensure that in pharmacy we can deliver an evidence-based service.

1.1 Evidence and Evidence-Based Healthcare and Service Redesign

It is important in healthcare decision-making that the treatment needs of both populations and individual patients are considered. Recommended treatments should be effective and represent good value for money. This is especially important at a time when in most of the countries in North America, Europe and Australia (that is the majority of what is known as the developed world) the demand on healthcare is increasing, and there is uncertainty how this increasing demand, and indeed need, will be met. This increase is due largely to changing demographic profiles with a greater proportion of older people living longer than was previously the case. As age increases there is an equivalent chance of poorer health and thereby requirement for treatment. There are also ongoing workforce challenges. There is further feminisation of the healthcare professional workforce, increasingly affecting medicine as well as the more traditional nursing and AHP professions which have always been dominated by the female gender. This means greater requests for career breaks for

C. Bond (✉)
Centre of Academic Primary Care, University of Aberdeen, Aberdeen, UK
e-mail: c.m.bond@abdn.ac.uk

© Springer Nature Singapore Pte Ltd. 2020
Z. Babar (ed.), *Pharmacy Practice Research Methods*,
https://doi.org/10.1007/978-981-15-2993-1_1

maternity, and increasingly paternity, leave. Further as societal norms change, there are more demands for part-time working. All of these present workforce planners with uncertainties and a need to consider developing a more flexible workforce with generic and interchangeable skills. A third factor also needs to be considered. Technological advances in treatment such as the use of robotics, artificial intelligence, pharmacogenomics and biologicals all bring their own benefits and challenges, in terms of financing and workforce capability.

All of the above represent both increased cost and opportunities for all countries, regardless of how their healthcare systems are funded—i.e. whether they have a Beveridge-based approach such as in the taxation-funded universal healthcare offered under the NHS in the UK; a Bismarck system, whereby healthcare costs are covered by third-party insurance systems, such as Germany or the USA; or a hybrid approach such as in Norway.

To ensure limited budgets are used efficiently and effectively, the central question is to identify treatments and services that are clinically effective and cost-effective. This knowledge can inform decisions, taken at both countrywide level by policymakers and at individual patient level jointly by the healthcare professional in partnership with the patient. Indeed the current drive towards more joint decision-making at patient level is driven by research findings which suggest that this leads to better clinical outcomes and more satisfied patients who are likely to adhere to treatments.

1.1.1   Multiplicity of Research

There is already much research conducted to address questions about clinically effective and cost-effective healthcare. As understanding and expertise grow in ensuring the robustness of this research, so does an awareness of the importance of involving specialist disciplines in its conduct (e.g. statisticians, health psychologists, health economists, sociologists, epidemiologists and triallists). Studies range from pharmaceutical industry pre-licensing drug studies and post-marketing surveillance, often not reported in peer-reviewed journals, through to rigorous independently conducted substantive studies. These studies may be of new approaches to delivering a service, such as prescribing by non-medical professionals or comparing an automated system with a manual one, for example, retinal screening. However not every change is always fully evaluated before it is implemented. Whilst the 'big' questions are often well researched, for example, the early studies demonstrating the value of reducing lipid levels in reducing morbidity and mortality from heart disease, some changes such as population-based public health initiatives are introduced without the underpinning research evidence. To some extent this is because the traditional 'gold standard' randomised controlled trial approach is harder to undertake in this context. Treatments for 'orphan' conditions—conditions of low prevalence—are also under-researched, although if taken together the totality of orphan diseases represent a large proportion of the healthcare workload. Therefore defining best available evidence is complex, and not always possible; the use of real-world data facilitated by the explosion in 'big data' may provide an alternative approach, and such methods are emerging as a discipline in their own right.

However even when studies are available, there remain challenges. Is there a generic way of accessing, collating, synthesising and interpreting results from the multiplicity of research reports in the peer-reviewed literature which can help 'answer' the question of finding the 'best treatment approach' for a particular population suffering a particular condition? Furthermore whilst at a first glance the published literature may seem to offer some understanding, studies often report conflicting results and may not be conducted in the exact context for which information is required. For example, do results of a study conducted in North America with a largely Caucasian population aged averagely 50 years and undertaken 10 years ago translate to a community in an area of Australia with a population of mixed ethnicity and aged over 65 years?

1.1.2 Quality of Research

The way research is conducted can also influence the bottom line as reported, potentially leading incorrect conclusions to be drawn. For example, a study conducted to explore whether taking an antidepressant relieves symptoms of depression conducted without a control group could lead to a gross overestimation of the effect of the medication, because of the now well-documented size of the placebo effect. Randomised controlled studies, regarded as the best study design, cannot however automatically always be judged as rigorous. If a study is not conducted well, its results might not be valid. For example, it is important that all participants allocated to a treatment group are analysed in that group and that those unable to be contacted for whatever reason at follow-up are classified as treatment failures. A good example of this would be in smoking cessation studies where those who are successful in stopping smoking are more likely to come back for follow-up assessment than those who have failed, leading to an overestimation of the effect of the smoking cessation intervention, be it a pharmacological or behavioural one. Therefore in deciding to what extent a single piece of research can contribute to informing policy, the study design and conduct of the study must all be critically evaluated. This is discussed in more detail below.

1.1.3 The Evidence-Based Medicines Movement

The conundrum therefore is how to develop techniques which allow the 'true' answer to the question of what is the most clinically effective and cost-effective choice to be distilled and synthesised from the published literature and then to be understood, articulated and translated into practice at the front line of service delivery.

One of the first people to think through the above issues systematically was Archie Cochrane, founder of the Cochrane Collaboration[1] and one of the fathers of evidence-based medicine. In later parts of this chapter, we will talk more specifically about evidence-based pharmacy, but for now the principles of evidence-based medicine apply equally to evidence-based pharmacy.

The classic logo of the Cochrane Collaboration[2] illustrates the dilemma that faces people trying to understand what a multiplicity of research reports tell us about a specific question. The Cochrane Collaboration logo is itself a schematic representation of one of the first questions answered by the collaboration. This was to identify the right way to manage a woman with a history of repeated premature births, to prevent this happening in subsequent pregnancies. Each of the horizontal lines in the logo represents the outcome of a trial in which pregnant women were treated with varying doses of corticosteroid and the confidence limits around the estimated odds ratio of a successful outcome. The vertical line is the line through an odds ratio of 1, namely, that there is no effect of treatment. Thus of the eight trials depicted, three show a benefit of using steroids. However the diamond at the bottom shows the overall beneficial effect of this treatment in reducing premature births when all the studies are combined as if in one big trial. In this technique now known as meta-analysis, all the individual studies are treated as one big study and one big population; increasing sample sizes in this way means the confidence interval around the estimated effect size are narrowed, and the robustness of the estimate is greater. Until this approach was understood, use of corticosteroids in pregnancy was only 20%. It steadily rose thereafter reducing rates of premature births, preventing much human suffering and reducing NHS costs.

The Cochrane Collaboration itself is now an international group of health service researchers, information scientists, statisticians and others who on a voluntary basis agree to conduct overviews of published literature to answer topical questions of relevance to healthcare providers. There are now 43 country groups and overall 11,000 members and 68,000 supporters from 130 countries (out of 195). There are 54 topic groups, ranging from Acute respiratory infection to Wounds and including condition-specific topics as well as generic topics such as public health or tobacco addiction. There are also 11 thematic fields including setting (e.g. primary care), type of consumer (e.g. children) or type of provider (e.g. nurses), but it is of relevance to this text to note that at the time of writing there is no pharmacy group, although there have been pharmacy-relevant reviews (see later). There are also 17 methods groups (e.g. adverse effects methods group, patient reported outcomes groups, statistics methods group, behaviour). The Cochrane Effective Practice and Organisation of Care group (studying the ways to encourage healthcare professionals to change their behaviour) is particularly relevant to this chapter and pharmacy, but it is hard to argue that pharmacist input would not be relevant to any of these groups.

---

[1] www.cochrane.org/ Accessed 19 Sept 2019.

[2] http://www.cochrane.org/about-us/history/our-logo Accessed 19 Sept 2019.

1.1.3.1 Systematic Reviewing and Critical Appraisal

Whilst meta-analysis is a widely accepted solution to synthesising the literature and informing policy decisions about the best treatment, as the scope of Cochrane reviews has expanded, it is realised that a statistical meta-analysis is not always possible and narrative reviews, meta-ethnography and realist reviews are all recognised approaches to synthesising and interpreting the body of literature. In addition, initial scoping reviews also have their place. Whichever approach is taken for reporting the review, it is critical, and core to the process, that all eligible studies have been systematically identified, using a precise method that can be described and replicated. This has led to an understanding of the way to search the electronic databases of published research in the topic area. Gone are the days of manually searching journals until sufficient articles had been identified which made the required point. In a systematic review, the aspiration would be to find and include all relevant papers, regardless of their final conclusion, although in practice this might be hard to achieve. Even highly skilled information scientists cannot find everything, but if there are omissions, these should be by chance and not by intent. Once papers are identified, they also have to be critically appraised. One of the issues to consider is the extent to which it is valid to combine the individual studies into one big virtual study. Are the studies similar enough in terms of characteristics of the population, the health service in which they were delivered, the co-morbidities and risk factors of the participants, the outcomes used and the follow-up period? All of this has to be taken into account when looking at the value of the final figure and its applicability to any single setting. Ideally to compare two treatments, a randomised controlled trial design should be used, to allow for the multiple confounders that might spuriously suggest a treatment will work when assessed by a simple before-and-after analysis.

1.1.3.2 Grades of Evidence

The Cochrane Collaboration have devised a set of quality rules and standards which, as far as they can, allow for the limitations in published studies to be systematically examined and reported. There are Cochrane standards for the conduct of studies of different study designs, including most recently standards for assessing qualitative research and combining the results using meta-ethnography. There are even standards for assessing systematic reviews of systematic reviews! Other organisations such as SIGN[3] and CASP[4] also have a range of similar tools. These widely accepted quality tools therefore allow a review to be judged or graded, both on the rigour of the study designs and the quality of the studies. For example, for an RCT, the Cochrane risk of bias tool assesses whether non-responders were included in the

---

[3] SIGN https://sign.ac.uk Accessed 1 Oct 2019.

[4] CASP https://casp-uk.net Accessed 1 Oct 2019.

follow-up, was an intention to treat analysis undertaken and were the assessors blind to group allocation.

Having assessed the quality of the identified literature, there are further decisions to be made. Should poor quality papers be excluded from final analyses? What is the cut-off to define 'poor'? Are there critical elements that must be met? What happens if there are no 'good' studies published on the topic of interest? Recent work has shown that studies related to pharmacy rarely meet all the requisite criteria and areas poorly conducted were mostly associated with randomisation, allocation concealment and blinding (Ritchie et al. 2019).

Amongst individual study designs, randomised controlled trials are the gold standard, followed by controlled trials, cohort studies, case studies and case reports. Both quality and study design can then be taken into account when assessing the importance which can be attributed to the bottom-line finding. Some of this decision-making is formalised in tools such as GRADE (Guyatt et al. 2008) which is a transparent simple system that classifies the quality of evidence as high, moderate, low and very low and allows recommendations based on the review to be categorised as strong or weak.

When undertaking a systematic review and reading an individual paper, it is sometimes hard to find information to know how to judge an item in the quality tool. To encourage better reporting, and ultimately better conduct of studies, the EQUATOR[5] network lists reporting guidelines for a multiplicity of research designs—the best known of which is the CONSORT[6] guideline for reporting an RCT.

1.1.4   Using Evidence to Influence Practice

Since the founding of the Cochrane Collaboration, the model of systematic reviewing and critical appraisal of the existing research has become the accepted approach to inform healthcare decision-making, and 'an evidence-based service' has become the mantra. Whilst the Cochrane Collaboration is an international movement and reviews are driven by researcher-led groups, individual countries have realised the need to develop their own organisations to undertake such reviews, answering questions driven by national priorities.

So, for example, in England and Wales, NICE (National Institute for Health and Care Excellence formally National Institute for Clinical Excellence)[7] was established in 1999. NICE undertakes and commissions reviews of the evidence for health and social care. Originally most activity was focussed on synthesising the evidence for choice of pharmacological agent, for example, should a newly launched, often expensive drug be used for a particular condition. Recently however

---

[5] http://www.equator-network.org/ Accessed 23 Sept 2019.

[6] http://www.equator-network.org/reporting-guidelines/consort/ Accessed 23 Sept 2019.

[7] www.nice.org.uk/ Accessed 27 Oct 2014.

guidelines are also produced making recommendations for the way care should be delivered, and as well as guidelines, there are NICE publications on quality standards and advice (evidence summaries and briefings).

Given increasingly constrained budgets and demands on the health service, there has also been a steady move towards considering not only effectiveness but costs. In order to compare different treatments for cost, the concept of the quality-adjusted life year (QALY) was born. The QALY is a measure of disease burden, including both the quality and the quantity of life lived, and provides a common standardised measure to allow comparisons between treatments, for example, between a new and an established treatment or between a drug and a non-pharmacological option. It provides an objective measure of the gains from a new treatment and can demonstrate whether possibly marginal health gains come at an unaffordable cost. Assessing health status is a key component of calculating the QALY. Whilst one of the earliest measures of health status was the SF36,[8] the Euroqol is now the measure of choice.[9]

The synthesis of the evidence to support NICE decisions may need to be commissioned. One centre which often undertakes this synthesis in the UK is the NHS Centre for Reviews and Dissemination[10] based at the University of York.

In Scotland, the Scottish Medicines Consortium[11] was established in 2001, prompted by a need to remove replication of decision-making across the then 15 individual Health Boards and to promote consistency in medicine use across Health Board boundaries. The SMC has been credited with providing more timely advice than NICE, but in practice the two groups work in tandem and complement each other's activities. In adopting evidence-based decision-making in this way, the UK is reflecting practice in other countries such as Canada and Australia. For example, there is a pan-Canadian process (CADTH Common Drug Review (CDR))[12] which reviews the clinical effectiveness and cost-effectiveness of drugs and provides recommendations for Canada's publicly funded drug plans. In Australia the Pharmaceutical Benefits Advisory Committee (PBAC) (Ritchie et al. 2019) recommends new medicines which can be provided under the Pharmaceutical Benefits Scheme (PBS) (medicines subsidised by the Australian Government). No new medicine can be listed unless the committee makes a positive recommendation. Reassuringly, a recent academic publication (Clement et al. 2009) demonstrated that conclusions about effectiveness and cost-effectiveness across the three countries were consistent but that there was also variation in final recommendation because of differences in other contextual factors such as agency processes, ability for price negotiation and social values.

---

[8] https://www.rand.org/health-care/surveys_tools/mos/36-item-short-form.html Accessed 23 Sept 2019.

[9] https://euroqol.org/eq-5d-instruments/eq-5d-5l-about/ Accessed 23 Sept 2019.

[10] www.york.ac.uk/inst/crd/ Accessed 27 Oct 2014.

[11] https://www.scottishmedicines.org.uk/ Accessed 27 Oct 2014.

[12] http://www.cadth.ca/ Accessed 27 Oct 2014.

As well as high-level use of evidence to inform policy, individual practitioners also need evidence-based guidance on managing individual patients with a particular condition, when they may be faced with a plethora of management and pharmacological treatment options. In Scotland the Scottish Intercollegiate Guideline Group[13] undertakes wide-ranging disease-based reviews, recognising that in some areas the level of evidence is not as strong as in others and making this clear in the final recommendations. The development groups include clinicians, researchers and lay representatives, and findings are disseminated as guidelines to inform practice, with an accompanying quick reference guide for professionals and good practice points highlighted. There are now 158 specific guidelines—the most recent one on the management of asthma. Guidelines over 10 years old are withdrawn. Without a full review of the evidence, it is not possible to be certain that these guidelines:

- Remain relevant to NHSScotland.
- Make recommendations based on the most up-to-date evidence for best practice.
- Do not recommend unsafe practice.
- Comply with current mandatory advice or government policy.

Condition-specific guidelines are also produced by specialist societies, e.g. for pain or hypertension, and sometimes organisations collaborate to produce a guideline. For example, the asthma guideline referred to above was produced in collaboration with the British Thoracic Society.

1.2 Evidence-Based Pharmacy

1.2.1 From Drugs to Services

As noted above the original focus of evidence-based medicine was mostly about choice of drug. There was an increasing recognition that similar techniques could also be applied to choices about different procedures, or diagnostic tests, and perhaps most recently different models of service delivery. This might include workforce changes, for example, pharmacists taking on advanced roles, or a change of setting in which treatment is offered, for example, should this be a specialist or generalist setting. These developments, and the need for appropriate methodologies to apply when moving from clinical research and studies of medicines, contributed to the development of the discipline of Health Services Research (HSR).[14] HSR investigates 'how social factors, financing systems, organizational structures and processes, medical technology and personal behaviours affect access to healthcare,

---

[13] www.sign.ac.uk/ Accessed 27 Oct 2014.

[14] http://en.wikipedia.org/wiki/Health_services_research Accessed 25 Sept 2014.

the quality and cost of healthcare and quantity and quality of life. Compared with medical research, HSR brings together social science perspectives with the contributions of individuals and institutions engaged in delivering health services'. It is a relatively new discipline whose methodologies are continually developing and becoming more sophisticated. Initially HSR focussed more on the different ways of understanding and delivering patient care from the perspective of the effectiveness of the medical workforce, in both secondary and primary care. However crucially it was not about whether a doctor could do something in a more effective or efficient way than another healthcare professional but more about the optimal way a doctor should work. For example, should a surgeon use technique 'a' or technique 'b' (Cooper et al. 2019), or should stroke patients be mobilised early or late after the acute event (Langhorne et al. 2017).

1.2.2 HSR and Pharmacy

In applying an evidence-based approach to pharmacy, a subspeciality within health services research has been developed known as pharmacy practice research. Its focus is on exploring how and why people access pharmacy services, the costs of pharmacy services, the outcomes for patients as a result of these services and comparison of these costs and outcomes to the same or similar services delivered by other providers. Its aim is to support evidence-based policy and decision-making with respect to pharmacist roles or the prescribing and use of medicines.[15] Pharmacy practice research often challenges traditional professional boundaries, reflecting the shift in the balance of care currently observed in healthcare delivery. For example, many conditions that were once primarily managed solely in a hospital setting are now managed in primary care settings, and many roles, particularly those delivered previously by doctors, are now being delivered by other healthcare professionals including pharmacists. Pharmacy research aims to understand the clinical, humanistic and economic impact of these changes from the perspectives of pharmacists, patients and other healthcare professionals. Internationally the term pharmacy practice research is not used, but the discipline is referred to as Social and Administrative Pharmacy, or Social Pharmacy. However all these terms suffer from a common failing which is that they are not generally recognised by the wider research community, either within the pharmacy profession or in wider healthcare research. There is a case now to revert to the more widely understood term health services research and refer to health services research in pharmacy (Bond and Tsuyuki 2019).

---

[15] http://en.wikipedia.org/w/index.php?title=Pharmacy_research&redirect=no Accessed 25 Sept 2014.

1.2.2.1 Quality of Research

The approaches taken in pharmacy practice research can be summarised under the broad areas of understanding and describing the way care is accessed and delivered, identifying areas for improvement and evaluating new service models using rigorous research approaches. However we should spend a moment now to reflect on the need, as in medicine, for rigorous approaches and to be critical of informing practice using research not conducted to a high standard.

As pharmacy practice research has developed, it has become inextricably linked to the move to change the whole paradigm of pharmacy from a technical supply function to a cognitive-based profession exploiting the unique expertise pharmacists have about medicines and their use, alongside the worldwide need to address the increasing demands on healthcare, financial constraints and predicted workforce shortages. Unfortunately, enthusiasm to demonstrate the contribution pharmacists can make to a wider role in healthcare has resulted in a multiplicity of small studies which were designed with the a priori assumption that a pharmacist could deliver a role effectively, for example, they could improve a patient's medication regime or increase their adherence, compared to current usual care. Critical also was the fact that with a few notable exceptions, much of the research was done by pharmacists themselves, generally with little insight into the increasingly sophisticated methodological approaches being used in HSR more generally. It is not surprising therefore that this body of research was widely criticised by the wider Health Services Research community and dismissed as not generating the necessary evidence for policy change. In response, in the UK, the Pharmacy Practice Research Resource Centre (based at the University of Manchester) commissioned a review of pharmacy practice research from Nicholas Mays, then Director of the Health and Health Care Research Unit at the Queens University Belfast. The results of the review were disseminated at a conference in 1994, but they made for uncomfortable reading for the majority of the pharmacy practice research community. The review concluded that the discipline of pharmacy practice research was largely immature and was limited to small descriptive and feasibility studies and most damningly that it was mostly designed and conducted by pharmacists with an apparent aim of demonstrating the value of pharmacy per se. The outcome was a plethora of studies, interesting in that they could be used as proof-of-concept studies, but of little value in providing generalizable data, often only reporting intermediate process outcomes rather than clinical or humanistic patient outcomes and with health economic input extremely rare. In summary, in an evidence-based age, such research could not inform policy.

A core recommendations made in the review by Nicholas Mays referred to above was that as pharmacy practice research integrates several research paradigms and perspectives, it should be delivered by multidisciplinary groups including not only pharmacists and other members of the clinical team but also statisticians, health psychologists, social scientists, health economists and epidemiologists, amongst others.

1.2.2.2 Systematic Reviews of Pharmacy-Related Research

Just as in other areas of science, evidence from pharmacy practice research should be formally collated using a systematic review approach, involving comprehensive identification of all papers addressing a topic, selecting them against predefined inclusion and exclusion selection criteria, quality assessing them and reporting them. Ideally for quantitative studies, this should be in a meta-analysis. The critical quality review is really important for highlighting deficiencies in studies which may tend to favour more positive outcomes such as lack of an objective outcome measure, evaluation of the study by the same person who delivered the intervention, small numbers, failure to follow up non-responders or failure to use an intention to treat analysis. A relatively recent paper in *Annals of Pharmacotherapy* has emphasised the value of systematic reviews for pharmacy practice (Charrois et al. 2009) and gives good guidance on searching, evaluating, interpreting and disseminating the findings. Systematic reviews of pharmacy roles are increasing, but readers need to critically consider the quality of the review method and the quality of the study inclusion criteria before quoting any conclusions. To take the profession forwards, only the highest level of evidence should be cited.

Conducting a systematic review is a piece of research in its own right, often referred to as 'secondary' research. Just as primary studies can be done to differing levels of quality so can a systematic review. As noted earlier there are quality criteria for assessing reviews and even for reviews of reviews. Publishing a systematic review through the Cochrane Collaboration is beneficial on several counts. Firstly all Cochrane reviews have a certain status; they are also easily found by those searching for evidence as one of the first actions is always to search the Cochrane library. Secondly and linked to the above is the fact that there is knowledge that Cochrane reviews have been conducted to the highest standards; in order to publish a review under the Cochrane banner, a detailed protocol must first be submitted and approved through a peer review and editorial process. Finally Cochrane reviews have a finite life and if not updated at regular predefined intervals, they are no longer considered valid.

There are currently 39 systematic reviews relevant to pharmacy in the Cochrane library, although often the pharmacist is not the main focus. Importantly the review team is almost always multidisciplinary, and there is therefore less likely to be a bias in favour of pharmacy in the interpretation and reporting. For example, a review of non-medical prescribing (Weeks et al. 2016) suggested that non-medical prescribers, practising with varying but high levels of prescribing autonomy, in a range of settings, were as effective as usual care medical prescribers, but did not separate out a conclusion for pharmacists and a conclusion for nurses.

At the time of writing, there are four reviews that look specifically at pharmacy services. One of the earliest was a review of the effect of outpatient pharmacists' non-dispensing roles on patient outcomes and prescribing patterns (Nkansah et al. 2010). In the most recent update of this review, the topic has been split into two reviews separating health promotion (Steed et al. 2014) and other services due to the proliferation of research papers in the field. The first of these reviews, the 'other services' one, was published in 2019 (de Barra et al. 2018). Despite the significant increase in number of studies, the conclusion of the updated review has not altered the bottom line of previous reviews. There is much heterogeneity across studies making meta-analysis difficult, and results tend to be inconclusive, i.e. not statistically significant. For example, there are suggestions that pharmacists could improve the care of patients with diabetes (5 trials, 558 participants, OR 0.29 (CI 0.04–2.22), low certainty of evidence) or can improve blood pressure control compared with usual care (18 trials, 4107 participants, OR 0.40 (CI 0.29–0.55), low certainty of evidence). Similar mixed results were found in a similar review including only low- and middle-income countries (Pande et al. 2013).

A study of smoking cessation advice provided by -trained community pharmacists (Sinclair et al. 2004), providing a counselling and record-keeping support programme for their customers, showed that this approach may have a positive effect on smoking cessation rates. The strength of evidence is again limited because only one of the trials showed a statistically significant effect.

Similarly in 2012, a Cochrane review on polypharmacy and the elderly (Patterson et al. 2012) including a range of study designs showed a reduction in inappropriate prescribing and drug-related problems but conflicting results on hospital readmissions, i.e. there was a difference in a process rather than a clinical outcome. The conclusion was therefore that it was unclear whether interventions to improve appropriate polypharmacy, such as pharmaceutical care, resulted in clinically significant improvements for patients.

Finally a 2013 review (Alldred et al. 2013), again on improving prescribing but this time in care homes only, could not come to a definitive conclusion due to heterogeneity in design intervention and outcomes! This review could have had the potential to be considered a stronger more robust review, as it only included RCTs. However individually few if any of these RCTs achieved high scores on the quality assessment. All of the eight studies remaining after selection from 7000 hits included a pharmacist as the main deliverer of intervention.

Systematic reviews are of course published in many places, additional to the Cochrane library. They are printed by academic journals, after going through appropriate peer review, and are prized by journal editors as they get cited frequently. Holland et al. undertook a review of papers evaluating the outcomes of pharmacist-led medication review in the elderly (Holland et al. 2008). Only RCTs were eligible for inclusion, and there was a meta-analysis for the main outcome of unscheduled hospital admissions. The authors comment on the steadily increasing quality of pharmacy practice research, but once again were not able to provide a definite answer on changes if any in the 'clinical outcome of hospital readmission or mortality'. Some process improvements, e.g. patient knowledge and adherence, were noted.

Finally, a review of the views of pharmacists, their staff and the public on a public health role for community pharmacy (Eades et al. 2011) concluded that overall whilst pharmacists were positive about providing public health services, these were secondary to medication-related and dispensing roles. Support staff were less confident and positive about providing a public health role, and whilst consumers were positive in principle about pharmacists providing such a service, they did not expect it and had rarely been offered it in practice. This review has identified descriptive studies such as surveys which are methodologically less challenging to conduct than intervention studies, yet the authors of the review once again comment on the poor quality of the studies.

One of the disappointing things for pharmacists reading these reviews is that often the data may suggest that the outcome of interest has improved but statistically it is declared inconclusive as the difference was not statistically significant. In an evidence-based age, non-significant findings, however positive, cannot be claimed as evidence. Studies do not only need to be well designed but also to have included an appropriate sample size calculation to ensure they are not underpowered. Indeed the importance of undertaking an iterative approach to intervention design and testing is now well accepted[16] by the research community who follow the MRC guidance on developing and evaluating complex interventions. Pilot work undertaken to assess likely effect size and provide factual data to guide the power calculation for the definitive study is now de rigueur, and without this, publication of studies in the leading journals is unlikely.

To conduct a strong study eligible for any of the reviews cited above would require an experienced team and a substantive grant. Accessing such funds for pharmacy-related research is becoming easier, but it still represents a formidable challenge if pharmacy-related studies are being assessed for prioritisation against studies of perhaps new surgical interventions. It is also sometimes difficult to get pharmacy colleagues in clinical practice to take part in research because they themselves are already very busy, and many funding arrangements do not pay for the pharmacists' time. Whilst they understand the need for research and recognise it is of value to the profession's future, lack of prioritisation in a busy pharmacy, perceived lack of time, motivation, confidence and competence are all contributory factors (Lowrie et al. 2015). There are limited initiatives introduced by the Royal Pharmaceutical Society and policymakers to embed research into every pharmacist's role, but progress remains slow especially compared to other professions such as medicine, where active research participation is an expected component of any *cv*. In Australia there have been moves to integrate pharmacy practice and research, and the community pharmacy contract global sum includes money to fund pharmacy-related research. An excellent example of how this has been put to good effect follows in the next section.

Small studies can of course be done to the highest quality, are a good training and, if well reported and done with an understanding that they are developmental or pilot studies, can make a useful contribution to the literature (Eldridge et al. 2016). However research cannot be a hobby, and those whose main role is clinical should always seek academic advice to ensure that small is good and publishable! Research that is not published for others to read and benefit from might as well not have been done.

---

[16] http://www.mrc.ac.uk/documents/pdf/complex-interventions-guidance/ Accessed 13 Oct 2014.

1.2.3   Importance of Right Outcome

In their Cochrane review, Nkansah et al. commented on the heterogeneity of many components of the research including variation in the types, intensity and duration of interventions or differences in timing of follow-up measurements. They also comment on the lack of detail in the papers on the development processes of the interventions, or how staff were trained to deliver the intervention, or the adherence—or fidelity—to the intervention as designed, or what constituted successful delivery of the intervention. All of these are important things for any researcher to consider in both designing, conducting and reporting a study (de Barra et al. 2019). The uncertainty around many of the aforementioned items could account for the conflicting results observed and also make it difficult to combine studies in a meta-analysis. However the main area of heterogeneity that the authors identify as requiring attention in the future is the need to select an appropriate outcome measure. At the study design stage, it should be possible to provide a theoretical reason for why the intervention in question is likely to change the selected primary outcome and whether the measure selected is likely to be sensitive enough to identify any changes. The gold standard choice of outcome to assess the clinical cost-effectiveness of intervention in general is a quality of life measure such as the SF36 or EQ5D which can be converted into QALY. Thus NICE and equivalent organisation can compare diverse interventions on the basis of a common unit, the QALY, to which they can also attach a price.

However in delivering pharmaceutical care, we need to realistically ask ourselves the likelihood of changing these broad brush measures which have several domains. For example, the EQ5D, now the favoured measure in the UK, has five domains covering mobility, self-care, usual activities, pain/discomfort and anxiety/depression. Whilst there is a youth version, there is no older people's version, and the scale itself has not been validated in every disease to which it has been applied. Nkansah et al. comment that in older people their likelihood of co-morbidities means that even improving outcomes in one of their conditions may not be sufficient to change the global assessment of overall quality of life, and they call for a new universal easily applied valid and reliable outcome to be developed to use in these populations, who because of polypharmacy regimes often comprise the majority of participants in pharmaceutical care interventions.

In a study of community pharmacist-led medicine management for patients with coronary heart disease (The Community Pharmacy Medicines Management Project Evaluation team (C. Bond Principal Investigator) 2007), there was no change in the primary outcome measure of patient quality of life as measured by the SF36, in the intervention group compared to the control. Yet there was significant increase in the patient satisfaction score for the care they received from the pharmacists. This leaves a conundrum of what is driving that increased satisfaction. Indeed there is a general move to begin to consider the use of more patient-centred outcomes such as discrete choice experiments (DCE), to quantify what it is the patient liked about the intervention. Early work has suggested that a DCE can be used in this way to value the pharmacy input and reverse the take-home policy message to be more positive (Tinelli et al. 2010).

However whilst the pharmacy profession and the research community all see the logic of this argument, a new pharmacy-delivered intervention is competing for funds with other new exciting developments. The rationale for the EQ5D and SF36 QUALY is that they can provide a single common unit of benefit to a heterogeneous mix of interventions—even including pharmacological and non-pharmacological therapies. At this present time, it is unclear how policymakers would view an alternative set of outcomes, and it remains unclear whether health services would be prepared to pay for more satisfied patients!

1.3   The Policy, Practice, and Research Triangle in Pharmacy

In 1986 the Nuffield report (Nuffield 1986) was the first to clearly identify in the UK that community pharmacists could play a more central role in healthcare delivery. It was particularly important because it was seen to be an objective pronouncement by opinion formers outwith the profession who would have little, if any, vested professional interest in its recommendations.

The overall message of Nuffield was embraced in the context of healthcare in general. It was immediately adopted by policymakers in a succession of publications,[17,18] which iteratively have been more ambitious in widening the scope of pharmacy practice and for moving the profession from having a predominantly technical medicine supply function to being a clinical profession with interfaces with both patients and other healthcare professionals. The extent of change in the intervening years has been groundbreaking. Whilst the UK has in many ways led the implementation of the extended role, this has also been happening elsewhere most notably in Canada and a lesser extent Australia. In an evidence-based healthcare system, it is interesting then to reflect on what has driven that change and to what extent it has been informed by research.

The reality is that to effect a change in role as significant as the one seen in pharmacy requires more than research. For such a change to happen, it has to be acceptable to society, the public, fellow healthcare professional and the pharmacy profession itself, it has to meet a policy need, and there has to be some evidence of feasibility and benefit.

As noted earlier in this chapter, and applying these ideas demographic changes will mean an inevitable increased future demand for healthcare, and thus there are external factors supporting workforce changes including advanced and extended pharmacy roles. Additionally technological advances mean that many conditions

---

[17] https://www.longtermplan.nhs.uk/publication/nhs-long-term-plan/

[18] https://www.gov.scot/publications/achieving-excellence-pharmaceutical-care-strategy-scotland/

previously treated surgically and requiring long stays in hospital can now be managed medically with pharmaco-therapeutic approaches or as day cases and needing pharmaceutical care. In other words we are seeing a secondary care-primary care shift, moving care out of hospitals and changing the optimal skill mix in the workforce. At the same time, there are medical workforce shortages, a move to have longer consultation times reducing patient throughput and a changing cultural expectation of the need to see a doctor for relatively minor symptoms, and increasing demand although arguably not need. The potential for other healthcare professions including pharmacy to fill that capacity gap has been recognised, and the ambition for pharmacy to extend its role has actually coincided with a policy need. Furthermore pharmacists have increasingly taken on new roles informally, for example, in hospitals advising medical staff of the best medicine regime for a patient and in the community issuing repeat prescriptions in advance of the formal form in the interest of continuity of supply for the patient and pursuing the long-held traditional role of providing advice to patients on the management of minor ailments. Today it is a formal role in a growing number of countries for pharmacists to prescribe prescription-only medicines; to prescribe on the NHS, or equivalent, pharmacy medicines rather than patients paying for them; to manage repeat dispensing; to advise on adherence; to provide a clinical medication review and make changes to drug regimens; to provide a multiplicity of public health roles including formal intensive advice to stop smoking, issuing emergency hormonal contraception, screening for chlamydia, giving brief interventions to address hazardous drinking, providing coronary heart disease health checks and administering flu vaccinations; and to provide travel advice, to give but a few examples. Finally these pharmacy-led services are being generally more recognised by the public and other members of the healthcare team meaning that extended pharmacy services are integrated into the NHS rather than being seen as a parallel service which remains the case in many other European countries, e.g. Spain and Italy. Most recent in the UK is the emergence of a rapidly increasing number of pharmacists working in general practice and care homes with an explicit role to improve prescribing.

Practice research can be categorised under four broad areas with respect to its role in relation to policy. The first category is where *research has informed policy* and has been the trigger for innovation (e.g. smoking cessation, repeat dispensing, new medicines service and PINCER) and where it was conducted before any explicit service need or service rollout. This could be regarded as blue sky research. The second is again where the research was undertaken before service rollout, but after a policy decision had been made, in other words it was to **support a planned policy** (e.g. medicine management). Thirdly there is research that has been conducted after a new service had been introduced to **confirm the appropriateness of implemented policy** (e.g. pharmacist prescribing). The final fourth category is where it has been used to evaluate an innovation or service in order to **understand the processes in place**, identify good and less good aspects and make recommendations for the future (e.g. evaluation of the new English community pharmacy contractual framework) and subsequent developments. Each of these will be considered in turn, but it will be clear as the descriptions are read that there is some overlap between groups and in many ways it is a continuum. Because much of the professional change has been spearheaded in the UK, and because the author is UK based, there is no apology that the following examples are all from that country.

1.3.1   Research Informing Policy

1.3.1.1   Smoking Cessation

In 1991, as part of a progressive trend in many countries to widen safe and convenient access to medicines, the first nicotine replacement therapy (NRT) (nicotine gum 2 mg) was deregulated in the UK from a prescription-only medicine to a pharmacy medicine. Since then many other nicotine replacement therapies at higher strength and in different formulations have been deregulated, and many are now freely available as a General Sales List medicine. The wider availability of NRT made it possible for pharmacists to take on a very clear public health function of supporting smoking cessation. This led to the idea that pharmacists and their staff could be trained to provide a formal smoking cessation service. A randomised controlled trial was designed and funded to test whether the smoking cessation outcomes of people attending trained pharmacies were any different than those attending community pharmacies providing advice on smoking cessation as per usual practice. In other words, could the quality of the service provided by community pharmacists be enhanced by training? A 2 h training package was developed for pharmacists and their staff, based on the theory of behavioural change. Smokers were followed up at 1 month, 4 months and 9 months after their first pharmacy visit. The study showed that smoking cessation rates at all three time points were better for those people attending trained compared to untrained pharmacies (Sinclair et al. 1998), and the cost of intensive pharmacist support was £300 per quitter, £83 per year of life gained (Sinclair et al. 1999). Despite this good evidence of benefit, endorsed by a Cochrane review (Sinclair et al. 2008), it was some time before smoking cessation advice became a core role for all community pharmacists in Scotland with appropriate recognition and a professional payment. First small local contractual arrangements were entered into, fighting professional turf wars on the way. Gradually pharmacists demonstrated that as a profession they could deliver on smoking cessation, and in 2008 the service became embedded in the national contract. Today in Scotland over 80% of all quit attempts go through community pharmacy, and community pharmacy supports over 70% of all successful attempts. Thus community pharmacy is tackling one of the biggest public health problems of this century. It is salutary to emphasise this long time line between the generation of the evidence and implementation into policy and also to remember it was not just the research that led the change. It also happened because society was ready to stop smoking and because smoking was suddenly identified as a priority public health policy issue.

1.3.1.2 Repeat Dispensing

With a similar time frame and in a similar way, a randomised controlled trial of pharmacists managing repeat dispensing conducted in the mid-1990s (Bond et al. 2000) led to repeat dispensing by pharmacists becoming embedded in both English and Scottish community pharmacy contractual frameworks. In the original RCT, when pharmacists managed repeat dispensing, they detected more medicine-related problems than were detected in the control group of usual care, they reduced the annual costs of drugs prescribed per patient in the system, and GPs, managers and patients liked the service. Once again in the years following the academic publication, small pilot projects of the service were implemented widely in various local areas, and ultimately the service became standard for all pharmacists, often integrated with more formal medication review as in the Chronic Medicine Service in Scotland.

1.3.1.3 New Medicines Service

The final example in this category is for the New Medicines Service recently introduced and evaluated in England. It is generally accepted that many people prescribed a new medicine stop taking it within a few weeks for a range of reasons. Indeed many people may even not take the first dose. A study published in 2006 (Clifford et al. 2006) showed that when patients who were prescribed a new medicine for a chronic condition were followed up by telephone there was an improvement in their positive beliefs about taking the medicines and there was reduced non-adherence and reduced problems compared to a control group who did not receive the follow-up call. This research underpinned the New Medicines Service introduced into English community pharmacy contracts on a 1-year pilot basis in 2012 and ultimately established into routine practice after a positive evaluation report. The New Medicines Service could also in fact fit into the next category of research confirming the appropriateness of a policy, as the way the service was implemented in practice was not through the centralised telephone service used in the original research but through individual pharmacists.

1.3.1.4 Pincer

PINCER (Avery et al. 2012) was a pragmatic randomised controlled trial in which pharmacists, based in general practices, identified patients at high risk of potentially serious errors and worked with the practice team (feedback, educational outreach and support) to reduce errors in these patients. The control group received simple computerised feedback. Data at 6 months showed that in the intervention group there was less likelihood of patients with a history of gastric ulcer being prescribed an NSAID without gastro-protection, a beta blocker if they had asthma and/or ACE inhibitor or loop diuretic without appropriate monitoring. The intervention was also shown to be cost-effective and as a consequence is being rolled out in England with dedicated finances attached.[19] To date 400 pharmacists have been trained to deliver the intervention and 2175 GP practices are involved.

1.3.2 Research to Support a Planned Policy

In the early 2000s, new community pharmacy contracts were being developed in the home countries of the UK, to reflect the aspirations of policy documents to move the pharmacy profession to a more cognitive role. Whilst most of the profession believed at the time that this was the future for the profession, whilst contractual payments were driven by volumes of items dispensed, it was unlikely that the focus of community pharmacy services would change. Building on the success of the practice-based primary care pharmacists, it was believed that community pharmacists could deliver at least some of these roles from their community pharmacy base, by delivering a holistic pharmaceutical care service. In pharmaceutical care, pharmacists would take responsibility for the management of a patient's medicines and their associated drug-related needs. Research was commissioned by the Department of Health to derive evidence of the benefits of a community pharmacy-led pharmaceutical care service for patients with coronary heart disease. At the time there was evidence from published studies of the benefits of individual components of a pharmaceutical care or medicine management service (e.g. lifestyle advice, blood pressure monitoring, adherence support), but there had been no studies of the whole service. A large definitive randomised controlled trial was conducted. This study has been previously referred to in this chapter as the one in which choice of outcome measure was critical. The study failed to show that there was an increase in appropriateness of treatment or patient quality of life although as noted earlier there was increase in patient satisfaction and observed individual improvements in prescribing. However whilst some community pharmacists identified many areas of improvement, others were less successful, so on average there was little change (Krska et al. 2007). When the new contract was implemented, it was emphasised that the Medicines Use Review component was about supporting the patient and not about improving appropriateness of care. This study also shows the challenges of generalising from small trials with self-selected participants to larger studies involving whole populations. The former are more likely to give positive results as the participants will be those who are more likely to have an interest in and commitment to the project. The larger whole population studies are more likely to reflect subsequent national implementation but may be more conservative in their estimate of benefit.

---

[19] https://www.nottingham.ac.uk/primis/pincer/pincer-intervention.aspx

1.3.3 Research to Confirm the Appropriateness of Implemented Policy

Research defending policy is often commissioned as a formal evaluation after a service has been introduced. In the UK this has been the case, for example, after the introduction of non-medical including pharmacist prescribing.

1.3.3.1 Pharmacist Prescribing

Non-medical prescribing was introduced in the UK after the Crown review (Department of Health 1999), a group established to review the supply and administration of medicines, recognising that much current practice was operating on the edge of the current regulations and legal frameworks. The Review recommended the implementation initially of non-medical supplementary prescribing, in which trained nurses or pharmacists, with the agreement of patients and medical staff, could continue to prescribe specified drugs for a patient, altering them as necessary within an agreed clinical management plan. Supplementary prescribing, introduced in the UK in 2003, was quickly followed by independent prescribing (2007) which gave trained nurses and pharmacists the right to prescribe any drug they wanted within their areas of professional competence including controlled drugs. More recently other healthcare professionals such as podiatrists and optician have also been given some prescribing rights. Accreditation criteria for undergraduate pharmacy degrees in the UK, introduced from 2015, will provide all pharmacy graduates with the requisite competencies to prescribe, although for now they won't be able to prescribe in practice until they have been qualified for 2 years. These significant changes were introduced without prior research evidence of safety or benefit. The rationale might have been that the stepwise introduction starting with supplementary and then followed by independent prescribing allowed a staged opportunity to reflect on the rollout supported by commissioned evaluations (Department of Health 2011). These evaluations focussed mostly on experiences and safety aspects and did not include evidence of effectiveness or efficiency compared to traditional approaches. There is now a considerable body of subsequent research on non-medical prescribing, mostly focussed on nurses and pharmacists. However the bulk of this research has been descriptive exploring the extent of implementation, the medical specialities where most non-medical prescribing is delivered and the views and experiences of patients, medical doctors and the new prescribers themselves. Few studies have looked at the clinical outcomes of non-medical prescribing. One exploratory study showed that in the field of chronic pain, pharmacist prescribing compared to traditional GP-led care for patients with chronic pain led to significantly improved pain outcomes at 6 months (as measured using the validated Chronic Pain Grade) but interestingly only some effect on the mental health subscale of the SF36. This again reflects earlier discussion in this chapter on the importance of choosing the right outcome measure.

1.3.3.2 Primary Care Pharmacy

In the late 1990s and early 2000s, the value of a pharmacist working closely with a general practitioner, based in the practice, became apparent. The role was purely advisory and based on the clinical pharmacy role then well established in the hospital setting. For most early post holders, it included reviewing practice prescribing and looking at a practice level at trends in prescribing, adherence to guidelines and formularies and making recommendations for changes to improve efficiency and effectiveness, at both practice and individual patient level. At individual patient level, some posts involved the pharmacist having face-to-face consultations with patients (McDermott et al. 2006), but until the advent of pharmacist prescribing (see previous example), any recommended changes had to be mediated by the medical prescriber.

The pharmacists working in general practice in the UK became known as primary care pharmacists, and over the course of approximately 10 years, the pharmacy profession evolved from being split into hospital and community pharmacists to having a third significant group of pharmacists delivering a clinical service. No large-scale definitive study was ever published of the added value that pharmacists brought to the practice team although small uncontrolled studies and case reports appeared to confirm that the pharmacists saved money for practices and brought prescribing into line with current guidelines. This is a very interesting example of a sea change in the pharmacy profession which emerged on the basis of a slowly building body of descriptive evidence and local rollout rather than a big study and national implementation. One systematic review of practice-based pharmacy services (Fish et al. 2002) including studies from North America (7), UK (5), Australia (2) and Sweden (1) showed that most published RCTs suggested benefits from the roles although studies were generally very small and not powered and did not include measures of cost-effectiveness. A more recent systematic review including 28 studies (Hayhoe et al. 2019) showed that there was reduced use of GP appointments and reduced use of emergency department attendances, but increased overall primary care use. There was some evidence of savings in overall health system and medication costs. The PINCER study described above is also of direct relevance here as it provided strong evidence for at least one aspect of a primary care pharmacist's role that was well evaluated and cost-effective, and as described above, this high-quality evidence has been recognised and the service implemented. Indeed in the last 5 years, introducing practice-based pharmacist has become national policy in all the devolved UK nations. In England, since the clinical pharmacists in general practice programme started in 2015, 1000 full-time equivalent posts have been introduced, and there are dedicated training programmes and interesting local evaluations. NHS England commissioned an independent evaluation of the scheme.[20] The evaluation comprised observational studies, one-to-one interviews with staff

---

[20] https://www.nottingham.ac.uk/news/pressreleases/2018/july/clinical-pharmacists-in-general-practice-improve-patient-care-new-report-finds.aspx

and patients, patient focus groups and case study site visits. It showed that clinical pharmacists significantly increase patient appointment capacity and reduce pressure on GPs.

1.3.4 Research to Inform Future Service Review

In this final category, the value of research in giving constructive feedback to providers and policymakers on how a service could be improved to support improved efficiency and effectiveness is illustrated. In 2005 a programme of work was commissioned to evaluate the introduction of the new community pharmacy contractual framework in England. As mentioned earlier this new contract represented a significant change from earlier contracts as it was structured to formalise, and recognise through remuneration, professional advisory services alongside traditional dispensing roles. The emphasis of the evaluation[21] was to describe implementation processes and provide constructive recommendations on addressing identified barriers to optimal service delivery. So, for example, one option introduced in the contract was for local organisations to commission advanced services from accredited community pharmacists. One such service was the Medicine Use Review (MUR) service. The research, which adopted a mixed methods approach, showed great variation in rate of uptake of the service in different local areas and by different pharmacists. The qualitative data revealed that there was misunderstanding on the part of general practitioners, pharmacists, patients and commissioners about the purpose of the MUR. GPs either expected and pharmacists delivered a full clinical review rather than providing supportive communication with the patient. There was also concern about the record keeping, inability to assess quality and communication with the GPs. Thus the report could highlight these areas and allow local solutions to address these to be put in place. Subsequently small studies of MURS have been able to demonstrate the benefits they can confer,[22] and the service has continued to be delivered by increasing numbers of pharmacists. However in the latest English policy document,[23] the MUR service is being phased out by 2020 but being replaced by a more clinical Structured Medication Review. This illustrates a possibly opportunistic and evolving approach to make pharmacy ever more integrated into the provision of core NHS services, with an increasing clinical remit, keeping other professionals and the public supportive as benefits are experienced and confidence grows. In a similar way, in the new contract, the Minor

---

[21] http://www.pharmacyresearchuk.org/waterway/wp-content/uploads/2012/11/National_evaluation_of_the_new_community_pharamcy_contract.pdf Accessed 14 Oct 2014.

[22] http://www.pharmaceutical-journal.com/news-and-analysis/news/inhaler-technique-murs-significantly-improve-outcomes/11107200.article

[23] Department of Health and Social Care The community pharmacy contractual framework for 2019/20 to 2023/24:supporting delivery for the NHS Long term plan July 2019 medicines and Pharmacy Directorate/DHSC/London.

Illness Service, which was based on the Care at the Chemist 'blue sky' study (Hassell et al. 2001) and subsequently shown to have proven benefits of clinical effectiveness and cost-effectiveness (Watson et al. 2015), is being subsumed within a new service, the NHS Community Pharmacists Consultation Service which will also take referrals from the out of hours help line NHS111, thus establishing pharmacy finally as the first port of call and an integral part of the NHS urgent care system.

1.3.5   An Integrated Example

In Australia the introduction of Home Medicine Reviews provides an interesting comparator and an example of excellent integration between service provision and research. Since the mid-1990s, the global sum allocated to fund professional pharmacy services under the 5-yearly Community Pharmacy Agreements (CPA) has increased from $5 m in the second CPA (1995–2000) to $663m in the fifth CPA (2010–2015). Several Commonwealth-funded research projects undertaken to evaluate the impact of pharmacist involvement in medication review, for consumers living at home, were conducted in the late 1990s, following a successful randomised controlled trial within the nursing home sector. This research subsequently informed negotiations within the third CPA to fund pharmacist and GP involvement in the Home Medicines Review (HMR) Program. A HMR[24] involves a comprehensive medication review conducted by an accredited pharmacist. The process begins with a referral from the patients' GP to either their preferred pharmacy or pharmacist. The pharmacist then conducts an interview with the patient, usually in their own home, before writing a report to the referring GP, documenting specific medication review findings and recommendations. The GP then meets with the patient to develop a medication management plan based on the pharmacist's report. This successful programme has been developed and iteratively refined by research, led by Professor Chen of the University of Sydney, Prof Gilbert from the University of South Australia and Prof Roberts from the University of Queensland. It is a real example of policymakers and researchers working together for the benefits of an improved service to patients.

1.4   Challenges

In the last decade, the volume of good-quality research on the cost-effective and clinically effective prescribing, supply and use of medicines has increased exponentially. However whilst acknowledging this improvement, this chapter has also shown that many shortcomings in the research remain. There is still a need to increase capability and capacity in this area in our profession. Regardless of the quality of the evidence,

---

[24] http://5cpa.com.au/programs/medication-management-initiatives/home-medicines-review/

there also remain challenges to bridging the policy research divide, and it is frustrating for researchers when policy is introduced for which there is no evidence, or where there is evidence that does not seem to have been taken into account. This reflects that in practice policy rarely uses just an evidence base, many decisions are based on political pragmatism, and many don't have any evidence or obvious logic!

Some of these challenges and reasons for them are considered briefly below.

1.4.1 Expertise, Time and Money!

A robust study that generates gold standard evidence requires an experienced team, appropriate iterative developmental and pilot work, time and substantive funding. All of these remain challenges for those working in the field of practice research. Capacity and expertise are being developed in universities and in the workforce, but it a steep learning curve until a researcher would be judged 'a safe pair of hands' to lead a substantive programme of work. Doctoral and post-doctoral experience are core to a research career as is the ability to network and link with those from relevant complementary disciplines. Commissioned research programmes addressing a national priority can often seem to have short deadlines between the initial call and its submission date, and unrealistic objectives to be addressed within the funding envelope, and tight timescales for when results should be available. It is better to argue the case to do part of the commission well than to spread efforts, expertise and resource too thinly.

1.4.2 Engaging Colleagues

Every pharmacists need to understand research and take part in research; a small proportion will be research leaders and career researchers who can network with the wider profession, generate ideas and design appropriate successful studies. Research of relevance to pharmacy frequently depends on peers in practice taking part in research collecting data, recruiting participants or delivering a new service, often referred to as an intervention. It is important that in all these roles adequate training and monitoring are in place to ensure accurate and consistent recording of data, nonbiased recruitment or delivery of the new service in the planned way. This requires patience from those on the research team and commitment from colleagues for whom maintaining services represents an ever-increasing workload to say nothing of the increased regulatory hurdles that are introduced. The Royal Pharmaceutical Society of Great Britain introduced a scheme called Research Ready for community pharmacists,[25] which accredited individual community pharmacies whose managers self-assessed their competence in these areas, but numbers who signed up were relatively small and matching them to a suitable project proved harder than anticipated.

---

[25] https://www.rpharms.com/development/research-and-evaluation/research-ready

1.4.3 Changing the Status Quo

Many new pharmacy roles are not new roles per se but are new to pharmacy. They will most likely have been delivered previously by medical colleagues, and there will be some resistance from those colleagues to another professional taking them on, especially if a transfer of funding would be involved. This attitude is slightly surprising and frustrating given that it is acknowledged by all, including the medical colleagues, that they currently do not have the capacity to deliver all that is demanded and that new ways of working need to be identified. Further there may initially be resistance from patients if they think that the move to transfer care is to 'save money', or that the new provider is not as well as qualified. Finally other non-medical colleagues may also be aspiring to take on the role that is being devolved, as in prescribing. The role of research therefore is to generate the evidence that shows that patients are not getting second best care, and to design the new service with stakeholder input so all concerns are addressed, and the new service is not seen to fail for the wrong reasons, for example, in the case of medication management or medicine use reviews that GPs are not referring patients to the service.

1.4.4 Public Patient Involvement (PPI)

In the last decade, there has been a culture change from a paternalistic paradigm of healthcare to one in which patients are at the centre of care, informed as far as possible and capable of shared decisions about their treatment This patient centred-approach also affects the development of new services and research design and conduct. However getting meaningful PPI can be difficult especially when considering that there is no single patient who can represent all patients even in a condition-specific category. Nonetheless understanding ways to do this meaningfully is important, and pharmacy studies should always think about the patient viewpoint during design and conduct. This will give brownie points when funding decisions are made too! Patient representatives can advise on things that are important to them to include as outcomes, ensure patient facing documentation is understood by the lay person and make comments on emerging findings (Massey 2018).

1.4.5 Negative Findings

Negative findings can be challenging to reveal especially if positive results had been central to implementation of a new service. This is where it is important at the design stage to think about incorporating a parallel strand of research which does not just focus on outcomes but is explanatory. For example, was the training sufficient to give the pharmacists the skills to deliver the new service, was the new service acceptable to patients, or did the GPs implement the recommendations?

Identify what, if anything, went wrong and provide recommendations for change. Most importantly, difficult though it might be, do not be persuaded to hide the negative findings, and ensure that at the project start the researchers have independence to publish findings. One of the identified frauds in publication is referred to as selective reporting when researchers only publish a proportion of the findings—the ones that make the point they hoped for! This is not only misleading but prevents others from learning from the issues. Increasingly this in-depth understanding of what has happened is given more status, and the MRC has issued guidance on how such process evaluations should be approached and reported (Moore et al. 2015).

1.4.6 Funding

Securing adequate funding is also a challenge. Whether applying to a dedicated call or applying for response mode funding (i.e. getting your own ideas funded) will always be within a competitive context. In general, pharmacy specific funds are modest so it is wise to try and access other funding streams and to collaborate with colleagues from other disciplines, packaging the research in more widely understood health services research language, using generalizable theoretical approaches and using the pharmacy as the setting not the aim. Persuading grant-giving bodies to prioritise funding on services such as aspects of medicine management (e.g. improving adherence, or improving appropriateness of prescribing) or symptom management compared to developing a new cancer treatment may also appear challenging. However at a time when patient safety is high on everyone's agenda, reducing prescribing errors is central, improving adherence is also a facet of medicines safety, and non-adherence leads to costs both in terms of medicines wastage and suboptimal treatment. Finally appropriate symptom management in the community pharmacy could lead to improved earlier diagnosis of serious diseases such as cancer and COPD, which when treated earlier have a better prognosis. There are also areas of national priority where pharmacy can provide a solution and where there is already evidence of benefit such as improving mental health services, reducing inappropriate polypharmacy, deprescribing of anti-cholinergic drugs, supporting harm reduction for drug misusers and antibiotic stewardship.

1.4.7 Duplication of Research

Finally to what extent is it necessary to repeat research done in one country in another country? Will policymakers acknowledge the relevance of generalising from a different healthcare setting, with different ethnic populations, and different cultural attitudes? The answer to this is not simple, as it will depend on the exact intervention or development in question, but nonetheless it is important to learn from others and draw on their experiences. A good example of this is the interest in

North America in the HMR service introduced in Australia. Whilst recognising that evidence in the USA about the value of extending pharmacists' roles in relation to medication management is increasing, authors of a recent paper have also explicitly drawn on evidence from elsewhere, namely, Australia (Zagaria and Alderman n.d.). The authors highlight that 'it is instructive to look at how similar practice models have been established and evolved in other countries'. This is an interesting example of where local research has been complemented by selected research from elsewhere generating a stronger body of evidence for the USA than could have otherwise been achieved in the same timescale.

1.4.8 Communicating with Policymakers

There is, as noted at the start of this chapter, a need to reconfigure health services if future need is to be managed within an affordable budget. However getting research into practice is notoriously difficult whether it be changing prescribing practice for a particular condition or service redesign involving pharmacists. Both involve changing professional and patient behaviours, and the emerging discipline of implementation science (Bauer et al. 2015) is key to ensuring essential evidence-based change happens. Those interested in generating evidence that identifies a role for pharmacy in this service redesign must reflect not only on the quality of their research but also on improving the way these findings are communicated to policymakers. This may not be just about recycling academic papers as policy briefings but is also about building real and virtual networks and using the social media to promote awareness and disseminate findings widely. Civil servants in relevant government departments are known to keep abreast of social media which by virtue of its format forces academics to distil their findings into short pithy and memorable pronouncements.

1.5 Conclusion

Pharmacy has come a long way in the last three decades in becoming a truly clinical profession. A recent paper (Mossialos et al. 2013) has described the expanded role for pharmacy as 'policy making in the absence of policy relevant evidence' and claims further research is needed. We would not argue with this but also would assert that there is a building body of evidence confirming the value to patients of this paradigm shift. However as we move forwards, more considerations need to be given to improving the quality of the evidence, ensuring that cost-effectiveness as well as clinical effectiveness is considered, making sure the right outcomes are chosen and finally opening up better lines of communication with policymakers to ensure greater partnership in planning a research strategy fit for the future.

References

Alldred DP, Raynor DK, Hughes C, Barber N, Chen TF, Spoor P. Interventions to optimise prescribing for older people in care homes. The Cochrane Library. 2013, issue 2 https://doi.org/10.1002/14651858.CD009095.pub2.

Avery AJ, Rodgers S, Cantrill JA, Armstrong S, Cresswell K, Eden M, Elliott RA, Howard R, Kendrick D, Morris CJ, Prescott RJ, Swanwick G, Franklin M, Putman K, Boyd M, Sheikh A. A pharmacist-led information technology intervention for medication errors (PINCER): a multicentre, cluster randomised, controlled trial and cost-effectiveness analysis. Lancet. 2012;379:1310–9. https://www.thelancet.com/journals/lancet/article/PIIS0140-6736(11)61817-5/fulltext

de Barra M, Scott CL, Scott NW, Johnston M, de Bruin M, Nkansah N, Bond CM, Matheson CI, Rackow P, Williams AJ, Watson MC. Pharmacist services for non-hospitalised patients. Cochrane Database Syst Rev. 2018;(9):CD013102. https://doi.org/10.1002/14651858.CD013102.

de Barra M, Scott CL, Scott NW, Johnston M, de Bruin M, Nkansah N, Bond CM, Matheson CI, Rackow P, Williams AJ, Watson MC Do Pharmacy Intervention Reports Adequately Describe Their Interventions? A Template for Intervention Description and Replication Analysis of Reports included in a Systematic Review. BMJ Open. 2019;(9):e025511. https://doi.org/10.1136/bmjopen-2018-025511.

Bauer MS, et al. An introduction to implementation science for the non-specialist. BMC Psychol. 2015;3(1):32. https://doi.org/10.1186/s40359-015-0089-9.

Bond C, Tsuyuki R. The evolution of pharmacy practice research—Part II: time to join the rest of the world. Int J Pharm Pract. 2019;27:219–20. https://doi.org/10.1111/ijpp.12545. This paper is jointly published by CPJ and IJPP

Bond CM, Matheson C, Williams S, Williams P. Repeat prescribing: an evaluation of the role of community pharmacists in controlling and monitoring repeat prescribing. Br J Gen Pract. 2000;50:271–5.

Charrois TL, Durec T, Tsuyuki RT. Systematic reviews of pharmacy practice research: methodological issues in searching, evaluating, interpreting, and disseminating results. Ann Pharmacother. 2009;43:1118–22.

Clement FM, Harris A, Li JJ, Yong K, Lee KM, Manns BJ. Using effectiveness and cost-effectiveness to make drug coverage decisions: a comparison of Britain, Australia, and Canada. JAMA. 2009;302(13):1437–43. https://doi.org/10.1001/jama.2009.1409.

Clifford S, Barber N, Elliott R, Hartley E, Horne R. Patient-centred advice is effective in improving adherence to medicines. Pharm World Sci. 2006;28(3):165–70.

Cooper K, et al. Laparoscopic supracervical hysterectomy versus endometrial ablation for women with heavy menstrual bleeding (HEALTH): a parallel-group, open-label, randomised controlled trial. The Lancet. 2019; https://doi.org/10.1016/S0140-6736(19)31790-8.

Department of Health. Review of prescribing, supply and administration of medicines. Final report. London: Department of Health; 1999.

Department of Health. Evaluation of nurse and pharmacist independent prescribing in England—key findings and executive summary. Final report, London: Department of Health; 2011.

Eades CE, Ferguson JS, O'Carroll RE. Public Health in community pharmacy: a systematic review of pharmacists and consumer views. BMC Public Health. 2011;11:582.

Eldridge SM, Lancaster G, Campbell M, Thabane L, Hopewell S, Coleman C. Christine Bond Defining feasibility and pilot studies in preparation for randomised controlled trials: using consensus methods and validation to develop a conceptual framework. PLOS One. 2016;11(3):e0150205. https://doi.org/10.1371/journal.pone.0150205.

Fish A, Watson MC, Bond CM. Practice based pharmaceutical services: a systematic review. Int J Pharm Pract. 2002;10:225–33.

Guyatt GH, Oxman AD, Vist GE, Kunz R, Falck-Ytter Y, Alonso-Coello P, et al. GRADE: an emerging consensus on rating quality of evidence and strength of recommendations. BMJ. 2008;336(7650):924–6.

Hassell K, Whittington Z, Coutrill J, et al. Managing demand: transfer of management of self-limiting conditions from general practice to community pharmacies. BMJ. 2001;323:146–7.

Hayhoe B, Cespedes JA, Foley K, Majeed A, Ruzangi J, Greenfiled G. Impact of integrating pharmacists into primary care teams on health systems indicators: a systematic review. BJGP. 2019;69(687):e665–74. https://doi.org/10.3399/bjgp19X705461. Accessed 1 Oct 2019.

Holland R, Desborough J, Goodyer L, Hall S, Wright D, Loke YK. Does pharmacist-led medication review help to reduce hospital admissions and deaths in older people? A systematic review and meta-analysis. Br J Clin Pharmacol. 2008;65(3):303–16.

Krska J, Avery AJ, on behalf of The Community Pharmacy Medicines Management Project Evaluation Team (including Jaffray M, Bond CM, Watson MC, Hannaford P, Tinelli M, Scott A, Lee A, Blenkinsopp A, Anderson C, Bissell P). Evaluation of medication reviews conducted by community pharmacists: a quantitative analysis of documented issues and recommendations. Br J Clin Pharmacol. 2007;65:386–96.

Langhorne P, Wu O, Rodgers H, et al. A Very Early Rehabilitation Trial after stroke (AVERT): a Phase III, multicentre, randomised controlled trial. Southampton (UK): NIHR Journals Library; 2017. (Health Technology Assessment, No. 21.54.) https://www.ncbi.nlm.nih.gov/books/NBK453581/ https://doi.org/10.3310/hta21540

Lowrie R, Morrison G, Lees R, et al. Research is 'a step into the unknown': an exploration of pharmacists' perceptions of factors impacting on research participation in the NHS. BMJ Open. 2015;5:e009180. https://doi.org/10.1136/bmjopen-2015-009180.

Massey K. Not just a 'tick box exercise'—meaningful public involvement in research. Int J Pharm Pract. 2018;26:197–8. https://doi.org/10.1111/ijpp.12450.

McDermott E, Smith B, Elliott A, Bond CM, Hannaford PC, Chambers WA. The use of medication for chronic pain in primary care, and the potential for intervention by a practice-based pharmacist. Fam Pract. 2006;23:46–52.

Moore GF, et al. BMJ. 2015;350. https://doi.org/10.1111/ijpp.12450. https://doi.org/10.1136/bmj.h1258 (Published 19 March 2015)

Mossialos E, Naci H, Courtin E. Expanding the role of community pharmacists: policy making in the absence of policy relevant evidence? Health Policy. 2013;111(2):135–48.

Nkansah N, Mostovetsky O, Yu C, Chheng T, Beney J, Bond CM, Bero L. Effect of outpatient pharmacists' non-dispensing roles on patient outcomes and prescribing patterns. Cochrane Database Syst Rev. 2010;(7):CD000336. https://doi.org/10.1002/14651858.CD000336.pub2.

Nuffield. Pharmacy: a report to the Nuffield Foundation. London: Nuffield Foundation; 1986.

Pande S, Hiller JE, Nkansah N, Bero L. The effect of pharmacist-provided non-dispensing services on patient outcomes, health service utilisation and costs in low- and middle-income countries. Cochrane Database Syst Rev. 2013;(2):CD010398. https://doi.org/10.1002/14651858.CD010398. Accessed 23 Sept 2019

Patterson SM, Hughes C, Kerse N, Cardwell CR, Bradley MC Interventions to improve the appropriate use of polypharmacy for older people (Review). The Cochrane Library 2012, Des Issues 5.

Ritchie A, Seubert L, Clifford R, Bond C. Do randomised controlled trials relevant to pharmacy meet best practice standards for quality conduct and reporting? A systematic review. Int J Pharm Pract. 2019. https://doi.org/10.1111/ijpp.12578.

Sinclair HK, Bond CM, Lennox AS, Silcock J, Winfield AJ, Donnan P Training Pharmacists and pharmacy assistants in the stage of change model of smoking cessation: a randomised controlled trial in Scotland. Tob Control. 1998;7:253–6.

Sinclair HK, Silcock J, Bond CM, Lennox AS, Winfield AJ. The cost effectiveness of intensive pharmaceutical intervention in assisting people to stop smoking. Int J Pharm Pract. 1999;7:107–12.

Sinclair HK, Bond CM, Stead LF. Community pharmacy personnel interventions for smoking cessation. Cochrane Database Syst Rev. 2004;(1):CD003698. https://doi.org/10.1002/14651858.CD003698.pub2.

Sinclair, H.K., Bond CM, Stead LF. Community pharmacy personnel interventions for smoking cessation (Review) 2008. The Cochrane Collaboration issue 2.

Steed L, Kassavou A, Madurasinghe VW, Edwards EA, Todd A, Summerbell CD, Nkansah N, Bero L, Durieux P, Taylor SJC, Rivas C, Walton RT. Community pharmacy interventions for health promotion: effects on professional practice and health outcomes. Cochrane Database Syst Rev. 2014;(7):CD011207. https://doi.org/10.1002/14651858.CD011207.

The Community Pharmacy Medicines Management Project Evaluation team (C. Bond Principal Investigator). The MEDMAN study: a randomized controlled trial of community pharmacy-led medicines management for patients with coronary heart disease. Fam Pract. 2007;24(2):189–200.

Tinelli M, Ryan M, Bond C. Discrete choice experiments (DCE's) to inform pharmacy policy: going beyond quality-adjusted life years (QALYs). Int J Pharm. 2010;18(S1):1.

Watson MC, Ferguson J, Barton GR, Maskrey V, Blyth A, Paudyal V, Bond CM, Holland R, Porteous T, Sach T, Wright D, Fielding S. A cohort study of influences, health outcomes and costs of patients'health seeking behaviour for minor ailments from primary and emergency care settings. BMJ Open. 2015;5:e006261. https://doi.org/10.1136/bmjopen-2014-006261.

Weeks G, George J, Maclure K, Stewart D. Non-medical prescribing versus medical prescribing for acute and chronic disease management in primary and secondary care. Cochrane Database Syst Rev. 2016;(11):CD011227. https://doi.org/10.1002/14651858.CD011227.pub2.

Zagaria MA, Alderman C. Community based medication management in the US and Australia. US Pharmacist. n.d. http://www.uspharmacist.com/content//d/senior_care/c/38678/. Accessed 16 Oct 2014.

Chapter 2
Qualitative Methods in Pharmacy Practice Research

Susanne Kaae and Janine Marie Traulsen

Abstract Qualitative research within pharmacy practice is concerned with understanding the behavior and underlying motives, perceptions, and ideas of actors such as pharmacy staff, pharmacy owners, patients, other health care professionals, and politicians to explore various types of existing practices and beliefs in order to improve them. As qualitative research attempts to answer the "why" questions, it is useful for describing, in rich detail, complex phenomena that are situated and embedded in local contexts. Typical methods include interviews, observation, documentary analysis, netnography, and visual methods. Qualitative research has to live up to a set of quality criteria of research conduct in order to provide trustworthy results that contribute to the further development of the area.

Qualitative approaches and methods are recognized as a positive addition to the health services research community. Simultaneously, scientific publications reporting qualitative studies in pharmacy practice research have grown exponentially in recent years (Guirguis and Witry 2019). Even research traditions based on natural science quantitative methods have recognized the need for qualitative approaches. These approaches allow for more nuanced insights into patient and prescriber behaviors and perspectives. This process of recognition is described in a recent textbook which devoted a chapter to the importance of qualitative methods in drug utilization research (Almarsdóttir and Rahmner 2016).

Going a step further, there is evidence of the usefulness of qualitative research impacting both practice and policy. One example of the impact of qualitative research is illustrated by a study inspired by the Antimicrobial Medicine Consumption Network at the WHO Regional Office for Europe. This qualitative study was carried out in several non-EU southeast European countries with the overall goal of reducing antimicrobial resistance. The purpose of the study was to reveal and understand patients' and health care professionals' perceptions and behavior prior to and during antibiotic treatment. Interviews were conducted with general practitioners, pharmacists, and patients. The results provided valuable data

S. Kaae · J. M. Traulsen (✉)
Research Group for Social and Clinical Pharmacy, Department of Pharmacy, Faculty of
Health and Medical Sciences, University of Copenhagen, Copenhagen, Denmark
e-mail: janine.traulsen@sund.ku.dk

© Springer Nature Singapore Pte Ltd. 2020
Z. Babar (ed.), *Pharmacy Practice Research Methods*,
https://doi.org/10.1007/978-981-15-2993-1_2

31

that made it possible to create better targeted awareness of the problem of antibiotic resistance for public campaigns and educational materials for health care professionals (Kaae et al. 2019).

Another example is a study by Wisell (Wisell and Sporrong 2016) whose use of qualitative methods explored in-depth the reasons behind and consequences of liberalization of community pharmacies in Sweden. Dissemination of the research results has led to invitations for the researchers to be included in political hearings and public debates about the optimal regulation of pharmacies in the Nordic countries. These are just two examples of research projects which were made possible by adapting a qualitative approach.

2.1 Why Qualitative Methods in Pharmacy Practice?

2.1.1 Introduction

Qualitative research within the health sciences has developed as a means to gather an in-depth understanding of human behavior as well as to find the underlying reasons, attitudes, and motivations that govern such behavior. Qualitative research has grown out of a variety of disciplines such as sociology, anthropology, history, education, and linguistics. The qualitative approach is concerned with the why and how of peoples' decision-making; this means that the studies usually consist of small and focused samples. There are a variety of qualitative research methods such as interviews, observation, documentary analysis, netnography, and visual methods which are often divided into different types.

In pharmacy practice research, qualitative methods are most often used in research whose goal is to identify, improve, and develop current practices, for example, to explore various types of existing practices and beliefs. This is done in order to understand attitudes, values, and perspectives underlying these practices (both by an individual or a group of people) by asking questions such as the following: What are the perceptions of the role of pharmacy/the pharmacist? How do practices work? Which don't work and why?

Typical research questions include the following:

- How is the collaboration of pharmacists with other health care professionals characterized?
- What are the facilitators and barriers to service implementations?
- What are the perceptions of pharmacy staff, of patients, and of other health care professionals with regard to existing practices?

The basic assumption among researchers who use qualitative methods is that people make sense out of their experiences, thus creating their own reality, and are capable of sharing those experiences with others. Further, it is assumed that what people say is valid, reliable, and meaningful. Qualitative studies are not seeking to verify some "truth." They assume that there are multiple truths, realities, and meanings, and the goal is to try to understand how people understand themselves.

For years, there has been a focus in research on patient-centered care. For pharmacy practice research, this means being aware of and trying to understand patients' needs and concerns related to medicines and how pharmacy practice is adequately meeting these needs. Further, what and who inform and influence the patient's views about medicine and treatment? Qualitative methods can contribute to answering questions such as the following:

- What are patients' perceptions and understanding of their needs of medicines?
- How is communication between pharmacy staff and patients characterized?
- What are appropriate means of communicating with patients?
- What are patients' perceptions of and experiences with pharmacy services?

Qualitative research is usually conducted in the subject's natural setting whenever possible; for example, the information is collected from the patient in the hospital or home or at the community pharmacy. Qualitative data comes in many and varied forms, including interviews, narratives, diaries, focus groups, online sources, and images.

In general, qualitative methods produce specific information on the particular cases studied. More general conclusions are only presented as propositions (informed assertions). When it comes to studying pharmacy practice, there is as such no right or wrong approach and no right or wrong method, and the rule of thumb is to find the appropriate method for answering the research questions. Often, a combination of quantitative and qualitative approaches is the most appropriate; this is known as method triangulation (Thurmond 2001). For example, a survey to explore and identify new trends in pharmacy practice could be followed by the thoughts and experiences of pharmacy personnel expressed through interviews with practitioners.

2.1.2 Steps in Qualitative Research

All scientific research consists of systematically gathering data on a specific topic in order to answer a specific question. Thus, research, including qualitative research, consists of various phases which can roughly be divided up into the conceptual phase, the design and planning phase, the empirical data generation phase (preparation and data gathering), the analytic phase, and the dissemination phase. Qualitative studies differ from all other research (quantitative as well as experimental) in the way the different phases are carried out with the exception usually of the dissemination phase.

There are four essential aspects of qualitative analysis, which ensure high research quality of both the individual phases and the link between. First, the participant selection must be well reasoned, and the inclusion must be relevant to the research question. Second, the methods must be appropriate for the research objectives and setting. Third, the methods which can include interviews, field observation, document analysis, and netnography must be comprehensive enough to provide rich and robust descriptions of the events studied. Fourth, the data must be appropriately analyzed and the findings adequately corroborated by using multiple sources of information, more than one researcher to collect and analyze the raw data, and another researcher checking to establish whether the participants' viewpoints were adequately interpreted or by comparing with existing social science theories and literature.

2.2 Interviews

Interviews are a common and useful method when investigating the subjective understandings, feelings, values, attitudes, experiences, and/or ideas of persons affected by or trying to change pharmacy practice (for example, patients, health care professionals including pharmacy staff, and policy makers). Through interviews, critical issues in current practices can be identified and thereafter addressed and resolved. Interviews can likewise detect well-functioning practices to support these further. Examples of topics in pharmacy practice covered by interviews include the experiences of pharmacy staff with newly introduced cognitive services or tools such as asthma services or programs for electronic transmission of prescriptions (Emmerton et al. 2012), the perception of pharmacy customers of the role of pharmacies and pharmacists (Cavaco et al. 2005), or patients' reasons for accepting cognitive services (Latif et al. 2011).

2.2.1 Types of Interviews

Interviews are a type of conversation between the researcher and one or several interviewees for the purpose of exploring the lifeworld perspective of the interviewee(s). Interviews vary according to the degree of structure, i.e., the extent to which the interviewee can influence the direction and content of the conversation. Interviews also vary according to the number of interviewees. Interviews with several participants at the same time are called group or focus group interviews.

2.2.1.1 Individual Interviews

Individual interviews are usually divided into three types: fully structured, unstructured, and semi-structured. There is no strict line between these, and depending on the research question, they can be mixed.

Structured interviews bare a strong resemblance to questionnaires with pre-defined questions and categories of answers of which there can be little or no deviation. When conducting a structured interview, the researcher will read aloud the questions and tick the answer boxes. A structured interview usually pertains to the methodological principles of quantitative research.

In contrast, unstructured interviews are characterized by the researcher asking as few questions as possible and avoiding steering the answers of the interviewee in a certain direction. Ideally, the flow of the interview is formed by the interviewee talking freely and in depth, i.e., creating a narrative about their experiences with the theme in question. The ultimate unstructured interview is thus the narrative. Narrative interviews are a method of collecting people's stories about their own experiences with as little interference from the researcher as possible. Telling stories about their experiences of health and illness is one way in which people make sense of their lives. As a method, narratives place people in the center of the research process, validating the meanings that they assign to their own stories (Anderson and Kirkpatrick 2016).

The most commonly used interview form is the semi-structured interview where the researcher focuses on relatively few, specific questions. However, the order and weight of the questions depend on the answers of the interviewee as the purpose is to explore the deeper perspective of the interviewee. Often, the researcher probes (asks the interviewee to elaborate further on an answer they have given) in order to get a better understanding of the issue at hand.

2.2.1.2 Focus Group Interviews

Originally conceived as a tool for market research, focus group interviews are a qualitative method which has increasing gained importance in health services research, also pharmacy practice (Frisk et al. 2019). Focus groups interviews are often preferred when the interaction between the different participants (ping-pong exchanges of opinions or provoking each other) is believed to produce data and insights that would be less accessible without the interaction found in a group. They provide nuanced data by asking open-ended questions about complex issues, for example, group norms such as pharmacy organization culture (Morgan 1988; Smith 1998). They can also stimulate nuanced reflections, which are otherwise difficult to catch, for example, patients' experiences of pharmacy visits. They are well suited for exploratory work.

To be able to stimulate group interaction, it is recommended that between six and ten persons participate (Hassell and Hibbert 1996); however, it is also possible to generate valuable knowledge by conducting focus group interviews with fewer participants. The form the group interview takes will often be a mixture of the unstructured and semi-structured interview. Although the researcher will probably have several research questions to be answered, they will allow the discussions between participants to move freely (Hassell and Hibbert 1996).

2.2.2   Preparing Interviews

Several methodological decisions have to be made before conducting the interview, for example, the structure of the interview guide, i.e., the themes including the number and types of questions and how many and which participants to recruit. In addition, consideration must also be taken as to how to record data for later analysis and where to conduct the interview. Finally, ensuring the consent of the interviewee is very important.

The interview guide is the tool used by researchers to organize and keep track of the development of the interview and to ensure that all relevant questions have been answered. The themes of the interview guide can come from a variety and mixture of different sources. Sources include literature reviews, theory, or expert knowledge. It is important that all themes in the interview guide can be justified.

2.2.3   Sampling

Participant sampling is another vital step to create valuable results. As interviews are characterized by creating substantial amounts of data, researchers often have to include a restricted number of participants. One purpose of qualitative research is to identify patterns with regard to similarities of feelings, attitudes, or experiences of people pertaining to a certain group. This requires a minimum number of participants in order to ensure that all relevant patterns are found and appear consistently. Hence, recruitment could continue until no new overall patterns are identified; this is known as data saturation, which requires that the analysis is carried out parallel to the data collection phase. For semi-structured interviews, approximately 20 interviews are often necessary in order to achieve saturation. It is, however, being debated whether saturation is in fact a true reflection of high-quality qualitative research.

The researcher must also reflect on who the interviewee represents. Does the researcher aim for maximum or minimum variation between the cases/interviewees? Does the participant illustrate a rare case, a critical case, or a typical case in relation to what is being investigated? Often, sampling is affected by practical issues including limited access; one option is "snowballing" whereby you ask participants and experts in the field if they could recommend potential participants who fulfill the inclusion criteria.

2.2.4   Conducting the Interviews

A narrative interview usually begins by the researcher asking the participant to tell "the story" of their illness, including details of their initial symptoms, the diagnosis, the treatment, the effects on their daily life, etc. Ideally, the researcher only rarely asks supplementary questions.

For both semi-structured and unstructured interviews, it is usually recommended to ask open-ended questions to stimulate rich and nuanced answers, perhaps followed by more closed questions in order to illustrate the specific perspective of the participant. Kvale (1996) describes nine types of questions that can be used during an interview including the technique of "silence" to give the interviewee time to reflect and express her-/himself. Asking "interpretation questions," i.e., clarifying whether the understanding of the researcher is aligned with the perceptions expressed by the interviewee, is also recommended (Kvale 1996).

As patients' accounts in unstructured narrative, semi-structured, focus group interviews are detailed and rich and often beyond the immediate comprehension of the researcher, noting down the interviewee's answers during the interview is not sufficient for capturing all the relevant information. This is why interviews should be audio-recorded. It is important to create a trusting environment during the interview in order to allow the interviewee to feel safe to express their true opinions. Therefore, reflecting about how to conduct the interview to create this atmosphere is crucial.

Conducting pilot studies is often not necessary if a sound interview guide has been developed. As lifeworld accounts are complex and not fully predictable, conducting interviews of an inductive nature, i.e., apply learning from one interview to the next to probe, for example, more accurately, is highly recommended.

2.2.5   Ethics

The ethics in doing interviews concerns, in particular, adequately informing the interviewee about the purpose of the research project. In addition, protecting the anonymity of the interviewee throughout the research process and being aware of the asymmetry of power in the interview situation where the researcher often defines the process, for example, to be sensible not to ask and probe about matters of which the interviewee feels uncomfortable talking about, are also central. It is also important to reflect about how the interview might influence the interviewee(s)—perhaps they themselves start thinking more or differently about certain topics because of the interview. One should also be aware of the recently introduced General Data Protection Regulations (GDPR) concerning storage of personal (and sensitive) data in the European Union and other national ethical requirements.

2.2.6   Analyzing Interviews

The first step in the analysis process is to transcribe the audio recordings into written data. Keeping the exact wording is essential as well as including supplementary notes in the transcribed text if the interviewee showed a special physical reaction at some point during the interview (body language). Smaller pauses and sounds like "oh…" and "hmm.." could be left out.

No matter what type of interview method is used, making sense of the qualitative dataset involves developing a coding framework in order to reduce the volume of data to more manageable sections, for example, themes. Hence, there is no strictly defined way to analyze transcribed interviews. Common approaches include meaning condensation/content analysis, thematic analysis, theoretical analysis, and grounded analysis. However, when analyzing narrative interview data, the analysis usually involves identifying a story across the dataset and is often also concerned with other aspects of the narrative such as how the account is structured and the use of language as well as metaphors (Anderson and Kirkpatrick 2016).

Meaning condensation, which according to Kvale (1996: p. 192) "entails an abridgement of the meanings expressed by the interviewees into shorter formulations," is, in practice, often linked to the developed and well-argued themes of the interview guide (illustrating the pre-understanding/prioritizations already made by the researcher). Within each theme of the interview guide for each of the interviewees, quotes pertaining to the particular theme are highlighted and moved to a special table in order to obtain an overview of the process (for example, using software). The researcher should at this point be open to new, interesting, and at times unexpected statements made by the interviewee that cannot directly be linked to the existing themes. When the entire interview has been coded in this way, the different quotes for one interviewee within one theme are condensed by the researcher, interpreting in her/his own words as briefly as possible the meaning expressed by the interviewee. When this process has been conducted for each individual participant, patterns of similarities or differences between participants can be identified (Kvale 1996).

Based on the initial coding, the researcher might also try to go beyond the self-understanding of the interviewee to understand, for example, which factors characterize or drive and influence the perspective of the interviewee. This type of analysis is known as "critical common sense" (Kvale 1996).

Other analytical approaches involve theoretical analyzing, i.e., interpretation of transcripts through the application of a specific and relevant theory or the technique of grounded theory which in a structured procedure generates new theory by viewing the transcripts without pre-assumptions. These hypotheses or ideas of patterns and the meaning of patterns can then be tested by applying them to all included cases in order to refine it or, if not fully consistent with the data material, to discard the idea and test others.

2.2.7   Strengths and Weaknesses of Interviews

The strength of the interview is to illustrate patterns of perceptions, attitudes, ideas, etc. of a group of actors, for example, within the field of pharmacy practice pinpointing similarities and differences between participants. Interviews reflect participants' own accounts of actions in real life which should not necessarily be understood as what actions actually take place (Kaae et al. 2010).

Interviews can help researchers to better understand people's experiences and behavior; however, there are drawbacks. For example, some people find it challenging and/or uncomfortable telling their story to a researcher as opposed to being asked in a (more anonymous) questionnaire. As is the case with all qualitative research, the small sets of interviews cannot be generalized. Interviews are ultimately subjective, so if the goal of the research is to describe actions taking place, methods such as observations may be more suitable.

2.3   Observation

Observation is increasingly gaining recognition within pharmacy practice research. As a research method, it entails the observation and description of a subject's behavior in their natural environment. In pharmacy practice, observations have been used to study, for example, pharmacy organization in relation to the impact of technology on the workflow of staff members (Walsh et al. 2003), communication between pharmacy staff and patients (van Hulten et al. 2011), and the behavior of patients when being in the pharmacy (Mobach 2007).

Observation pertains to both quantitative and qualitative methodology. When using observations for qualitative research purposes, studies are often engaged with describing details of behavioral patterns of actors within the pharmacy practice field. This could be characterizing the leadership style of a pharmacy owner (Kaae et al. 2011) or communication behavior, i.e., "the roles" of the pharmacist and patient during the interaction or "how the two parties interact" (Murad et al. 2014).

2.3.1 Types of Observation

Different types of qualitative observation exist, depending on whether or not the researcher takes part in the activities being observed. Hence, the researcher can choose to be fully covert from the action taking place; the researcher can choose to be overt/visible but not participating in the activities, or they can engage in and take an active part of the actions to be investigated.

2.3.1.1 Nonparticipatory Observation

The idea of nonparticipatory observation is to capture the way certain behaviors take place in the real world without the researcher exerting any influence. This type of observation can be covert or overt according to whether the participants are aware of being observed. Non-interfering covert observation raises many practical and ethical challenges which must be addressed and resolved.

If choosing overt observation, practicalities such as where to stand in order to hear and see all relevant aspects must be considered. The risk of the so-called "Hawthorne effect" must be considered, i.e., the influence the presence of the researcher has on the actors' behavior. According to the Hawthorne effect, people try to live up to the existing norms or the assumed expectations of the researcher. It has, however, been shown that participants display different reactions when being observed; hence, it is difficult to foresee exactly if and how the observer influences the behavior of participants (McCambridge et al. 2014). It has been suggested that when possible, the researcher should spend time with participants prior to the observation in order to get them accustomed to the presence of the observer (Smith 1998). Using audio or video recordings as observation tools could be an option in order to reduce the Hawthorne effect.

2.3.1.2 Participant Observation

To get a more in-depth understanding of the behaviors taking place, participant observation is relevant. An ideal opportunity for participant observation in pharmacy practice exists for the pharmacist researcher. However, observing while at the same time acting in the environment is challenging and thus according to Robson (2002) requires extensive training.

A special type of covert participant observation has been used in pharmacy practice in the case of mystery shoppers. This method is often used to assess the communication behavior of the staff at the pharmacy counter. It is mainly used for quantitative purposes.

2.3.2 Preparing the Observation

Preparing an observation study includes decisions regarding the sampling setting, i.e., where the behaviors under observation will take place, how to collect data, and what data will be collected as well as the period of time necessary to collect sufficient amounts of data.

Typical representative or unique cases could be included depending on the research questions (see also "Preparation of the Interview"). The number of different settings as well as settings within a setting should be considered before starting the observation. If, for example, exploring communication at the counter, it should be decided what the number and characteristics of included pharmacies should be (for example urban or rural) and, additionally, how many and what members of staff should be observed. It is also important to decide the time of day when the observations will take place. Finally, the number of different encounters at the counter or when to stop observation has to be determined. This often necessitates parallel data collection and analysis.

The collection instrument for observation can take several forms. Based on the works of Spradley, Robson (2002) suggests nine dimensions to observe, all of which have to be described thoroughly initially in order to obtain rich and nuanced data. The levels include Space, Actors, Activities, Objects, Acts, Events, Time, Goals, and Feelings. Hence, the description includes both physical elements as well as the immediate interpretation of goals and feelings of the people under investigation. The advantage is that the context of the behaviors is then registered along with the behaviors themselves. As behaviors are indisputably dependent on the context in which they take place, this factor can then be described and analyzed.

The scheme designed by Robson (2002) will in most cases have to be supplemented with new categories/dimensions pertaining to specific elements of interest. For example, when observing communication at the pharmacy counter, nonverbal behavior, spatial behaviors (if actors move closer or further away from each other), extralinguistic behavior (for example, speed of speaking or loudness), and linguistic behaviors (actual content and structure of talk) could all be integrated (Robson 2002). Use of audio or video recordings might also provide useful supplementary data. These tools will inevitably register a variety of details during the action which could never be obtained to the same degree when taking notes by hand (Murad et al. 2014).

2.3.3 Analyzing the Observation

When using audio or video recordings, the first step in the analysis could be to transcribe actions into written accounts. Coding directly on recordings is also feasible. Then the nine categories developed by Robson (2002) could be used as the first step in the analysis.

Units of behavior are then defined. The unit can be defined in many ways—one patient-staff encounter at the counter, the actions of the pharmacy owner during 1 day, etc. The next step is either to select verbal statements or/and contemporary behavior within the unit and start coding these to be able to characterize the typical nature of the observed behavior within the unit.

After coding the data according to the first set of categories, the researcher can then start looking more into the meaning of the content of the different codes. Which codes are linked and in which ways? What really defines the actions within one code? Contextual factors can be considered here as well. Do behaviors differ according to differences in the context? New meanings and codes are then developed and renamed and finally turned into a total understanding of the characteristics of the first unit. The unit can then be compared with other units to explore similarities and differences between them.

2.3.4 Strengths and Weaknesses of Observations

Observations are useful to explore what people actually do instead of relying on what people say they do. In some cases, peoples' perceptions of their actual actions coincide with what others register (Fedder et al. 1998). In case of discrepancies, observations are often believed to be "truthful" compared to self-reported practices reported in questionnaires or interviews. However, expressed perceptions should never be discarded as false but rather understood to represent another angle to the case, i.e., how people perceive or want to be perceived in a certain situation. As people are often unaware of their actions or can never explain in detail how they actually act, observations are useful in registering this.

Observation is only a limited resource for initiating practice improvements because they don't allow the practitioners to reflect on their own behavior, for example, the opportunity to provide reasons and arguments for acting in a particular way. Hence, the reasoning and perceptions of the involved actors of their behavior hold very useful information as to how they can be motivated into changing practices in the future. A very fruitful way of triangulation is first to carry out observations and then ask interviewees to comment directly on the observations made (Kaae et al. 2010).

2.4   Documentary Methods

A document is a piece of written, printed, or electronic matter that provides information or evidence which relates to some aspect of the social world and often serves as an official record. Documents reveal what people do or did and what they value. Often, the behavior revealed in the document occurred in a natural setting which gives this type of data a strong validity.

Document analysis is the method of using documents as the object of study. The goal of the analysis is to find and interpret patterns in data, to classify patterns, and (when possible) to generalize the results. Documentary methods have been useful within pharmacy practice to explore the development of policies influencing practice. Examples include the analysis of how and why publicly reimbursed cognitive services are agreed upon (Kaae et al. 2009) and society's expectations of pharmacist-patient medical communication as expressed in the legislation (Svensberg et al. 2015).

A documentary study can either be quantitative or qualitative; it all depends on the research questions. Qualitative methods of document analysis involve interpreting the information provided in the material through descriptive and analytic means, in particular studying the context and the multiple meanings that can be found in the documents. Document analysis as a research method often avoids ethical issues in that most often the documents being analyzed are in the public domain.

2.4.1   Types and Sources of Documents

The document sources are many, are varied, and can be found in a variety of places; one example is literature reviews, which are the process of reading, analyzing, evaluating, and summarizing scholarly literature. Another example is medical documents (including patient journals) which are frequently the object of study in pharmacy practice studies. In research that focuses on the patient perspective, personal documents can be used such as patient diaries and copies of their correspondence with health professionals.

Official documents such as government publications, legal documents, documents of public hearings, guidelines, and reports are often the source of policy analysis in pharmacy practice. For example, document analysis of a particular pharmaceutical policy—such as the problem of counterfeit drugs—might include white papers or reports produced by the ministry of health as well as position papers produced by the World Health Organization or other international organizations. The intention of most official documents is to be read as objective statements of fact; however, in research, documents are regarded as socially produced and serve as evidence or proof and therefore can reveal some of the underlying meanings and motives. One should, however, be aware that there can also be opinions and perceptions that actors deliberately do not want to display publically.

2.4.2   Preparing for the Documentary Analysis

Most important when preparing document studies is to identify and then decide on exactly what documents you need/want to analyze, in other words, based on your research question(s), what documents can provide answers, or at least partial answers, to these questions.

Further, it is important to keep order in your documents and your notes. Sometimes, it is useful to scan the documents onto a computer and use a qualitative analysis software package.

2.4.3   Analyzing Documentary Material

The first step in analyzing the documentary material is to roughly sort out the documents, weeding out those that are not relevant. Then, it is a good idea to summarize the contents of the relevant documents.

Next, go back to your main and supplementary research questions to see if you have found answers. You move from raw data (the documents themselves) to an understanding and/or interpretation of the material by looking for repetition and trying to find patterns (Hodson 1999).

A useful tool in document analysis is a worksheet. Basic categories include the title of the document, the author, the potential for author bias, the source, and the date published. There should be space in the worksheet for notes whereby you address the following questions: What are the important facts? What inferences can be made from this document? What is the main point/idea? How can this be used in my research question? (Does it in any way answer my research questions or contribute to this?) Was there any unexpected, yet relevant, information? The goal is to find an explanation and understanding of the questions addressed in your project. The answer can take many forms. For example, an analysis of package inserts for a particular medicine could reveal that the majority of the problems with package inserts are most likely due to communication problems—in other words, customers do not understand the advice provided in the inserts because the language is perhaps very technical.

2.4.4 Strengths and Weaknesses of Document Analysis

In general, documentary studies are useful when a document exists that is relevant to your research question; when you reach the realization that if you did not analyze this (these) document(s), you would have a hole in your research; and when it is not possible to observe or do interviews with your population. Although computers can be useful to help organize and sort data, no computer can manage your data—it is up to you to devise a system of filing and recalling for all your documents and notes (Traulsen and Klinke 2005).

2.5 Netnography

Netnography is an online research method which has its roots in ethnography (the term combines "network" with "ethnography") and has gained popularity and impetus in the field of marketing research. Robert V. Kozinets, a professor in marketing and social media, defines it as the use of online communities, such as newsgroups, blogs, forums, social networking sites, podcasting, video casting, photo sharing communities, and virtual worlds, for research purposes (Kozinets 2010). Some call netnography a method and others a discipline; basically, it is using the computer as a tool to support research and the Internet as a source of generating/providing data. Examples of netnography related to pharmacy practice are analyses of public opinions about pharmacists prescribing hormonal contraceptives (Irwina et al. 2018) and studying the online presence of community pharmacies (Domínguez-Falcón et al. 2018).

Initially devised as a tool to explore consumer behavior, netnography is a useful tool/method in pharmacy practice research for studying online cultures and communities such as patient groups and organizations or to do marketing and consumer research.

Netnography is more naturalistic and unobtrusive than other qualitative methods such as focus groups or interviews (however, other ethical dilemmas exist). Netnography explores cultural phenomena (such as blogs, Facebook groups, and other Internet-based social media, tweets, etc.) where the goal of the research is to observe communities and social groups from the point of view of the subject of the study, what some call "writing the culture of the group." Netnography can also be used to understand infrastructures, groups, and networks by providing information on the symbolism, meanings, and behavior patterns of online consumer groups, pharmacy staff, etc.

2.5.1 Analyzing Netnographic Material

In general, data obtained through the Internet can be analyzed the same way as other documentary material (see "Documentary Methods"). Whereas data basically consists of discrete entities that are described objectively without interpretation (for example, transcriptions of interviews or text found in a document), the data must be organized, structured, and interpreted. It must thereafter be synthesized so that interrelationships can be identified and formalized.

2.5.2 Strengths and Weaknesses of Netnography

The social media opens great opportunities for pharmacy practice research, making it easy to contact and establish dialogues with patients, patient associations, as well as pharmacists and health care professionals. For example, if the research is concerned with understanding the increase in use of antidepressants among young women, one could set up a blog and/or a "chat room" and invite young women to join. One recent initiative includes a study which set up a pharmacy-based nationwide online tele-pharmacy chat service offering free pharmacy counseling to all followed by an analysis of the types of inquiries in order to identify the needs of customers and therein improve pharmacy services for citizens (Ho et al. 2014).

There are ethical issues in netnography which, very much like observation, concern whether or not participants are aware of your presence. For example, if you investigate the discussions of a Facebook group, are the members of the group aware that they are being followed? If yes, they might hold back information that they would otherwise have disseminated. As with other types of research, you need informed consent from participants to use quotes, etc. However, one particular aspect about using quotes from Internet sources in publications is that they can relatively easily be traced, thereby compromising the anonymity of participants (Eysenbach and Till 2001).

One way to manage some of the ethical dilemmas linked to netnography is to supplement data from online sources with off-line research methods. Hence, using online social groups, blogs, etc. can be a way to get inspiration on specific topics and tendencies that you can then explore more in depth, for example, by conducting interviews off-line.

2.6 Visual Research/Visual Methods

Today, a large part of the social world is visual, reflected in the social sciences in recent decades by rapid growth in the use of visual methods in qualitative (and quantitative) research. It is often suggested that this phenomenon is somehow related to the increasing importance of visual images in contemporary social and cultural practice (Rose 2013). Visual research methods are built on a history of early participatory needs assessment work in health care, health education, and health promotion.

An academically recognized method, visual research originated in anthropology and sociology and then spread into psychology and health studies. This thriving academic field has resulted in numerous books and journals dedicated to publishing the results of social scientific visual research.

These methods use various forms of visual materials as part of the research process of generating evidence in an attempt to answer the research question(s). These methods are diverse with regard to the types of visual materials used as well as the procedures to which those materials are subjected.

2.6.1 Types of Visual Methods

While photos, posters, and film were originally the object of analysis, with the introduction and spread of social media, today many would say that we have moved into a predominately visual social world in which we are bombarded with visual images on a daily basis. This development has provided the researcher with a variety of visual media on which to focus. Examples of visual materials used in academia include photographs, films, video-diaries, collages, drawings, photo voice, and photo diaries, just to name a few.

Sometimes, the visual materials are generated by the researcher: visual material developed exclusively for research. Other times, materials are created by research participants: Children may be asked to "draw" their illness or illustrate how they use their medicine. Sometimes, visual materials are "found": Participants may be asked to describe/interpret the meaning of a health promotion poster. All types of visual materials can be theorized, contextualized, and analyzed in different ways (Rose 2013).

Although there is limited space to consider every type of visual material, one is worth mentioning here due to its current popularity. This is photo voice, a visual method that provides participants with a camera and asks them to produce visual accounts of their experiences and/or those things that are important to them in a particular context. Photo voice was promoted as a participatory health promotion strategy in as early as the 1990s (Wang et al. 1998) and successfully used in the fields of education, disability studies, and public health research, indicating its vast applicability.

The photo voice method is based on the assumption that increased participant control of data generation through production of visual images will help highlight important aspects of lived experience among participants who might otherwise have been overlooked or ignored by researchers. Photo voice is typically used with marginalized populations that have been silenced in the political or public arena. The method is often used in social science and health research as a means of catalyzing personal and community change. Photo voice has been described as an effective tool for carrying out participatory needs assessment, conducting participatory evaluation, and reaching policy makers (Wang and Burris 1994).

2.6.2   Preparing Visual Methods

In preparing to carry out visual methods, most important is to identify and decide on exactly the form of the material you will use. When using existing images—such as posters/photos/videos—be sure you have them available and in good shape prior to the encounter with participants. In cases where participants will be asked to create visual images—such as photos, photo voice, or drawings—it is important to make the necessary equipment available. For drawings, this means making sure there are ample supplies, i.e., paper, pens, inks, and paints. When asking participants to take photos or carry out a photo voice exercise, three things are essential: first, securing and testing the necessary equipment (cameras, audio equipment); second, giving participants training in the basic techniques of documentary photography and the use and care of the equipment; and third, providing participants with support, time, and opportunity to show and discuss their photos/videos. It is important to provide a safe and supportive environment in which participants can learn new skills and gain confidence in their ability to express ideas and opinions.

2.6.3   Analyzing Visual Methods

Most academically trained researchers will agree that all observations and studies are theory laden; in other words, there are no theory-free views of the world. Although not all research makes a clear explicit theoretical claim, upon further analysis, a trained academic will be able to locate the "implicit" (not mentioned) theoretical basis (Lau and Traulsen 2017). Many would agree that choosing a theory can be difficult. It is well known that an explicit theoretical framework sets the agenda for the types of researchable questions that can be addressed in the study. That being said, it is these explicit theoretical relevancies that establish the frame for analysis. Thus, how to analyze visual phenomena is structured by the theoretical framework the study has adopted.

There are numerous ways of analyzing data produced by visual methods. Textual analysis is intended to grow out of close attention to the visual data in the tradition of content analysis. Answering the research question(s) is the main point of entry into the analysis, together with the framework established by the theoretical approach, which may be structuralism, cognitive anthropology, and ethnomethodology. In all cases, attention to the symbolic meaning of the visual representation is crucial.

2.6.4   Strengths and Weaknesses of Visual Methods

One of the major strengths of visual methods is that they do not rely on a specific language. Therefore, researchers can choose participants from a large sample pool, making it possible to recruit persons who are illiterate, uneducated, or disabled. Further, participants can include persons who have difficulty communicating due to severe mental illness or persons who do not share the same language, including accents and colloquialisms, as the research team.

The limitations of most visual methods are that they often require the researcher to budget for the necessary equipment, such as cameras, audio equipment, ink, and printing costs. Another potential problem can be the question of who owns the photos. Although the research team may be providing the equipment, the participants are taking the photos. This should be taken into consideration when the researchers obtain informed consent in order to avoid potential problems.

It is particularly important to think carefully about informed consent in our era of digital dissemination and open-access publication. Images can be reworked, redistributed, and recirculated in the digital economy in ways that may not have been envisaged at the time of the research study (Mannay 2014).

2.7   Validity and Transferability in Qualitative Studies

As in all scientific research, qualitative studies have to live up to the quality criteria of research conduct within the research community (Malterud 2001). These criteria are neither rigid nor fixed; they include validity, transferability of the research process, and results. Qualitative research is not a unified field; several published criteria exist for producing good qualitative research, guiding the research process, and providing trustworthy results. As pharmacy practice research is situated within different research traditions including natural sciences, social sciences, and humanities, several conflicting or supplementary perceptions of exactly which quality criteria to apply and how to apply them exist. Therefore, the appropriate criteria for each individual study should come from within the theoretical and methodological framework from which the study emerges (Cohen and Crabtree 2008). In the end, it is important to remember that certain guidelines may help improve the quality and the credibility of the study results; however, adopting them does not guarantee high quality.

Aside from adhering to quality criteria, research in pharmacy practice should also be assessed by its contribution to the development of the field. This depends on the purpose of the research questions which are often driven by either an in-depth knowledge of the field coupled with a desire to gain more knowledge and understanding or, in the case of exploratory research, a desire to embark on a new area of inquiry. A good research question does not necessarily result in good-quality research; however, a poorly conceived or constructed question will inevitably create problems that affect all subsequent stages of a study (Agee 2009).

2.7.1 Validity

Validity is an indication of the soundness of the study and applies to both the design and the methods. Validity is measured by whether or not the researcher has managed to do what they proposed to do, i.e., adequately presenting the reality (s)he intended to investigate. Ensuring validity includes validation of every step of the research process from formulating relevant research questions to the dissemination of results. How this is managed is again a question of which research tradition the researcher identifies with.

Transparency is a crucial element in building up validity as no process undertaken in a study is justified by itself. To obtain transparency, a thorough description of all relevant actions undertaken during the project is required including solid arguments for the choices made. Solid argumentation ought to include a description of the pre-understanding of the researcher, i.e., the prior understanding, beliefs, attitudes, etc., previously acquired by the researcher(s). Eliciting understandings and decisions made during the research project also helps to bridge the different phases to each other in order to ensure, for example, that the data collection tool is in line with the research questions as well as with a relevant theory and review of the literature in the field.

Another important quality element in qualitative research is obtaining richness of data which allows for interpretation that goes beyond purely descriptive accounts. This calls for research methods which are sensitive to details including good interviewing skills.

Finally, being open to finding and acknowledging unexpected patterns in the data is also important for the validity of a qualitative study.

2.7.2 Transferability

Transferability refers to the degree to which the results of qualitative research can be generalized or transferred to other settings or contexts. It is important always to consider the context of the study when attempting to generalize or transfer the results. The transferability of results is relevant because one of the main purposes of research is pooling knowledge in order to get a better insight into relevant areas in order to develop these further. Results in pharmacy practice research often show strong resemblances between different countries, which make the issue of transferability highly relevant. One example is the implementation of pharmaceutical care where barriers such as the attitude of the pharmacist (Mak et al. 2012; Gastelurrutia et al. 2008) and lack of recognition by other health care professionals (McDonough and Doucette 2001; Bradley et al. 2012) have been identified independently in several countries across different continents.

Transferability is of course directly linked to the cases included in the study—the pharmacists, patients, pharmacies, etc. Who exactly was involved in the study? Whom do they represent? Can it be argued that other actors with similar profiles exert the same behavior, ideas, and perceptions? It has been argued that the reader of the study and not the writer/researcher is often better at assessing whether results of one setting are transferable to another as the reader often knows best what the relevant comparable setting is. This requires transparency by the researcher in order for the reader to make an adequate assessment.

As the goal of sampling in qualitative observation is not to generalize results but to explore different views/experiences, identify patterns, etc., one well-chosen case could in theory demonstrate features and categories that are relevant for a number of other cases (Mays and Pope 1995). Selection bias, i.e., including cases and people who are more engaged in the topic than those abstaining from participating, is often unavoidable. Rather than trying to change what can't be circumvented, it is important to describe the biases when writing up the results and then try to assess the influence they exert over the results.

In closing, it is important to remember that evaluating the quality of research is essential if the results are to be utilized in practice and incorporated into pharmacy practice.

2.8   Strengths and Limitations of Qualitative Studies

2.8.1   Strengths

Qualitative research attempts to answer the "why" questions and is therefore useful for describing, in rich detail, complex phenomena that are situated and embedded in local contexts. For example, what are the reasons underlying the inappropriate use of antibiotics? When used combined with and parallel to quantitative data collection, qualitative methods help explain why a particular response was given, and they provide in-depth details by unveiling attitudes, feelings, and behaviors, thus creating a detailed picture about why people act in certain ways and their thoughts and feelings about these actions (Denzin and Lincoln 2010).

The openness and flexibility of qualitative research has one major advantage. It creates openness since it is carried out in an informal, relaxed atmosphere that invites participants to be open and honest, encouraging them to expand on their responses. This in turn can open up new areas of interest not initially considered with the added advantage of allowing respondents to answer questions in as much detail as they want.

Qualitative research collects data in naturalistic settings making it possible to get more valid information about respondents' attitudes, values, and opinions since it opens the possibility for people to explain. Qualitative approaches are especially responsive to local situations, conditions, and stakeholders' needs.

2.8.2 Limitations

The major limitation of qualitative research is that fewer people are usually studied. This has several consequences; for example, the results are unlikely to be representative of a particular population. This means that the results can be difficult to directly compare or generalize to other people/patient types, other settings, or other research findings.

Qualitative research is extremely dependent on the skills of the researcher, particularly when conducting interviews. There is always the danger that the results can be easily influenced by the researcher's personal biases and idiosyncrasies. For this reason, transparency of the research process is encouraged.

With regard to resources, qualitative studies are time-consuming and labor-intensive—in terms of both data collection and data analysis. Critics say that qualitative research has lower credibility among some administrators and policy makers who often prefer percentages, statistics, and tables.

2.9 Summary

Qualitative research answers the "why" questions by establishing close personal contact to the person(s) being studied; it emphasizes understanding through the in-depth study of people's words, actions, and records (written as well as visual). Qualitative research is responsive to local situations, conditions, and stakeholders' needs. In spite of the fact that it is time-consuming and labor-intensive and the objects/persons studied are limited in number, qualitative research provides a more complete, detailed description of respondents' attitudes, values, and opinions, therein providing nuanced information that can lead to valuable improvements in pharmacy practice.

References

Agee J. Developing qualitative research questions: a reflective process. Int J Qual Stud Educ. 2009;22(4):431–47.

Almarsdóttir AB, Rahmner PB. Qualitative methods in drug utilization research. In: Drug utilization research: methods and applications. Wiley; 2016.

Anderson C, Kirkpatrick S. Narrative interviewing. Int J Clin Pharm. 2016;38:631–4.

Bradley F, Ashcroft DM, Noyce PR. Integration and differentiation: a conceptual model of general practitioner and community pharmacist collaboration. Res Soc Adm Pharm. 2012;8:36–46.

Cavaco AM, Dias JP, Bates IP. Consumers' perceptions of community pharmacy in Portugal: a qualitative exploratory study. Pharm World Sci. 2005;27(1):54–60.

Cohen DJ, Crabtree BF. Evaluative criteria for qualitative research in health care: controversies and recommendations. Ann Fam Med. 2008;6(4):331–9.

Denzin NK, Lincoln YS. The SAGE handbook of qualitative research. London: Sage; 2010. isbn:978-1-41297-417-2.

Domínguez-Falcón C, Verano-Tacoronte D, Suárez-Fuentes M. Exploring the customer orientation of Spanish pharmacy websites. Int J Pharm Healthcare Marketing. 2018;12(4):447–62.

Emmerton LM, Smith L, LemAy KS, Krass I, Saini B, Bosnic-Anticevich SZ, Reddel HK, Burton DL, Stewart K, Armour CL. Experiences of community pharmacists involved in the delivery of a specialist asthma service in Australia. BMC Health Serv Res. 2012;12:164. https://doi.org/10.1186/1472-6963-12-164.

Eysenbach G, Till JE. Ethical issues in qualitative research on internet communities. BMJ. 2001;323:1103–5.

Fedder DO, Levine DL, Russell RP, Lewis C, Lamy PP. Strategies to implement a patient counseling and medication tickler system—a study of Maryland pharmacists and their hypertensive patients. Patient Educ Couns. 1998;11:53–64.

Frisk P, Holtendal C, Bastholm-Rahmner P, Sporrong SK. Competence, competition and collaboration: Perceived challenges among Swedish community pharmacists engaging in pharmaceutical services provision and research. Int J Pharm Pract. 2019;27:346. https://doi.org/10.1111/ijpp.12518.

Gastelurrutia MA, Benrimoj SI, Castrillon CC, de Amezua MJ, Fernandez-Llimos F, Faus MJ. Facilitators for practice change in Spanish community pharmacy. Pharm World Sci. 2008;31(1):32–9.

Guirguis LM, Witry MJ. Promoting meaningful qualitative research in social pharmacy: moving beyond reporting guidelines. Int J Pharm Pract. 2019;27:333–5.

Hassell K, Hibbert D. The use of focus groups in pharmacy research: processes and practicalities. J Social Adm Pharm. 1996;14(4):169–77.

Ho I, Nielsen L, Jacobsgaard H, Salmasi H, Pottegård A. Chat-based telepharmacy in Denmark: design and early results. Int J Pharm Pract. 2014;23(1):61–6.

Hodson R. Analyzing documentary accounts. London: Sage Publications; 1999.

van Hulten R, Blom L, Mattheusens J, Wolters M, Bouvy M. Communication with patients who are dispensed a first prescription of chronic medication in the community pharmacy. Patient Educ Couns. 2011;83(3):417–22.

Irwina AN, Stewart OC, Nguyena VQ, Bzowyckyj AS. Public perception of pharmacist-prescribed self-administered nonemergency hormonal contraception: an analysis of online social discourse. Res Social Adm Pharm. 2018; https://doi.org/10.1016/j.sapharm.2018.08.003.

Kaae S, Traulsen JM, Søndergaard B, Haugbølle LS. The relevance of political prestudies for implementation studies of cognitive services in community pharmacies. Res Social Adm Pharm. 2009;5(2):189–94.

Kaae S, Søndergaard B, Haugbølle LS, Traulsen JM. Development of a qualitative exploratory case study research method to explore sustained delivery of cognitive services. Pharm World Sci. 2010;32:36–42.

Kaae S, Søndergaard B, Haugbølle LS, Traulsen JM. The relationship between leadership style and provision of the first Danish publicly reimbursed CPS—a qualitative multi-case study. Res Social Adm Pharm. 2011;7:113–21.

Kaae S, Ghazaryan L, Pagava K, Korinteli I, Makalkina L, Zhetimkarinova G, Tentiuc E, Ratchina S, Zakharenkova P, Yusufi S, Maqsudova N, Druedahl L, Sporrong SK, Cantarero LA, Nørgaard LS. Knowledge, attitudes and behaviors around antibiotics in six countries in the Eastern WHO European region: Armenia, Georgia, Kazakhstan, Moldova, Russia and

Tajikistan—a qualitative, comparative analysis. Res Social Adm Pharm. 2019;16:238. https://doi.org/10.1016/j.sapharm.2019.05.014.

Kozinets RV. Netnography: doing ethnographic research online. London: Sage; 2010.

Kvale S. Interviews: an introduction to qualitative research interviewing. London: Sage Publications, Inc.; 1996. isbn:0-8039-5819-6.

Latif A, Boardman H, Pollock K. Reasons involved in selecting patients for a Medicines Use Review (MUR): exploring pharmacist and staff choices. Int J Pharm Pract. 2011;19(Suppl 1):31–3.

Lau SR, Traulsen JM. Are we ready to accept the challenge? Addressing the shortcomings of contemporary qualitative health research. Res Social Adm Pharm. 2017;13(2):332–8.

Mak VS, Clark A, Poulsen JH, Udengaard KU, Gilbert AL. Pharmacists' awareness of Australia's health care reforms and their beliefs and attitudes about their current and future roles. Int J Pharm Pract. 2012;20(1):33–40.

Malterud K. Qualitative research: standards, challenges, and guidelines. Lancet. 2001;358(11): 483–8.

Mannay D. Story telling beyond the academy: exploring roles, responsibilities and regulations in the Open Access dissemination of research outputs and visual data. J Corp Citizenship. 2014;2014:109–16.

Mays N, Pope C. Observational methods in health care settings. BMJ. 1995;311:182–4.

McCambridge J, Witton J, Elbourne DR. Systematic review of the Hawthorne effect: new concepts are needed to study research participation effects. J Clin Epidemiol. 2014;67(3):267–77.

McDonough RP, Doucette WR. Developing collaborative working relationships between pharmacists and physicians. J Am Pharm Assoc. 2001;41(5):632–92.

Mobach MP. Consumer behavior in the waiting area. Pharm World Sci. 2007;29(1):3–6.

Morgan DL. Focus groups as qualitative research. London: Sage Publications, Inc.; 1988.

Murad MS, Chatterley T, Guirguis LM. A meta-narrative review of recorded patient-pharmacist interactions: exploring biomedical or patient-centered communication? Res Social Adm Pharm. 2014;10:1–20.

Robson C. Real world research. A resource for social scientists and practitioner-researchers. In: Observational methods. Oxford: Blackwell; 2002.

Rose G. Visual methodologies: an introduction to researching with visual materials. 3rd ed. London: Sage; 2013.

Smith F. Focus groups and observation studies. Int J Pharm Pract. 1998;5:229–42.

Svensberg K, Sporrong SK, Bjornsdottir I. A review of countries' pharmacist-patient communication legal requirements on prescription medications and alignment with practice: Comparison of Nordic countries. Res Social Adm Pharm. 2015;11(6):784–802.

Thurmond V. The point of triangulation. J Nurs Scholarship. 2001;33(3):254–6.

Traulsen JM, Klinke BO. Project handbook—from idea to project—a handbook for pharmacy projects: The Danish University of Pharmaceutical Sciences; 2005. isbn:87-990703-1-6.

Walsh KE, Chui MA, Kleser MA, Williams SM, Sutter SL, Sutter JG. Exploring the impact of an automated prescription-filling device on community pharmacy technician workflow. J Am Pharm Assoc. 2003;51(5):613–8.

Wang C, Burris M. Empowerment through photo novella: portraits of participation. Health Educ Q. 1994;21:171–86.

Wang CC, Yi WK, Tao ZW, Carovano K. Photovoice as a Participatory Health Promotion Strategy. Health Promot Int. 1998;13(1):75–86.

Wisell K, Sporrong SK. The Raison D'être for the community pharmacy and the community pharmacist in Sweden: a qualitative interview study. Pharmacy (Basel). 2016;4(1):3. https://doi.org/10.3390/pharmacy4010003.

Wisell K, Winblad U, Sporrong SK. Stakeholders' expectations and perceived effects of the pharmacy ownership liberalization reform in Sweden: a qualitative interview study. BMC Health Serv Res. 2016;16(1):379.

Further Reading

Almarsdottir AB, Kaae S, Traulsen JM. Opportunities and challenges in social pharmacy and pharmacy practice research. Res Social Adm Pharm. 2014;10(1):252–5.

Almarsdóttir AB, Traulsen JM. Multimethod research into policy changes in the pharmacy sector—the Nordic case. Res Social Adm Pharm. 2009;5:82–90. https://doi.org/10.1016/j.sapharm.2008.04.005.

Denzin NK, Lincoln YS. The SAGE handbook of qualitative research. Thousand Oaks: Sage Fifth Edition; 2017.

Flick U. An introduction to qualitative research. London: Sage Publication, Inc.; 2009. isbn:978-1-84787-323-1.

Giacomini MK, Cook DJ. Are the results of the study valid? For the Evidence-Based Medicine Working Group. JAMA. 2000;284(3):357–62. https://doi.org/10.1001/jama.284.3.357.

Kozinets RV. The field behind the screen: using netnography for marketing research in online communities. J Marketing Res. 2002;39(1):61–72.

Kozinets RV. Netnography initial reflections on consumer research investigations of cyberculture. Adv Consum Res. 1998;25:366–71.

Rolfe G. Validity, trustworthiness and rigour: quality and the idea of qualitative research. J Adv Nurs. 2006;53(3):304–10.

Chapter 3
Action Research in Pharmacy Practice

Lotte Stig Nørgaard and Anna Bryndís Blöndal

Abstract Action research (AR) is based on a collaborative problem-solving relationship between the researcher and client. The chapter describes how data collection methods are used in AR. Concepts related to AR are mentioned, including the multifaceted role of the researcher. Strengths, weaknesses, and data quality in AR studies are described, along with the four AR steps and their related key features. The chapter then describes experience-based recommendations for how to run an AR study and concludes with suggestions for how to move forward with AR. Last, three concrete AR studies carried out in three different countries are described.

3.1 Introducing Action Research (AR)

If you do research which (1) is educative; (2) deals with individuals as members of social groups; (3) is problem-focused, context-specific, and future-oriented; (4) involves interventions; (5) aims at improvement and involvement; (6) involves cyclic processes (in which research, action, and evaluation are linked); and (7) is founded on an approach by which those involved in research are participants in a change process where they collaborate with researchers, then you are presumably doing action research (AR) (Hart and Bond 1995).

AR is defined as a methodology (or approach) that is based on a collaborative, problem-solving relationship between the researcher and the client/participant, aiming at both solving a problem and generating new knowledge. The key idea is that AR

L. S. Nørgaard (✉)
Faculty of Health and Medical Sciences, Department of Pharmacy,
University of Copenhagen, Copenhagen, Denmark
e-mail: lotte.norgaard@sund.ku.dk

A. B. Blöndal
Faculty of Health and Medical Sciences, Department of Pharmacy,
University of Copenhagen, Copenhagen, Denmark

Faculty of Pharmaceutical Sciences, University of Iceland, Reykjavík, Iceland

© Springer Nature Singapore Pte Ltd. 2020
Z. Babar (ed.), *Pharmacy Practice Research Methods*,
https://doi.org/10.1007/978-981-15-2993-1_3

uses a scientific approach to study the resolution of important social and organizational issues together with those who experience these issues directly (Coghlan 2019).

In AR both qualitative and quantitative research methods are typically used. Furthermore, AR is often described as a methodology that strives toward filling the gap between practice and theory (Meyer 2000; Reason and Bradbury 2007). It is a methodology that is somewhat different from other methodologies because traditionally researchers tend to conduct research "on" people, whereas action researchers conduct research with people (McNiff 2010). In short, it includes action, reflection, and partnership. Its purpose is not solely to understand social layout but to facilitate change while empowering stakeholders (Bradbury-Huang 2010; Brydon-Miller et al. 2003). The overall characteristic of AR is the use of ongoing cycles, which allows the change to be thoroughly monitored, analyzed, and evaluated to solve the problem. The process steps are well-known as diagnosing and analyzing problems, planning, implementing/taking action, and evaluating. After evaluation, a new cycle can begin based on the new situation and the change adapted accordingly.

Over the last few years, a good deal of cases have been described in international journals on processes and outcomes of AR studies involving pharmacists and pharmacy practice (Blondal et al. 2017c; Bradley 2013; Donovan et al. 2019; Elliott et al. 2017; Mc Namara et al. 2019; Meijer et al. 2004; Sørensen and Haugbølle 2008; Stupans et al. 2015) and generally within the healthcare system (Bate 2000; Montgomery et al. 2015). Books and chapters about theoretical thoughts and practical guidelines have also been published in recent years, on both action research in general (Coghlan 2019; McNiff 2013; Reason and Bradbury 2007) and especially its application in the healthcare (Babar 2015; Koshy et al. 2010).

In this chapter, we discuss the history and related concepts of AR, viewed explicitly from a pharmacy practice research point of view. We address strengths, limitations, and the challenges faced by the AR researcher. Core features of AR methodology are discussed and illustrated by a description of each step of the abovementioned cyclical process. In the end, we describe recommendations on how to plan an AR study and provide some examples from the pharmacy practice field.

3.2   History and Related Concepts

AR in its traditional sense has its origins in the behavioral sciences, but it has since developed in a more organizational context. This approach comes from the work of the social psychologist Kurt Lewin (1890–1947) who is recognized as the founding father of AR. Action research has many origins and methodologies though and has developed from approaches organizations take regarding their environmental and social impact to a more democratic and empowering approach to change. Related developments have been occurring both in organizational research and in community development, education, and nursing (Waterman et al. 2001).

Another approach from AR has developed from the field of sociology and focuses on how communities as sociopolitical systems enact social change. This approach is participatory action research (PAR). PAR focuses on the concern of power and powerlessness. It investigates how the powerless are excluded from decision-making and moves to empower people to construct and use their knowledge. Fals-Borda is one of the founding fathers of this approach (Fals-Borda 2001).

Participatory research is explained as the co-construction of research through partnerships between researchers and people affected by and/or responsible for action on the issues under study (Elliott et al. 2017; Jagosh et al. 2012; Lalonde et al. 2014; van Buul et al. 2014).

Community-based participatory research (CBPR) takes place in community settings and involves community members in the design and implementation of research projects. Examples of CBPR are to be read in Tapp et al. (2014) and Rudolph et al. (2010).

Other similar approaches to AR are "co-construction," "action learning," "action science," and "reflective practice" (Coghlan and Brannick 2009).

3.3 Strengths, Weaknesses, and Data Quality in AR

The strengths of AR relate to its participatory and democratic components and its power to address practical problems in specific situations. Because it is educative and enables participants to handle complex problems, in actuality, many "researchers" do the job. In addition, the diversity in knowledge and skills in a project group can be an essential ingredient for the success of an AR study. In an AR study, there is, namely, room for learning and especially learning from mistakes.

However, there are of course also weaknesses connected with AR. None of the participants in a steering group, for instance, make decisions autonomously. Rather, the process is collective, which makes decision-making procedures relatively complicated. Collective decision-making by the various parties is consequently much more time-consuming compared to traditional project management. That also means that project leaders must be aware of when it is necessary to use the collective form of decision-making and when to make decisions in a smaller forum.

One might wonder what type of quality criteria can and should be followed and strived to be fulfilled in AR studies—different as they are compared to a lot of other studies. Reason and Bradbury (2007) have argued that an AR study can be judged by the following questions:

- Is the study explicitly both aimed at and grounded in the world of practice?
- Is the study both explicitly and active participative: research with, for and by people, rather than on people? Does it have meaning for all involved?
- Does the study draw on a wide range of knowing—including intuitive, experiential, presentational, as well as conceptual knowing—and does it link to form theory?
- Is the study worthy of the term significant?
- Does the study emerge toward a new and enduring infrastructure? Toward changes? Does it make change happen in political systems, etc.?

Change, especially sustainable change, is often difficult to achieve. Therefore, an AR study should be judged solely not only by the changes produced but also by what has been learned from the experience of undertaking the work. Thus, it is crucial to document and describe all steps in an AR study in sufficient detail (Meijer et al. 2004).

Action researchers must also consider how their findings can be validated and tested for reliability in the best possible way (Tanna et al. 2005). This can be achieved by answering the following questions to create a detailed data quality description of their study (Waterman et al. 2001):

- Were the different phases of the study clearly outlined?
- Were the participants and the stakeholders clearly described and justified?
- Was consideration given to the local context while implementing change?
- Was the relationship between researchers and participants adequately considered?

3.4 Core Features of AR Methodology

The primary contrast between AR and other types of research is the role of the researcher and the constant use of the problem-solving cycles. AR projects often form a continuous and overlapping spiral of cycles (see Fig. 3.1).

Different models of AR cycles are available in the literature (Bradbury-Huang 2010; Coghlan 2019; McNiff 2013; Reason and Bradbury-Huang 2013). However, the core steps in all of them are (see Fig. 3.2):

1. Diagnosing and analyzing problems—purpose, goals, aims, and vision
2. Planning—plans and strategy
3. Taking action—implementation and performance
4. Evaluating—results, consequences, and effects

Fig. 3.1 Spiral of action research cycles

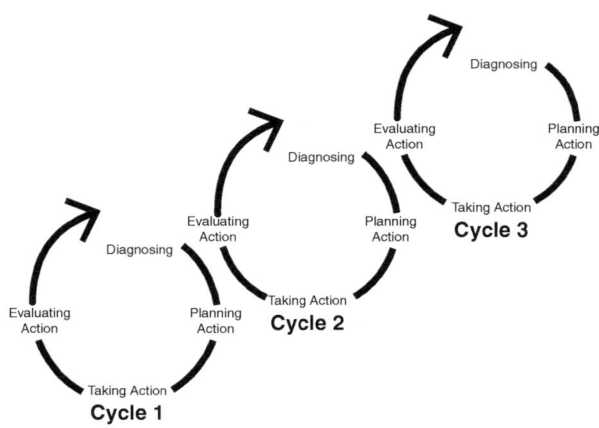

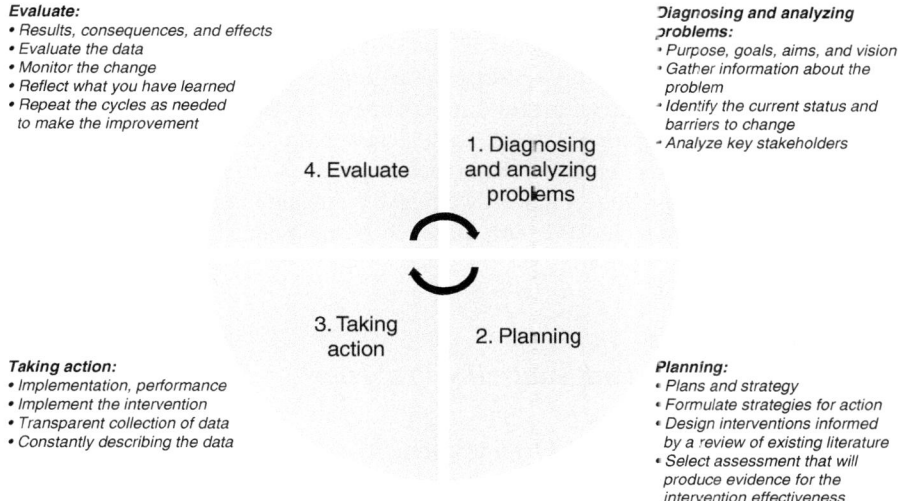

Evaluate:
• Results, consequences, and effects
• Evaluate the data
• Monitor the change
• Reflect what you have learned
• Repeat the cycles as needed
  to make the improvement

Diagnosing and analyzing problems:
• Purpose, goals, aims, and vision
• Gather information about the problem
• Identify the current status and barriers to change
• Analyze key stakeholders

4. Evaluate

1. Diagnosing and analyzing problems

3. Taking action

2. Planning

Taking action:
• Implementation, performance
• Implement the intervention
• Transparent collection of data
• Constantly describing the data

Planning:
• Plans and strategy
• Formulate strategies for action
• Design interventions informed by a review of existing literature
• Select assessment that will produce evidence for the intervention effectiveness

Fig. 3.2 Action research circle with key features of each step (Coghlan 2019; Hart and Bond 1995; McNiff 2013; Reason and Bradbury-Huang 2013)

AR is never a straightforward linear process toward an ending. On the contrary, it is a process of continual review and readjustment. In many ways, the AR is continually going back- and forward between different phases. This aspect makes it particularly useful in pharmacy research to gain new knowledge within healthcare settings, which are often complicated, pharmacist roles that are different, and the need for collaboration with other healthcare professionals. AR studies enable pharmacists to do ongoing evaluation and improvement within a study period and therefore support healthcare delivery development much better than other traditional methodologies (Tanna et al. 2005). Understanding the elements of AR is essential for any researcher to avoid common problems in data collection and analysis. AR is about real-time changes, and all choices need to be clear and transparent for all participants.

3.4.1   The Role of the Action Researcher

The action researcher conducts research with people not on people and therefore rejects the notion of an objective value-free approach (McNiff 2013). Instead of trying to achieve an unrealistic aim for the researcher to remain impartial by observing and being unbiased to the research outcome, the action researcher is actually a participant in the study. The primary purpose of an AR study always involves participation and can be related to personal development of the participants or organizational changes. This focuses the researcher on any reform, and by working in collaboration with others, their research leads not only to organization changes but also to personal improvement (Brydon-Miller et al. 2003). Being a reflective practitioner is an essential part of the process. A reflective practitioner is someone who, at regular intervals, looks back at the work they have done, and the work process, and considers how they can be improved (Verma and Paterson n.d.). Since AR is always done in company with others, an action researcher's role is also to implement the AR in such a manner as to produce a mutually agreeable outcome for all participants in a domain or organization and for the process to be maintained by them afterward (O'Brien 2001).

3.4.2   Diagnosing and Analyzing Problems

The first step of the cycle unfolds in real time by gathering information about the problem and seeking to gain understanding of the project. Why is this research necessary, and what are we trying to accomplish? For a problem to be developed into the subject for an AR study, it needs to be made into a more detailed research plan, so that it becomes susceptible to change or improvement. In this round, it is essential to analyze who the key stakeholders are and to get them on board with the research (Hart and Bond 1995). It is critical to establish collaborative relationships with those who have an ownership or need to have ownership so that they will maintain the outcome of the research afterward. By combining research knowledge and local knowledge, results are more valid for stakeholders and more likely to lead to changes in peoples' practices or the situation in which people practice (Reason and Bradbury-Huang 2013).

Key Features of Step 1:

- *Purpose, goals, aims, and vision*
- *Gather information about the problem*
- *Identify the current status and barriers to change*
- *Analyze key stakeholders*

3.4.3   Planning

Now that the problem has been identified, the second step is to formulate systematic strategies for action, which include measurable results on how to successfully solve the problem. By reviewing the pertinent literature, a plan of action is made based on the best possible data (Bradbury-Huang 2010). Both quantitative and qualitative or mixed research methods, which have been described in detail in other chapters, are typically used depending on the specific issue. The action researchers have to make sure that data used to justify their actions are both valid and reliable. In AR studies, the personal reflections of researchers are one of the components used.

Therefore, qualitative data collection is always in some way part of AR. What separates AR from other research is that an action researcher's personal reflections and analysis can be used as qualitative research data (Meyer 2000).

Table 3.1 provides an overview of data collection and producing methods that either have been or might be applied in AR. Inspiration for the table was found in Bradbury-Huang (2010), McNiff (2010), Coghlan and Brannick (2009), Reason and Bradbury (2007), Bradley (2015), and University of Copenhagen (2019) ("Methods—Innovation and entrepreneurship in education," n.d.). The presumed less well-known methods and tools are defined in Table 3.1.

Key Features of Step 2:

- *Plans and strategy*
- *Formulate strategies for action*
- *Design interventions informed by a review of existing literature*
- *Select assessment that will produce evidence for the intervention effectiveness*

Table 3.1 Overview of data collection and producing methods that either have been or might be applied appropriately in AR

The "How might we…?" method (A phrase used for framing effective ideation)	Documentary analysis
Observations (direct or indirect)	Surveys
Interviews (individual or focus groups)	Experiments
Etnoraid (an ethnographic method used to study people's cultural behavior)	Mechanical observation
Researcher personal reflections	Simulation
Photovoicing (a qualitative method used for documenting and reflecting reality through a combination of photography and grassroots social action)	Challenge mapping (a qualitative method pinpointing specific challenges from fieldwork by the use of pictures of and quotations from users, as well as an explanatory text that addresses a problem, barrier, or theme)
Problem trees (structured ways of collectively unpacking levels of problems)	Life histories, narratives, and storytelling
Social/participatory mapping (map drawing of study setting noting physical/social characteristics)	Idea selection by dot voting or by weighed criteria
Venn/spider diagrams (drawing of relationships)	Stakeholder analysis
SWOT analysis	The FIVE WHYS tool (analysis tool used to find a single base cause of a problem or to multiple reasons for the same problem)
Brain writing/brain walking (variants of traditional brainstorming)	The ECOSYSTEM method (provides an overview of complex relationships and graphically represented point of departure for group discussion)
CONFUSION TOLERANCE tool (creating 100 ideas in 15 minutes!)	The MINDMAPPING tool (mind maps are used to harness the input and thoughts inspired by a theme and to visualize their relationships)

3.4.4 Taking Action

The third step is to act and implement the intervention based on what was planned in phase 2. For the AR study to meet the standards of high-quality research, data collection has to be clear and transparent. Quality assessment criteria must be adopted and adhered to accordingly to achieve credibility, validity, and reliability in order to establish trustworthiness for the AR results (Bradbury-Huang 2010). Therefore, research performance and both collecting and constantly describing data are vital.

Key Features of Step 3:

- *Implementation and performance*
- *Implementing the intervention*
- *Transparent collection of data*
- *Constantly describing the data*

3.4.5 Evaluate

At this stage, data are evaluated, and the research outcome is reflected. In this step, all data is analyzed (also the researcher's personal data) in a search for identification of both positive and negative changes. Is the initial problem solved, or is another cycle needed to improve? If so, steps 1 to 4 are repeated as required (Bradbury-Huang 2010; Coghlan 2019; McNiff 2013; Reason and Bradbury-Huang 2013).

Key Features of Step 4:

- *Results, consequences, and effects*
- *Evaluate the data*
- *Monitor the change*
- *Reflect what you have learned*
- *Repeat the cycles as needed to make the improvement*

3.5   Recommendations for How to Plan an Action Research Study

On the back of our own AR-based experiences, we have made the following list of recommendations and comments for how to conduct an action research study. The first version of the list was made by Haugbølle and Sørensen (2006) together with 13 participants from 9 different European countries at a workshop entitled "Developing participatory action research in pharmaceutical care" (Haugbølle and Sørensen 2006).

When planning a pharmacy practice research study, a standard project description needs to be written (introduction, background, aim, research questions, design, methods, and plan for the project). What sets this apart from other forms of research, however, is that in an action research-based study, it is recommended to involve the participants or stakeholders from the very beginning when the aim and research questions are being formulated.

1. *Swear the stakeholders in*

    Start the project by describing a preliminary purpose and background of the study. The next step for the researcher is to find out about the context, meaning, the setting, the people, and institutions: who are involved in the study, who will support but not directly participate in the project, and what arrangements need to be put in place for the study. The researcher must also assess stakeholders or conflicting priorities that could obstruct the study. Once this has been determined, a decision can be made about who to invite into a project group. For achieving research goals, each project leader needs to have a motivation strategy to create and maintain the spirit of enthusiasm among participants. For members to fully contribute and be willing to make change, incentives and rewards must be considered and made clear These can include, for instance, personal development and positive organizational changes.

2. *Start at the right time (and continuously pay attention to when "time is ripe")*

    When should the study be initiated? The researcher's timeline must be aligned with the hospital ward's or pharmacy's priorities, expectations, and capabilities. This is to ensure, for example, that the clinical teams will be able to start producing data at the time convenient for all parties.

3. *Map the organizational structure*

    It is vital to map the organization in which the action research study is being conducted: who the leaders are (formal and informal), what the purposes and tasks of the organization are (the ward, the community pharmacists, etc.), staff competencies, and is there any cooperation with other parts of the organization. Other activities with whom the action research study might be "competing" with are also needed, because time commitments for this new study will be required and it must be aligned and coordinated with other activities in the organization.

4. *Involve, share, let go of control, divide tasks, and compromise*

    The researcher is working together as part of a project group to diagnosis the problem and formulate the research questions and issues. This is in contrast to other types of research studies. Moreover, the nature of this collaboration will require a certain level of detachment and flexibility on the part of the researcher to potentially "kill their darlings." This is because some issues, which may be important for the researcher, may not be considered useful from the participants' point of view. Nevertheless, it is important to bear in mind that action researchers sometimes may have to proceed even though all participants are not fully satisfied with the process. This is when decision-making is in a smaller forum becomes necessary.

5. *Use existing structure*

It is always time-consuming, especially for the participants such as health-care professionals, to put in new meetings in the busy daily work. Therefore, it is wise to figure out how to integrate sharing information and discussions about the study in current existing communication channels of the work of the clinical teams. This could be in monthly or weekly meetings, in newsletters or minutes, etc.

6. *Set up milestones*

It is overwhelming to plan changes in an organization which will run over a long period of time—maybe even years. Therefore, it is essential to divide the project into smaller milestones, which can easily be detected and celebrated at every breakthrough.

7. *Plan-do-observe-reflect (make room for reflection)*

The action research cycle elements are diagnosing, planning, action, and evaluation. This cycle is an important part of the action research concept. Problems and methods for solving them are formulated as the study moves along. Several cycles may need to be implemented in order for progress to be made. In the first cycle, the pilot, what is possible in the daily life for the practitioners may first be tried. What has been learned from this will enable the project team to make the tests in the next cycle better to suit all participants.

8. *Answer the question: what are the engines for change?*

Find out how motivated the participants are, either the individual, being engaged in their professional career and the development of the pharmacist professional role, or motivation coming from the environment, e.g., third-party payment of pharmaceutical services. Such influence can be a powerful motivation for the change process if they go hand in hand.

9. *Focus on Disseminating Products*

An essential task for the action researcher is to plan the dissemination of various kinds of information about the study, not only papers in international journals or an educational thesis for the researcher but also by informing participants, supporters, staff, community members, and others about the research results.

10. *Be aware: it is time-consuming*

Though we are very enthusiastic about the action research-based way of doing research, we acknowledge that an action research-based study takes more time and typically lasts years.

The pilot cycle may sometimes achieve disappointing results because at such an early stage of the study, neither the researcher nor the practitioners have reached the expectations established at the beginning of the study. However, once the plan and actions have been re-evaluated and gain a better understanding of the situation, the team becomes more accustomed to this way of working.

3.6   Moving Forward

AR has been around for several decades now, as well as within pharmacy practice research (Blondal et al. 2017c; Bradley 2013; Donovan et al. 2019; Elliott et al. 2017; Mc Namara et al. 2019; Meijer et al. 2004; Sørensen and Haugbølle 2008; Stupans et al. 2015). Although this approach may not be widely published, it does not mean that the core components of AR have vanished from the pharmacy practice researcher's mindset. On the contrary, related concepts, theories, and methodologies such as innovation, co-construction, patient engagement, and involvement have become part of the pharmacy practitioner's vocabulary and toolbox; how you "name the child" is not really important. What is essential, in our view, is that practice-based research is participatory and democratic, based on stakeholder views and patient preferences, and that it solves at least some of the complex problems experienced by patients and/or healthcare professional in the real world. Also, often-times it is quite challenging to conduct structured, conventional pharmacy research in the healthcare system, notably within the hospital setting. This is because patient groups are diverse, many professionals are involved, and the timeframe of the study is not definite. Furthermore, it is important to recognize that complicated circumstances can occur in such an environment, that staff day to day work to meet the constantly changing demands of the service and patients, is always a priority. This has led to fewer published articles from pharmacy hospital settings even though the material is qualified. Implementing more action research studies in a hospital setting is perhaps an approach to publish more articles in such surroundings, which will also benefit practice since healthcare organizations and hospitals, in particular, are highly resistant to change.

Action research is thus a valuable methodology for producing collaborative knowledge and action required for addressing today's societal, political, economic, and environmental changes. As stated previously, action research is a methodology with a strong stakeholder involvement, something which increases the likelihood of action research-based results to be implemented in every day practice and policy when the project period has ran out. After study 1 below was completed, a real impact remained within the primary care clinics in Iceland. The research pharmacist was appointed to develop pharmaceutical care in collaboration with general practitioners. The development is currently ongoing within the primary care clinics in Iceland. As to study 2 below, both managers and pharmacists involved in the research mentioned the positive contribution of the participatory action research in assisting them with the transition of pharmacists into new management positions through shared understanding of pharmacist managers' new roles and required competencies. At the time, it specifically helped in the development of new job descriptions for pharmacy managers. The pharmacy managers in these posts have developed significantly in these new roles over the past few years since research was conducted, a key feature being their active involvement in the district and sub-district management teams. Study 3 below paved the way for the inclusion of obligatory medication reviews tasks being part of pharmacy curriculum in Denmark, just as the study influenced positively the way medication reviews are now carried out in Danish pharmacies, almost 10 years after the completion of the study.

The many and varied methods used in all these action research studies might seem unnecessarily complex, but implementing, for instance, sustainable cognitive services in a primary healthcare system in constant change is in itself a complex process, something which has to be mirrored in the choice of methods. For all three studies described below, the partnership benefited from contextual and practice experiences of health services stakeholders and research experience of the researcher. Especially in study 2, the broad stakeholder group was important for shared learning and understanding, and the approach facilitated translation into action and change in the organizations.

The core components of action research such as democratization, ownership, involvement, and co-construction of research through partnerships between researchers and people affected by and/or responsible for action on the issues under study (such as healthcare professionals) are increasingly viewed as pivotal for all activities in the healthcare system.

3.7 Examples of Action Research in Pharmacy Practice

3.7.1 Study 1: Introducing Pharmaceutical Care to Primary Care in Iceland: An Action Research Study (Blondal et al. 2017c)

3.7.1.1 Objective

In Iceland, pharmaceutical care services are provided in hospitals but not in other care settings, despite the requirement for pharmaceutical care provision being written into legislation in 1994. The main challenge in Iceland is that currently there is little communication between community pharmacists and general practitioners (GPs) on clinical issues. GPs do not recognize pharmacists as healthcare providers, nor do they have any experience with pharmacist-led clinical services (Blondal et al. 2017b). To date, studies have not focused on the actual process undertaken when pharmacists develop a new outpatient service in close collaboration with GPs. The problem was how to introduce and adapt pharmaceutical care service into Icelandic primary care clinics. Therefore, the aim of this study was to use action research to introduce and study pharmacist-led pharmaceutical care in primary care in collaboration with GPs, testing different settings and models of care, aiming at meeting specific local and Icelandic needs.

3.7.1.2 Materials, Methods, and Settings

It was expected that several action research cycles would be needed to get to a process that was feasible for the existing organization and at the same time be beneficial to patients. By involving and making GPs active in decisions about the implementation, it was expected that they would be more willing to accept pharmacist-led pharmaceutical care. An active participation strategy was used; the first author was active in introducing and starting the service, i.e., being a practitioner, while at the same time being a researcher. The process started by understanding GPs' perspectives and introducing a service, which was then modified throughout the action research cycles. The study settings were a primary care clinic in the Reykjavik area and homes of patients who received the pharmacist-led pharmaceutical care.

Five GPs from the primary care clinic and 125 of their patients participated in the action research process. The GPs chose participants who were over 65 years of age based on the criteria established by the Home Medicines Review (HMR) program in Australia (Ageing AGD n.d.). GPs then made a referral to the pharmacist for pharmaceutical care service.

Data was collected from pharmaceutical care interventions with patients, research notes, meetings, and in-depth interviews with GPs throughout the study, which ran from September 2013 to October 2015.

Pharmaceutical care intervention: The researcher provided pharmaceutical care as defined in the pharmaceutical care literature (Cipolle et al. 2012) to 125 patients throughout the study. Twenty-five patients received care in the pilot phase followed by 50 elderly home-dwelling patients in the first round of the action research process who did not have access to their medical records, and finally in the second round, 50 elderly home-dwelling patients who were receiving dose-dispensed medicines received pharmaceutical care services at the primary care clinic where the pharmacist had access to the patients' medical records (Blondal et al. 2017a).

In-depth interviews with GPs: Three in-depth interviews with each of the five GPs were conducted. Interviews were audio-recorded, transcribed verbatim, and thematically analyzed independently by the first and last authors. Themes were finally discussed among the researchers for agreement. Coding and thematic analysis were undertaken using conventional content analysis and NVivo 11 software. The first round of in-depth interviews studied the GPs' perspectives on various issues such as the past decade's development of primary care in Iceland, today's status regarding medicine use and monitoring, GPs' use and perception of pharmacists, and their vision for primary care in the future. In the second and third rounds, GPs were asked about the advantages and disadvantages of the service provided and their views on collaboration with the pharmacist on clinical issues. Additionally, in the third round, the GPs' views on differences between the two ways of providing pharmaceutical care, their ideas about the best way to provide this service in primary care in the future, and their current opinion of pharmacists and their role in patient care were sought.

Meetings: Throughout the duration of the project, three meetings were held between the participating pharmacist and the participating GPs. The meetings were conducted to explore the progress of the project and to find common ground on which to move forward. The meetings were not recorded, but minuted including ideas, discussions, and decisions made.

Research notes: Throughout the entire project, the participating researcher kept notes of her experience. These notes consist of descriptions of events relating to the project's process and progress, which supplemented the data and were used to further understand the project, interventions, GP meetings, and interviews. The participating researcher continuously reflected on the data by reflecting on the issues, what had been planned, discovered, and achieved during the process.

3.7.1.3 Results

Throughout the process of the study period, two cycles emerged (see Fig. 3.3).

The main findings of this study are that GPs did not seem to understand the role of pharmacists in patient care and their knowledge about pharmacists as patient care providers developed during the research period. The GPs accepted the pharmacists' recommendations and comments about their patients' drug therapy almost entirely. They were supportive of working side by side with pharmacists in clinical decision-making, and they wanted to have access to a pharmacist on a daily basis. Lastly, it became apparent that pharmacist access to medical records is necessary for an optimal service.

By using action research methodology, it was possible for the research intervention to adapt to the context and setting, making the success of implementation more probable. Those aspects were crucial in this study because it allowed the project to

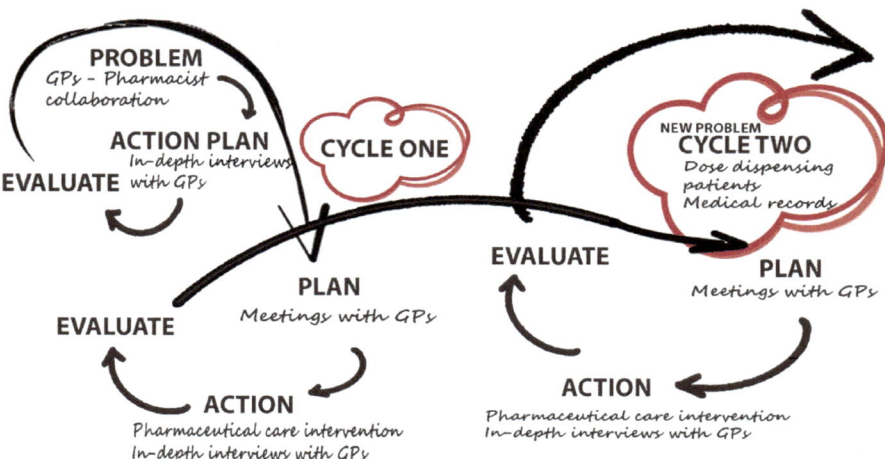

Fig. 3.3 Overview of the two action research cycles in the study

constantly develop in the primary care clinic and to change along the way. Also, by collaborating with the GPs, different perspectives were presented, and this increased the project's validity and efficiency.

3.7.1.4 Conclusions

When implementing pharmaceutical care practice, many barriers have been noted in the literature. In Iceland, the lack of communication between GPs and pharmacists was one of them. This research study indicated that action research is a useful methodology to promote and develop a relationship between those two healthcare providers in primary care. The most efficient collaboration is when pharmacists and GPs work side by side at the primary care clinic.

3.7.2 Study 2: Roles and Competencies of District Pharmacists: A Case Study from Cape Town (Bradley 2013)

Objective: The aim of this study (a Ph.D. thesis) was to explore the contribution of sub-structure and sub-district pharmacists to health system development, how to support them in their roles, by considering their roles and related competencies in the South African health system and by piloting an intervention to enhance their competencies. *Setting:* The managers in Cape Town City Health and Metro District Health Services together with the district and sub-district pharmacists in the period between 2008 and 2011. *Methods:* Participatory action research (PAR). The partnership benefitted from the contextual and practical experiences of the health services stakeholders and the researcher's evolving research expertise. Including a broad stakeholder group was considered to be important for developing the shared learning and understanding what would translate into action and change in the organizations. The flexible and emergent approach of PAR was considered to be suited for studying a complex health system in the midst of change. After an initiation stage, the research evolved into a series of five iterative cycles of action and reflection, each providing increasing understanding of the roles and related competencies of sub-structure and sub-district pharmacists, and their experiences as they transitioned into these new management positions in the two organizations. The research centered on two series of three interactive workshops facilitated by the researcher and attended by both pharmacists and managers. Semi-structured interviews and focus groups were conducted at various stages during the research, to inform conceptualization and supplement workshops and, later on, to reflect on the experiences of sub-structure and sub-district pharmacists. *Results and conclusion:* The research identified five main roles each for sub-structure and sub-district pharmacists. Four of these roles were the same for each: (1) sub-structure (sub-district) management; (2) planning, coordination, and monitoring of pharmaceuticals, HR, budget, and infrastructure; (3) information and advice; and (4) quality assurance and clinical governance. Their fifth roles were different: research for sub-structure pharmacists and dispensing at clinics for sub-district pharmacists. Although they looked similar, there were substantial differences between sub-structure and sub-district pharmacist roles in the two organizations. Five competency clusters were identified for both cadres, each with several competencies: professional pharmacy practice, health system/public health, management, leadership, and personal, interpersonal, and cognitive. Although the competencies appear similar, there were differences between the roles, so the different cadres required different competencies within these competency clusters. Transitioning into these new management positions was an emergent process, which entailed pharmacists changing from performing technical and clinical functions associated with professional pharmacy practice to coordinating pharmaceutical services across the sub-structure or sub-district. They moved from working in a pharmacy to being a member of a multi-professional team in a sub-structure or sub-district. Adjusting to these new management positions took time and was facilitated by several personal and organizational factors which varied in the two organizations. Managers and pharmacists mentioned the positive contribution of the PAR in assisting with this transition through the development of shared understanding of the DHS and the roles and functions of pharmacists working in these management positions.

3.7.3 Study 3: MEDISAM: Implementation of a Home Medicines Review (HMR) Collaboration Model for Pharmacists, Pharmacy Interns, and Doctors

In Denmark, a successful way of developing clinical tasks in community pharmacy has been through launching educational initiatives at university level in collaboration with pharmacy interns, their pharmacy supervisors, and other relevant collaboration partners (Sørensen and Haugbølle 2008). The *objective* of the MEDISAM study which ran from 2008 to 2010 was thus to develop, implement, and evaluate a collaboration model for home medicines reviews (HMRs) and medicine reconciliations in Denmark through the involvement of pharmacy internship students, their pharmacy supervisor, and physicians. The *design* used for development and implementation was action research (AR). The four AR phases, diagnosis/research questions, planning, action, and evaluation, were followed throughout the study. Methods used were dialogue meetings, interviews, and questionnaires with physicians, pharmacists, and pharmacy interns, minutes from meetings with external partners, and discussion and input from internship pharmacies during the early supervisor days. Data were registered, among other things, changes and learning for all parties, drug-related problems, pharmacist recommendations, and physician's acceptance of pharmacist recommendations. *Results*: In 2008, 20 internship phar-

macies, 21 general practitioners (GPs), and 52 type 2 diabetes patients participated
in the study. In 2009, 27 internship pharmacies, 2 hospital pharmacies, 22 GPs, and
118 type 2 diabetes patients participated. In 2010, all 91 Danish internship pharmacies (including 11 hospital pharmacies) and 308 patients (from different patient
groups) participated in the study. Alone in 2010, 749 drug-related suggestions were
identified (2,4/patient), and the pharmacy provided 601 intervention suggestions to
physicians, of which 17% were accepted and implemented. Another result relates to
the development of the so-called Copenhagen HMR model, which ended up com-
prising patient interviews in patient's home and written collaboration expectation
agreements between participating pharmacist and physician, describing their roles
and responsibilities (Kaae et al. 2014). As to specific changes, the study paved the
way for making HMRs an obligatory task at the pharmacy internship. Several different cooperation models between GPs and pharmacists were developed following
the study (Krabbe et al. 2013). *Conclusion*: The MEDISAM study did over a 3-year
period result in the development and implementation of an HMR collaboration
model involving patients, pharmacy interns, pharmacists, and physicians. By focusing on the development of an HMR cooperation model, the study contributed to the
establishment of a cohesive course of treatment for patients and a reduced number
of drug-related problems for patients.

Acknowledgments This chapter is an updated version of the chapter "Action Research in
Pharmacy Practice" written by Lotte Stig Nørgaard and Ellen Westh Sørensen in 2015 in the book
Pharmacy Practice Research Methods by Zaheer-Ud-Din Babar. We are very thankful for contributions made by Ellen Westh Sørensen in that chapter and surely acknowledge that we stand on her
shoulders in our efforts toward making and improving the updated version of the chapter. We are
also very thankful for constructive comments made by Hazel Bradley to study 2.

References

Ageing AGD. (n.d.). Home medicines review program qualitative research project final report.
    http://www.health.gov.au/internet/main/publishing.nsf/Content/hmr-qualitative-research-
    final-report
Babar ZUD. Pharmacy practice research methods. Cham: Springer International Publishing AG;
    2015.
Bate P. Synthesizing research and practice: using the action research approach in health care set-
    tings. Soc Policy Adm. 2000;34(4):478–93. https://doi.org/10.1111/1467-9515.00205.
Blondal AB, Almarsdottir AB, Gizurarson S, Jonsson JS. Lyfjafræðileg umsjá á Heilsugæslunni í
    Garðabæ—greining á fjölda og eðli lyfjatengdra vandamála eldri einstaklinga [Pharmaceutical
    care in primary care in Gardabaer—types and number of drug therapy problems identified
    among elderly patients]. 2017a;103(11):481–6.
Blondal AB, Jonsson JS, Sporrong SK, Almarsdottir AB. General practitioners' perceptions of
    the current status and pharmacists' contribution to primary care in Iceland. Int J Clin Pharm.
    2017b;39:1–8. https://doi.org/10.1007/s11096-017-0478-7.
Blondal AB, Sporrong SK, Almarsdottir AB. Introducing pharmaceutical care to primary care
    in Iceland—an action research study. Pharmacy. 2017c;5(2):23. https://doi.org/10.3390/
    pharmacy5020023.

Bradbury-Huang H. What is good action research?: Why the resurgent interest? Action Res. 2010;8(1):93–109. https://doi.org/10.1177/1476750310362435.

Bradley H. Roles and competencies of district pharmacists: a case study from Cape Town. 2013. http://etd.uwc.ac.za/xmlui/handle/11394/3255

Bradley H. Participatory action research in pharmacy practice. In: Barbar Z, editor. Pharmacy practice research methods. 2015. https://www.springer.com/gp/book/9783319146713

Brydon-Miller M, Greenwood D, Maguire P. Why action research? Action Res. 2003;1(1):9–28. https://doi.org/10.1177/14767503030011002.

van Buul LW, Sikkens JJ, van Agtmael MA, Kramer MHH, van der Steen JT, Hertogh CMPM. Participatory action research in antimicrobial stewardship: a novel approach to improving antimicrobial prescribing in hospitals and long-term care facilities. J Antimicrob Chemother. 2014;69(7):1734–41. https://doi.org/10.1093/jac/dku068.

Cipolle RJ, Strand L, Morley P. Pharmaceutical care practice: the patient-centered approach to medication management. 3rd ed. New York: McGraw-Hill Medical; 2012.

Coghlan D. Doing action research in your own organization. London: Sage; 2019.

Coghlan D, Brannick T. Doing action research in your own organization. London: SAGE Publications; 2009.

Donovan G, Brown A, Von Hatten E, Armstrong C, Hardisty J. Introducing pharmacy students to the structure and function of general practice through undergraduate placements. Curr Pharm Teach Learn. 2019;11:1055. https://doi.org/10.1016/j.cptl.2019.06.013.

Elliott RA, Lee CY, Beanland C, Goeman DP, Petrie N, Petrie B, et al. Development of a clinical pharmacy model within an Australian home nursing service using co-creation and participatory action research: the Visiting Pharmacist (ViP) study. BMJ Open. 2017;7(11):e018722. https://doi.org/10.1136/bmjopen-2017-018722.

Fals-Borda O. Participatory (action) research in social theory: origins and challenges. In: Bradbury H, Reason P, editors. Handbook of action research. London: Sage Publications; 2001.

Hart E, Bond E. Action research for health and social care. Buckingham: Open University Press; 1995.

Haugbølle LS, Sørensen EW. Workshop IV: developing participatory action research in pharmaceutical care. In: 4th international working conference on pharmaceutical care research—beyond the pharmacy perspective. Workshop leadership and lectures, Hillerød, February 2005; 2006.

Jagosh J, Macaulay AC, Pluye P, Salsberg J, Bush PL, Henderson J, et al. Uncovering the benefits of participatory research: implications of a realist review for Health Research and Practice. Milbank Q. 2012;90(2):311–46. https://doi.org/10.1111/j.1468-0009.2012.00665.x.

Kaae S, Sørensen EW, Nørgaard LS. Evaluation of a Danish pharmacist student–physician medication review collaboration model. Int J Clin Pharm. 2014;36(3):615–22. https://doi.org/10.1007/s11096-014-9945-6.

Koshy E, Koshy V, Waterman H. Action research in healthcare. London: Sage; 2010.

Krabbe T, Sørensen E, Nørgaard L, Kirkeby B. Den multimedicinerede patient—En samarbejdsmodel for medicingennemgang og –afstemning mellem praktiserende læge og apotek (The poly-pharmacy patient—a cooperation model for medication reviews and medication reconciliation between the GP and the pharmacy). 2013. p. 28–32.

Lalonde L, Goudreau J, Hudon É, Lussier MT, Bareil C, Duhamel F, et al. Development of an interprofessional program for cardiovascular prevention in primary care: a participatory research approach. SAGE Open Medicine. 2014;2:2050312114522788. https://doi.org/10.1177/2050312114522788.

Mc Namara KP, Krass I, Peterson GM, Alzubaidi H, Grenfell R, Freedman B, Dunbar JA. Implementing screening interventions in community pharmacy to promote interprofessional coordination of primary care—a mixed methods evaluation. Res Soc Adm Pharm. 2019;16:160. https://doi.org/10.1016/j.sapharm.2019.04.011.

McNiff J. Action research for professional development and experienced. 1st ed. Poole: September Books; 2010.

McNiff J. Action research: principles and practice. 2013. https://doi.org/10.4324/9780203112755

Meijer WM, DJde S, Jurgens RA, de Berg LTW d J. Pharmacists' role in improving awareness about folic acid: a pilot study on the process of introducing an intervention in pharmacy practice. Int J Pharm Pract. 2004;12(1):29–35. https://doi.org/10.1211/0022357022980.

Meyer J. Using qualitative methods in health related action research. BMJ. 2000;320(7228):178–81. https://doi.org/10.1136/bmj.320.7228.178.

Montgomery A, Doulougeri K, Panagopoulou E. Implementing action research in hospital settings: a systematic review. J Health Organ Manag. 2015;29(6):729–49. https://doi.org/10.1108/JHOM-09-2013-0203.

O'Brien R. Overview of action research methodology. 2001. http://www.web.ca/~robrien/papers/arfinal.html. Accessed 1 July 2019.

Reason P, Bradbury H. The Sage handbook of action research participative inquiry and practice. London: SAGE; 2007.

Reason P, Bradbury-Huang H, editors. The SAGE handbook of action research: participative inquiry and practice. 2nd ed. Los Angeles: SAGE Publications Ltd; 2013.

Rudolph AE, Standish K, Amesty S, Crawford ND, Stern RJ, Badillo WE, et al. A community-based approach to linking injection drug users with needed services through pharmacies: an evaluation of a pilot intervention in New York City. AIDS Educ Prev. 2010;22(3):238–51. https://doi.org/10.1521/aeap.2010.22.3.238.

Sørensen EW, Haugbølle LS. Using an action research process in pharmacy practice research—a cooperative project between university and internship pharmacies. Res Soc Adm Pharm. 2008;4(4):384–401. https://doi.org/10.1016/j.sapharm.2007.10.005.

Stupans I, McAllister S, Clifford R, Hughes J, Krass I, March G, et al. Nationwide collaborative development of learning outcomes and exemplar standards for Australian pharmacy programmes. Int J Pharm Pract. 2015;23(4):283–91. https://doi.org/10.1111/ijpp.12163.

Tanna NK, Pitkin J, Anderson C. Development of the specialist menopause pharmacist (SMP) role within a research framework. Pharm World Sci. 2005;27(1):61–7.

Tapp H, Kuhn L, Alkhazraji T, Steuerwald M, Ludden T, Wilson S, Dulin MF. Adapting community based participatory research (CBPR) methods to the implementation of an asthma shared decision making intervention in ambulatory practices. J Asthma. 2014;51(4):380–90. https://doi.org/10.3109/02770903.2013.876430.

University of Copenhagen. Methods—innovation and entrepreneurship in education. n.d. https://innovationenglish.sites.ku.dk/metoder/. Accessed 17 July 2019.

Verma S, Paterson M. Action research in health sciences interprofessional education. n.d. https://www.academia.edu/14398325/Action_Research_in_Health_Sciences_Interprofessional_Education.

Waterman H, Tillen D, Dickson R, de Koning K. Action research: a systematic review and guidance for assessment. Health Technol Assess (Winchester, England). 2001;5(23):iii–157.

Chapter 4
Quality Improvement Methods in Pharmacy Practice Research

Amie Bain and Debra Fowler

Abstract Quality improvement is a problem-based approach to pharmacy practice research with the explicit aim of improving the services delivered from an individual or organisation. As quality improvement science advances, so do the opportunities to assess, monitor and improve services in a rigorous way for the benefits of service users, individual pharmacists and organisations. This chapter introduces some of the approaches taken to the assessment of quality in pharmacy practice and outlines a selection of commonly used models and tools for quality improvement. This is followed by a brief discussion on how to report quality improvement work for the benefit of the wider pharmacy community.

4.1 Introduction

The improvement of services provided by an organisation has long been a subject of interest in the business community and is an important element of quality management. In recent years the concept of quality improvement has pervaded the healthcare sector and has evolved into a practice that employs rigorous scientific methods in order to bring about positive change to the delivery of patient care and health outcomes. Quality improvement aims to 'close the gap' between the expectations and reality of what a service delivers and, as such, is often highly contextualised to a local site. Quality improvement research differs from other pharmacy practice

A. Bain (✉)
School of Applied Sciences, University of Huddersfield, Queensgate, Huddersfield, UK

Pharmacy Department, Royal Hallamshire Hospital, Sheffield Teaching Hospitals NHS Foundation Trust, Sheffield, UK
e-mail: A.Bain@hud.ac.uk

D. Fowler
Pharmacy Department, Royal Hallamshire Hospital, Sheffield Teaching Hospitals NHS Foundation Trust, Sheffield, UK

© Springer Nature Singapore Pte Ltd. 2020
Z. Babar (ed.), *Pharmacy Practice Research Methods*,
https://doi.org/10.1007/978-981-15-2993-1_4

research approaches in that its focus is local improvement of processes and services rather than the generation of new, generalisable scientific knowledge (Ogrinc et al. 2008).

Quality improvement research often involves smaller samples and iterative changes to dynamic processes over time, which would be incongruent with standard research review processes involving fixed research protocols, or strictly controlled experimental approaches (Lynn 2004). The quasi-experimental, non-linear methods associated with quality improvement research are, however, necessary to meet the aims of quality improvement, which fundamentally concern organisational behaviour and change.

This does not mean that quality improvement initiatives do not need to carefully consider possible ethical implications or the current available literature or have robust methods and reporting standards for wider dissemination. Indeed, well-reported quality improvement research often generates valuable new knowledge about systems of care and organisational change that the wider pharmacy community can benefit greatly from. A sound understanding of quality theory and the variety of improvement methods available will therefore facilitate a more informed and robust change process for the benefit of organisations, pharmacists and service users.

Much has been written about the philosophy of quality improvement in healthcare, as well as its associated methodologies and methods, and an in-depth exposition and critique would be beyond the scope of this chapter. Here we provide a brief overview of quality improvement methods in pharmacy practice by critically examining selected quality theories, improvement models and tools. In order to illustrate the application of tools and models to pharmacy practice, specific examples of how these tools have been used in the context of pharmaceutical service improvement are given throughout.

4.2   What Is Quality and How Do We Improve It?

There is no universal definition of what 'quality' is in healthcare, despite its ubiquitous use and currency, perhaps due to its intrinsically subjective nature. The Health Foundation regards quality as 'the degree of excellence in healthcare' but acknowledges that excellence is multidimensional (The Health Foundation 2013). Quality, or excellence, may be viewed differently depending on what exactly is being measured and by whom, and this can be particularly pertinent when considering patient experience alongside cost-effectiveness in order to improve pharmacy services.

Adequate assessment of the quality of a service is important to benchmark and improve services, as well as for accountability purposes. Despite its nebulous and abstract nature, quality must therefore be defined, at least in some capacity, in order to be measured. Quality theory seeks to define and describe quality in healthcare, with several proposed frameworks containing multiple and various dimensions with which to measure and assess quality. Two of these contrasting theories will be considered in order to illustrate the diversity in approaches to quality assessment.

4.2.1 Quality Theory

One of the first to define quality with respect to healthcare, Avedis Donabedian, suggested that quality assessment involves structure, process and outcome (Donabedian 1988). These essential elements are important to consider together due to their dynamic and interdependent relationship (see Fig. 4.1). Although the model originally represented a linear relationship between structures, processes and outcomes (as shown), adaptations and interpretations of the model incorporate dynamism to increase its utility in complex systems (e.g. in Carayon et al. 2006).

Although this framework is widely accepted and used in practice, some argue that relationship between the important and interconnected dimensions of quality (structure, process, outcome) can be difficult to establish, and some factors can be difficult to categorise where overlap occurs (Liu et al. 2011; Gardner et al. 2014; Ayanian and Markel 2016; Dwyer et al. 2017). Nevertheless, its flexibility and broad applicability make it a very useful model for assessing quality in the healthcare setting (Donabedian 1982). Shiyanbola and colleagues used this framework in order to describe older people's perceptions of pharmacy service quality (Shiyanbola et al. 2016), and a worked example of how the Donabedian framework could be applied to assess the quality of insulin prescribing in hospital is given in Table 4.1.

Maxwell (1984) offers a more comprehensive framework comprised of the following elements: accessibility, relevance (to the whole community), effectiveness, equity, social acceptability, efficiency and economy. This quality theory arguably has a greater external focus than Donabedian's model, although lacks the essential structure and process elements (Clarke and Rao 2004). By considering the wider population, rather than primarily the individual care-provider perspective, application of Maxwell's framework lends itself to a broader assessment of quality. One crucial element for pharmacy services that is not explicitly mentioned in Maxwell's model is patient safety, although this is addressed in adaptations of this model by both the World Health Organization (2006) and the Institute of Medicine (2001).

The focus on individual patients' needs in the assessment of quality is also of upmost importance and is reflected in the commonly cited Institute of Medicine's 6 Domains of Healthcare Quality. Any change to a system must consider the impact and importance to patients and service users and not be concerned with making efficiency savings alone. Indeed, quality in the United Kingdom's National Health Service (NHS) is defined simply in terms of patient safety, experience and clinical effectiveness, with quality standards, indicators and improvement strategies currently reflecting this (Department of Health 2008).

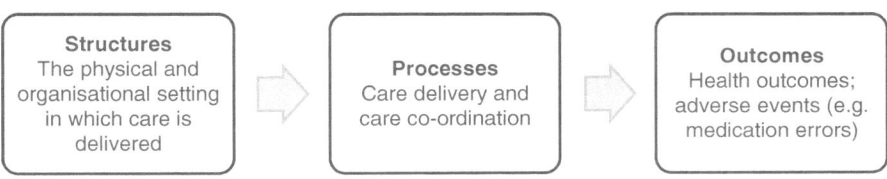

Fig. 4.1 The Donabedian quality framework, adapted from the depiction in McDonald et al. (2007)

Table 4.1 Application of Donabedian's framework to assess the quality of insulin prescribing in hospital

Structure	Process	Outcome
Accessibility and reliability of information systems for medicines reconciliation/history taking	Medicine history taking by clerking doctor	Accuracy and completeness of drug history/medicines reconciliation
Resources to record medicines reconciliation/history (electronic vs. paper)	Medicines reconciliation by pharmacist or medicines management technician	Number of prescribing errors
Medical and non-medical prescriber availability, experience, competence	Patient availability and ability to give an accurate history	Number and severity of adverse events (e.g. hypoglycaemia, hyperglycaemia)
Similarity between names of insulin products and brands	Access to and availability of prescriber to rectify any discrepancies Timely, complete, clear and accurate prescription amendments made	Number and type of pharmacist/nurse/patient interventions to prevent erroneous drug administration
Self-administration or self-management policy	Access to case notes and/or computer systems needed for prescribing	Blood glucose range appropriate for clinical situation
Dispensing for discharge policy (patient use of own medicines, which can also aid initial prescribing if present and valid)	Prescribing verification by pharmacist timely, complete and accurate	Self-administration or self-management of insulin by patient where appropriate
	Provision of medicine if required by pharmacy (also dependent on other supporting systems and access/availability of patient's own drugs)	

The differences in quality theories or frameworks may somewhat reflect the fundamental differences in conceptualising the measurement of quality depending on one's perspective (the practitioner may have a different view to the patient or the manager). Therefore, although useful, one must be mindful of the viewpoint and potential benefits and limitations of any quality assessment undertaken of a particular pharmacy service (Clarke and Rao 2004).

Once quality is adequately defined in terms of a service area, attention must be given to how one can go about improving it. This should start with a comprehensive review of the relevant quality improvement literature in order to learn from similar initiatives and to ensure that the approach is evidence-based.

It is also essential to consider the involvement of service users throughout quality improvement initiatives, as their unique insight can provide an invaluable contribution to effective service design (Ocloo and Matthews 2016). Collaboration with other healthcare professionals is also important in the improvement of pharmacy services, as very rarely will change to a pharmacy service have minimal impact on services provided by other healthcare professionals (e.g. the provision of medicines to a hospital ward directly impacts the nursing staff who access and administer medicines).

Along with considering insights from the literature, service users and other health-care professionals, the consideration of service improvement theory can help describe how quality improvement can be achieved, assessed, recorded and monitored.

4.2.2   Service Improvement Theory

Boyne (2003, p. 223) defines service improvement as:

a closer correspondence between perceptions of actual and desired standards of public service.

Because many stakeholders will determine what quality is and impose varying criteria for success, which themselves may change over time or context and may even conflict with each other, concepts and measures in service improvement have been described as 'political rather than technical and contingent rather than universal' (Boyne 2003). In order to measure the 'gap' between expected and realised standards of service provision, Ashworth et al. (2010) outline three different approaches that may be taken: outcome/goal attainment, output measures and process/practices. These approaches are described in Table 4.2, along with examples relevant to the current practice of prescribing insulin prescribing in hospitals in the United Kingdom.

Table 4.2 Approaches to the measurement of standards for service improvement (Ashworth et al. 2010)

Measure	Features	Considerations	Example
Outcome/ goal attainment	All public services are expected to fulfil policy goals Change in performance judged in terms of realisation of outcomes framed in specific policy interventions (e.g. mortality data)	Potential subjectivity in outcome reporting Timescale of measure related to outcome Attribution of outcome to change is difficult	Reduced admissions/ readmissions/inpatient episodes of/due to hypo–/hyperglycaemia in patients with diabetes All patients undergo medicines reconciliation within 24 h of admission to hospital
Output	Quantity, quality of efficiency of a service (e.g. targets, CQUIN)	Attribution of outcome to change is difficult Distortion of target data Sustainability Unintended consequence (e.g. time pressures on discharge prescribing may negatively affect quality of information conveyed to community services)	Number of insulin-prescribing errors recorded (e.g. patient safety reports, audit) Percentage of prescriptions verified by pharmacist Time taken to complete discharge prescription
Process/ regulation	Following correct procedures or best practice leads to improvement of outputs/ outcomes (e.g. CQC, NICE)	Process of benchmarking may not be evidence-based or capture a true reflection	Adherence to medicines code and hospital-prescribing guidelines

In the United Kingdom, previous government policy emphasis on output and process/regulatory measures, targets and performance management led to improvements in NHS services, including shorter waiting times in emergency departments (Ashworth et al. 2010; The King's Fund 2016). However, the application of these 'extrinsic' top-down approaches to improving quality has not been without criticism (Øvretveit 2009). For example, performance management has been accused of creating a culture of compliance and risk aversion, as well as stifling innovation and disempowering staff (The King's Fund 2016). Subsequent reviews of NHS reforms concluded that in order to achieve further improvements in quality, a culture of learning and improvement needed to be built, led by sufficiently equipped and supported organisations and frontline staff rather than relying on centrally imposed reforms (Department of Health 2008).

These 'intrinsic' approaches to service improvement are supported by Seddon (2008), who appeals to the self-motivation of staff within individual organisations to lead improvements with continued, co-operative commitment, rather than reactive compliance to externally imposed targets. Engaging frontline staff and service users in developing, designing and implementing quality improvement interventions has previously been shown to result in more sustainable change than using 'command and control' models, and the NHS Institute for Innovation and Improvement's Sustainability Model and Guide reflects this in its recommendations for increasing sustainability of particular projects (Maher et al. 2010; The King's Fund 2016).

Engaging frontline staff in the improvement of the services they provide is not always straightforward, however. Limited understanding of local system dynamics as well as quality improvement concepts and methods, different perceptions of quality care, lack of authority and colleague endorsement have all been reported in the literature (Davies et al. 2007). Nevertheless, organisational approaches to quality improvement have the power to be transformative if they harness the combined efforts of everyone to make changes that will lead to better patient outcome, better system performance and professional development (Batalden and Davidoff 2007).

Pereira and Aspinwall (1997) highlight the need for a sound understanding, analysis and selection of different processes for quality improvement based on the mission and goals of the organisation. There are various models that may be used to translate quality and service improvement theory in order to help understand problems and processes and plan, implement and evaluate quality improvement interventions. A selection of these models will be discussed below in relation to pharmacy practice.

4.3 Quality Improvement Models

4.3.1 Business Process Reengineering

Business process reengineering (BPR) is defined as:

> *the fundamental rethinking and radical redesign of business processes to achieve dramatic improvements in critical, contemporary measures of performance, such as cost, quality, service and speed.* (Hammer and Champy 1994)

Proponents of BPR suggest that such a dramatic improvement in performance may be achieved by completely rethinking service processes in a way that making continuous small, incremental changes might not. The use of BPR in pharmacy practice involves significant 'top-down' changes to systems such as the introduction of automatic dispensing systems or electronic prescribing (also known as computerised physician order entry (CPOE)) across an organisation. These changes are often time-consuming due to the radical, cross-functional, cultural and structural change to current practice involved. One example of the explicit use of BPR in pharmacy practice involves the reengineering of the dispensing process to reduce waiting times in an outpatient pharmacy (Chou et al. 2012).

Although application of BPR has been very successful in enhancing quality in some healthcare settings, the wider literature shows that more than half of BPR initiatives fail to deliver the expected results, which may be due to inadequate appreciation of the human dimension and organisational change management (Khodambashi 2013; Pereira and Aspinwall 1997).

4.3.2   Plan-Do-Study-Act

In contrast to the high-risk, radical change of organisational practice involved in BPR, the plan-do-study-act (PDSA) model of service improvement involves repeating small cycles of iterative tests of change as part of a continuous improvement approach (Fig. 4.2). Many quality improvement approaches adopt this model, including the Model for Improvement (Langley 2009), and it has been widely used and studied in healthcare (Boaden 2009).

The emphasis on the responsibility of frontline staff to lead rapid small-scale tests of change in this approach may liberate healthcare professionals to lead change and improvement in their locality and has been embraced as a pragmatic approach

Fig. 4.2 The plan-do-study-act model for quality improvement

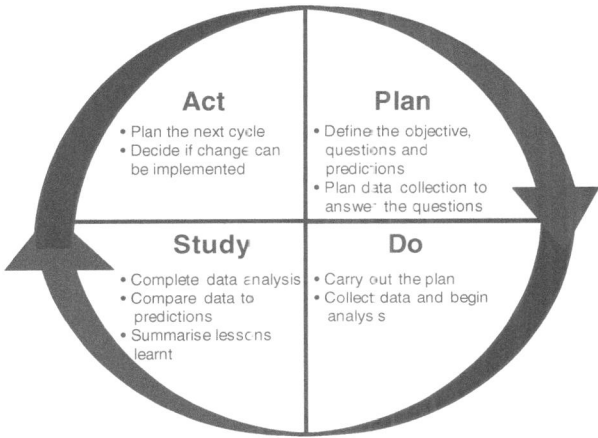

by many (Reed and Card 2016). A PDSA approach is well suited to drive incremental local change in a shorter space of time, and its application to improve pharmacy services is more widely reported in the literature. Examples include the use of PDSA to improve insulin prescribing to patients on admission to hospital (Tully et al. 2018) and communication of patient information regarding NSAID use in rural community pharmacies (Morrison et al. 2018).

However, some argue that not all problems are tractable to PDSA, particularly more significant problems on a larger scale, unless it is used as a part of a suite of methods by staff who are adequately resourced, supported by leadership, and trained in its appropriate use (Dixon-Woods et al. 2014; Reed and Card 2016). Furthermore, despite its widespread use in healthcare, there is little evidence to suggest PDSA is more cost-effective than any other approach (Boaden 2009; Taylor et al. 2014). Some of the criticisms of the PDSA approach, particularly those relating to sustainability issues, have been addressed with the subsequent use of SDSA (standardise-do-study-act) cycles to help standardise processes once the desired aims have been achieved. The combination of approaches may therefore help embed long-term continuous improvement and maintain performance over time (Gitlow 2000).

4.3.3   Lean and Six Sigma

Lean and Six Sigma are concerned with the elimination of 'waste' from service processes and redirecting resources in order to reduce costs, improve efficiency and increase the consistency of care. Lean and Six Sigma are often used together to consider the 'flow' of a process, uncover root causes of inefficiencies, reduce variation through standardisation and improve repeatability in a service (Rotter et al. 2018).

Lean considers the 'eight wastes' that add costs but negate value, defects (requiring rework), overproduction, waiting, under-utilised talent, unnecessary transportation of materials, excess inventory, unnecessary movements by people and over-processing, most of which have been reported in the activities of clinical pharmacists (Green et al. 2015).

Six Sigma seeks to analyse the root causes of problems and improve processes by using the DMAIC methodology (Fig. 4.3).

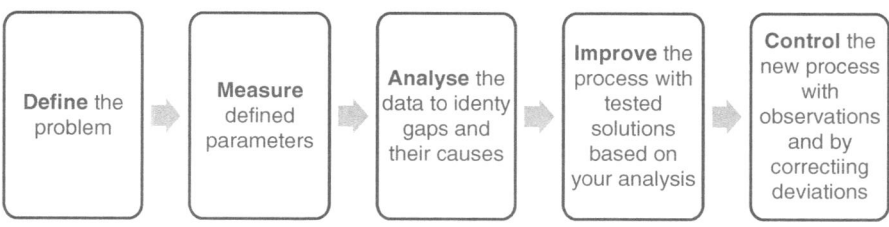

Fig. 4.3 DMAIC framework in Six Sigma

Together, Lean and Six Sigma provide a structured approach to rapid transformation and cost-saving (Yaduvanshi and Sharma 2017). Examples of where these approaches have been used in pharmacy practice include a hospital pharmacy sterile production unit, where errors were reduced by 50% (Hintzen et al. 2009), an inpatient dispensary where rework was reduced by 25% (Smith 2009) and improving efficiencies in clinical pharmacy work in hospital (Shiu and Mysak 2017).

Criticisms of the Lean and Six Sigma approach involve the view that human factors are often not prioritised; the 'top-down' strategy involved may jeopardise the sustainability of improvements when frontline staff are not the agents of change. Often, significant infrastructure investment is required, and the approach often involves scrutinising processes in isolation without consideration of how other systems interact (Hines et al. 2008).

For any given improvement project, a combination of strategies may be required due to the complex and diverse processes and contexts in which a service is often delivered. For example, with respect to improving the quality of insulin prescribing in an organisation, a top-down, organisation-wide BPR approach (e.g. successful implementation of electronic prescribing) may be used alongside locally driven and sensitive PDSA approaches in a co-ordinated, rigorous and complementary way. Whichever approach, or combination of approaches, is used for any given project, due consideration should be given to the choice of methods used to collect and analyse data for the purposes of quality improvement.

4.4 Quality Improvement Methods and Tools

Quality improvement projects may utilise an array of traditional qualitative and quantitative research methods, including semi-structured interviews, questionnaires, randomised cluster trials, uncontrolled before-and-after studies and interrupted time series studies, amongst others. Other methods are more exclusive to quality improvement and are often called 'quality improvement tools'. There are many tools available to assist with quality improvement and assessment, which vary in style and complexity. For any given improvement project, a suitable complement of methods and/or tools should be selected according to the available literature, the resource, the model/approach used and the problem in question. As the more traditional methods have been discussed elsewhere in this book, this section will provide a brief overview of a selection of the more commonly used quality improvement tools in pharmacy practice.

4.4.1 Audit

The use of clinical and nonclinical audit is possibly the most frequently used tool to contribute to improvement efforts in pharmacy practice. The measurement of practice or a process against agreed, predefined quality criteria (or 'standards' which may be derived from evidence-based clinical guidance) enables shortfalls to be easily measured and monitored on an ongoing basis throughout improvement efforts (Benjamin 2008). Audit proformas are designed to comprise measurement of the predefined standards, and a snapshot review of a convenient defined sample over a specified timeframe is conducted either prospectively or retrospectively. Specific strengths and shortfalls in practice against the standards are identified following data analysis, and subsequent action plans are made to address and drive improvement accordingly. Repeat audits are then conducted at appropriate intervals according to the problem in question so that change can be monitored following any interventions made.

Audits are frequently performed in pharmacies at a local level in order to drive improvements relevant to the individual practice. Larger-scale audits are also performed where and improvement efforts involve regional or national priority areas. Examples include the Community Pharmacy Contractual Framework National Clinical Audit and the annual National Diabetes Inpatient Audit in the United Kingdom (NaDIA 2018). The effectiveness of audits has been questioned, however, as they are often very time-consuming and demanding, with greater emphasis usually being put on the initial data collection rather than making improvements (Boyle and Keep 2018). When used as part of a quality improvement effort that emphasises more targeted data collection, rapid change and testing of interventions (such as the PDSA approach described above), audit is arguably more useful than as a stand-alone method for improvement. Another criticism of audit is its inadequacy to describe variation and improvement between two snapshots in time. This may be addressed with the use of control charts to monitor data over time (see Sect. 4.5).

4.4.2   Root Cause Analysis

Root cause analysis (RCA) is commonly used to retrospectively examine the quality of service provision at a local level after the occurrence of an adverse event or audit findings revealing shortfalls in the quality of care or a process. The process is structured and designed to investigate the human, physical and latent factors that may have contributed to the event. A fishbone diagram (also known as an Ishikawa or 'cause and effect' diagram) is often used in order to help identify the source of a problem so that improvement efforts may be directed towards the cause of the issue (see Fig. 4.4).

The process of an RCA should ideally involve multidisciplinary input from all stakeholders depending on the adverse event identified, and associated planning for system modifications, re-audit to prevent recurrence of the event. Patient safety events are often the subject of RCAs, with examples in pharmacy practice including investigating transcription errors in community pharmacy (Knudsen et al. 2007). Undertaking RCAs of individual events is, however, labour intensive and may suffer from hindsight bias and may have limited applicability to the wider context. Nevertheless, it is a widely used and useful tool. A comprehensive guide to undertaking RCAs with respect to medication errors is given by Jhugursing et al. (2017).

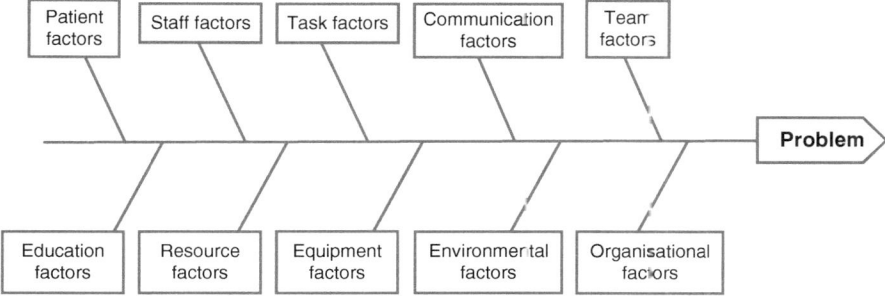

Fig. 4.4 Example of a fishbone diagram, adapted from Fereday and Malbon (2015)

4.4.3 Failure Modes and Effects Analysis

Failure modes and effects analysis (FMEA) differs from RCA in that it does not require a particular event to have occurred in order to examine failures in a process and as such may be more broadly applicable. High-risk processes are the most common subjects of FMEA as 'failure modes' may be identified, prioritised and mitigated before errors occur and potentially cause patient harm. FMEA requires a proactive, collaborative, multidisciplinary team to assign scores (out of 10) for occurrence, severity and detection of these modes in order to generate a Risk Priority Number. This may be particularly useful for evaluating new processes prior to implementation and has been previously used as a successful method for assessing the process of insulin prescribing in hospital as part of a continuing improvement strategy (Berruyer et al. 2016).

The use of FMEA may be limited by the subjectivity and knowledge of the team undertaking it, who may not identify issues outside of their practice nor suggest adequate resolutions for issues identified. The mathematical validity of FMEA methodology has also been questioned, in particular the use of ordinal scales to prioritise failure modes (Magnezi et al. 2016; Shebl et al. 2012). Furthermore, failure modes may never be eliminated and may require further and repeated actions in order to be mitigated in an environment that is dynamic and variable.

4.4.4 Process Mapping

A tool widely used in Lean and Six Sigma approaches is that of process mapping, whereby the staff or patient journey through a process or service is mapped in order to identify inefficiencies and 'wastes' such as unnecessary movement, variation and discrepancies. By outlining the process in step-by-step detail, opportunities for improvement are identified, and potential solutions can be discussed and 'designed out' of the system. A 'high-level' process map may give insight to the process overview and help to identify areas to develop the detailed process map, including identifying specific aims and areas for improvement. Process mapping is usually a collaborative effort between multi-departmental stakeholders in a process (ideally involving patients and their representatives) and, as such, provides a broader insight into the process, minimises researcher bias and considers the 'whole system' more effectively than other tools might. An example of process mapping in community pharmacy practice is given by Weir et al. (2018).

4.4.5   Control Charts

Control charts (or run charts) are often used in quality improvement interventions to visualise and analyse the performance of a process over time using measurements appropriate to the intervention aims and outcomes. Longitudinal data are then subject to analysis to determine if a change to the system reflects random variation or a 'real' change as a result of an intervention. Control charts are a key tool used as part of statistical process control approaches to quality improvement and draw many similarities to quasi-experimental interrupted time series analysis methods (Kontopantelis et al. 2015). Control charts are easily understood and interpreted, and are useful in providing contemporaneous information to support decision-making, but require statistical knowledge and software to compose and analyse in a rigorous way (Fretheim and Tomic 2015). One example of a practice utilising control charts to improve the acceptance and consistent use of prescription processing guidelines is given by Al-Hussein (2009).

4.5   Reporting Quality Improvement Studies

An important component of quality improvement is critical reflection and evaluation of the entire process and outcomes achieved (or not achieved). Although many pharmacists undertaking quality improvement may be required to write a project report for their organisations, few will progress to peer-reviewed publication for wider dissemination. Well-designed and well-executed quality improvement reports may be publishable as research, and as the science of improvement work advances, so does the need for this to be reflected in the literature. There are now dedicated journals for the publication of quality improvement research, such as the *Journal of Healthcare Quality* and *BMJ Open Quality*. As quality improvement research is highly contextual and often involves multiple interventions over time, detailed contextual and organisational details that are often excluded in original research outputs should be included in improvement reports in order to facilitate interpretation of the results. Reference to the 'Standards for Quality Improvement Reporting Excellence' (SQUIRE) guidelines is strongly encouraged to further enable high-quality report writing for quality improvement interventions (Ogrinc et al. 2008).

In addition to the SQUIRE reporting guidelines, it may also be useful to refer to the Quality Improvement Minimum Quality Criteria Set (QI-MCQS) (Hempel et al.

2015). The QI-MCQS is a tool to aid the critical appraisal cf quality improvement reports and as such would prompt project leads and authors to consider and include the information required for a high-quality report. This tool also helps reviewers of quality improvement literature identify and learn from higher-quality studies prior to planning their project. An example of where this tool has been used for the quality assessment of improvement research as part of a systematic review of insulin-prescribing interventions is provided by Bain et al. (2019).

4.6   The Importance of Quality Improvement for Pharmacy Practice

In a time where pharmacy services are required to be increasingly safe, efficient and patient-centred with increasingly limited resources, quality improvement methods and tools provide an important and helpful means of service development. Pharmacists and pharmacy researchers have unique insights and critical skills to make a positive contribution to quality improvement and evaluation, both within the pharmacy sector and as part of the wider healthcare organisation. Pharmacists should therefore consider engaging in involvement in quality improvement research wherever the opportunity presents. Quality improvement research is accessible and practice-based and encourages vital collaboration between pharmacy and other healthcare professionals, patients and service users.

Indeed, all staff should be engaged in the decisions that affect them and the services they provide and should be empowered to innovate and improve the quality and safety of services (Department of Health and Social Care 2015). In order to do this, however, a culture of learning and improvement needs to be built, and staff capabilities for identifying and undertaking improvement work need to be strengthened (The King's Fund 2016).

Where possible, collaboration with academic pharmacists with an interest in implementation or action research can help support rigorous quality improvement efforts in clinical settings. Pharmacist researchers will be required to be competent in using mixed methods as part of a collaborative and participatory approach in order to achieve the research aims of quality improvement (Almarsdottir and Babar 2016). The involvement of pharmacists in larger quality improvement initiatives can also help increase the visibility of pharmacy's contribution to patient care and the wider healthcare framework.

4.7   Conclusions

Quality improvement science is a growing field cf pharmacy practice research, and researchers, frontline pharmacists as well as managers are encouraged to consider undertaking quality improvement interventions as part of their dedication to provide high-quality services to patients. The wide variety of approaches, methods and tools available provide a rich repertoire that could facilitate improvement projects of any size and context. When undertaking improvement projects, it is important to give due consideration to the service users, the wider context in which the 'problem' or process is situated, and those affected. Methods that are well suited to the approach taken should be chosen, and if possible, improvement projects should be published for the benefit of the wider community and the advancement of the profession.

References

Al-Hussein FA. Guideline implementation in clinical practice: use of statistical process control charts as visual feedback devices. J Fam Community Med. 2009;16(1):11–7. http://www.ncbi. nlm.nih.gov/pubmed/23012184

Almarsdottir AB, Babar ZUD. Future methods in pharmacy practice research. Int J Clin Pharm. 2016;38(3):724–30. https://doi.org/10.1007/s11096-016-0300-y.

Ashworth R, Boyne GA, Entwistle T. Public service improvement: theories and evidence. Oxford: Oxford University Press; 2010. https://global.oup.com/academic/product/ public-service-improvement-9780199545476?cc=gb&lang=en&

Ayanian J, Markel H. Donabedian's Lasting Framework for Health Care. N Engl J Med 2016; 375:205–7. https://doi.org/10.1056/NEJMp1605101.

Bain A, Hasan SS, Babar Z-U-D. Interventions to improve insulin prescribing practice for people with diabetes in hospital: a systematic review. Diabetic Med. 2019;36:13982. https://doi. org/10.1111/dme.13982.

Batalden PB, Davidoff F. What is "quality improvement" and how can it transform healthcare? Qual Saf Health Care. 2007;16(1):2–3. https://doi.org/10.1136/qshc.2006.022046.

Benjamin A. The competent novice: audit: how to do it in practice. Br Med J. 2008;336(7655):1241. https://doi.org/10.1136/BMJ.39527.628322.AD.

Berruyer M, Atkinson S, Lebel D, Bussières J-F. Utilisation de l'insuline en établissement de santé universitaire mère–enfant : analyse des modes de défaillance. Arch Pediatr. 2016;23(1):1–8. https://doi.org/10.1016/j.arcped.2015.09.033.

Boaden R. Quality improvement: theory and practice. Br J Healthcare Manage. 2009;15(1). http:// content.ebscohost.com/ContentServer.asp?T=P&P=AN&K=105637529&S=R&D=rzh&Ebsc oContent=dGJyMNHX8kSeqLI4xNvgOLCmr1Cep7JSsam4SrSWxWXS&ContentCustomer =dGJyMPGprky0qLFPuePfgeyx44Dt6fIA

Boyle A, Keep J. Clinical audit does not work, is quality improvement any better? Br J Hosp Med. 2018;79(9):508–10. https://doi.org/10.12968/hmed.2018.79.9.508.

Boyne GA. What is public service improvement? Public Adm. 2003;81(2):211–27. https://doi. org/10.1111/1467-9299.00343.

Carayon P, Schoofs Hundt A, Karsh BT, Gurses AP, Alvarado CJ, Smith M, Brennan PF. (2006). Work system design for patient safety: The SEIPS model. Quality and Safety in Health Care. BMJ Publishing Group. https://doi.org/10.1136/qshc.2005.015842.

Chou YC, Chen BY, Tang YY, Qiu ZJ, Wu MF, Wang SC, et al. Prescription-filling process reengineering of an outpatient pharmacy. J Med Syst. 2012;36(2):893–902. https://doi.org/10.1007/ s10916-010-9553-5.

Clarke A, Rao M. Developing quality indicators to assess quality of care. Qual Saf Health Care. 2004;13(4):248–9. https://doi.org/10.1136/qhc.13.4.248.

Davies H, Powell A, Rushmer R. Healthcare professionals' views on clinician engagement in quality improvement. The Health Foundation. 2007. http://www.health.org.uk/publication/ healthcare-professionals'-views-clinician-engagement-quality-improvement

Department of Health. High quality care for all. 2008. http://webarchive.nationalarchives.gov.
    uk/20130105061315/http://www.dh.gov.uk/prod_consum_dh/groups/dh_digitalassets/@dh/@
    en/documents/digitalasset/dh_085828.pdf

Department of Health and Social Care. NHS constitution for England. 2015. https://www.gov.uk/
    government/publications/the-nhs-constitution-for-england

Dixon-Woods M, Martin G, Tarrant C, Bion J, Goeschel C, Pronovost P, et al. Safer Clinical
    Systems: evaluation findings Learning from the independent evaluation of the second phase of
    the Safer Clinical Systems programme Evaluation. 2014. health.org.uk. http://www.health.org.
    uk/sites/health/files/SaferClinicalSystemsEvaluationFindings_fullversion.pdf

Donabedian A. The criteria and standards of quality. Health Administration Press. 1982.
    https://books.google.co.uk/books/about/The_criteria_and_standards_of_quality.
    html?id=o7hpAAAAMAAJ

Dwyer T, Craswell A, Rossi D, Holzberger D. Evaluation of an aged care nurse practitioner ser-
    vice: quality of care within a residential aged care facility hospital avoidance service. BMC
    Health Serv Res. 2017;17(1):33. https://doi.org/10.1186/s12913-017-1977-x.

Donabedian A. The quality of care: how can it be assessed? JAMA. 1988;260(12):1743–8. https://
    doi.org/10.1001/jama.1988.03410120089033.

Fereday S, Malbon N. A guide to quality improvement methods. Healthcare Quality Improvement
    Partnership. 2015. p. 347. https://doi.org/10.1136/bmj.f7617

Fretheim A, Tomic O. Statistical process control and interrupted time series: a golden opportunity
    for impact evaluation in quality improvement. BMJ Qual Saf. 2015;24(12):748. https://doi.
    org/10.1136/BMJQS-2014-003756.

Gardner G, Gardner A, O'Connell J. Using the Donabedian framework to examine the qual-
    ity and safety of nursing service innovation. J Clin Nurs. 2014;23(1–2):145–55. https://doi.
    org/10.1111/jocn.12146.

Gitlow HS. Quality management systems: a practical guide. St. Lucie Press. 2000. https://books.
    google.co.uk/books?id=O5aq0HMyXOcC&pg=PA15&lpg=PA15&dq=gitlow+sdsa&source=
    bl&ots=DscSVXkhGk&sig=ACfU3U0bSCD9J3otLqJSg5zcNJOSCZbNYg&hl=en&sa=X&v
    ed=2ahUKEwinpNvrvd3jAhXSEcAKHQHMCGgQ6AEwAHoECAgQAQ#v=onepage&q=g
    itlowsdsa&f=false

Green CF, Crawford V, Bresnen G, Rowe PH. A waste walk through clinical pharmacy: how do
    the 'seven wastes' of Lean techniques apply to the practice of clinical pharmacists. Int J Pharm
    Pract. 2015;23(1):21–6. https://doi.org/10.1111/ijpp.12106.

Hammer M, Champy J. Reengineering the corporation: a manifesto for business revolution.
    New York: Harper Business; 1994.

Hempel S, Shekelle PG, Liu JL, Sherwood Danz M, Foy R, Lim Y-W, et al. Development of the
    Quality Improvement Minimum Quality Criteria Set (QI-MQCS): a tool for critical appraisal
    of quality improvement intervention publications. BMJ Qual Saf. 2015;24(12):796–804.
    https://doi.org/10.1136/bmjqs-2014-003151.

Hines P, Martins AL, Beale J. Testing the boundaries of lean thinking: observations from the legal
    public sector. 2008;28(1):35–40. https://doi.org/10.1111/j.1467-9302.2008.00616.x.

Hintzen BL, Knoer SJ, Van Dyke CJ, Milavitz BS. Effect of lean process improvement techniques
    on a university hospital inpatient pharmacy. Am J Health Syst Pharm. 2009;66(22):2042–7.
    https://doi.org/10.2146/ajhp080540.

Institute of Medicine (US) Committee on Quality of Health Care in America. Crossing the quality
    chasm: a new health system for the 21st century. Washington, DC: National Academies Press;
    2001. https://doi.org/10.17226/10027.

Jhugursing M, Dimmock V, Mulchandani H. Error and root cause analysis. BJA Educ.
    2017;17(10):323–33. https://doi.org/10.1093/bjaed/mkx019.

Khodambashi S. Business process re-engineering application in healthcare in a relation to
    health information systems. Procedia Technol. 2013;9:949–57 https://ac.els-cdn.com/
    S2212017313002600/1-s2.0-S2212017313002600-main.pdf?_tid=23c8b8c9-9533-45c2-
    b4ca-8abbcc9970d4&acdnat=1522444944_6f77f14eda61e422522b56a88f981ad3

Knudsen P, Herborg H, Mortensen AR, Knudsen M, Hellebek A. Preventing medication errors in community pharmacy: root-cause analysis of transcription errors. Qual Saf Health Care. 2007;16(4):285–90. https://doi.org/10.1136/qshc.2006.022053.

Kontopantelis E, Doran T, Springate DA, Buchan I, Reeves D. Regression based quasi-experimental approach when randomisation is not an option: interrupted time series analysis. BMJ (Clin Res Ed.). 2015;350:h2750. https://doi.org/10.1136/bmj.h2750.

Langley GJ. The improvement guide: a practical approach to enhancing organizational performance. San Francisco: Jossey-Bass; 2009.

Liu SW, Singer SJ, Sun BC, Camargo CA Jr. A conceptual model for assessing quality of care for patients boarding in the emergency department: structure-process-outcome. Acad Emerg Med. 2011;18(4):430–5. https://doi.org/10.1111/j.1553-2712.2011.01033.x.

Lynn J. When does quality improvement count as research? Human subject protection and theories of knowledge. Qual Saf Health Care. 2004;13(1):67–70. https://doi.org/10.1136/qshc.2002.002436.

McDonald KM, Sundaram V, Bravata DM, et al. Closing the Quality Gap: A Critical Analysis of Quality Improvement Strategies (Vol. 7: Care Coordination). Rockville (MD): Agency for Healthcare Research and Quality (US); 2007 Jun. (Technical Reviews, No. 9.7.) Available from: https://www.ncbi.nlm.nih.gov/books/NBK44015/.

Magnezi R, Hemi A, Hemi R. Using the failure mode and effects analysis model to improve parathyroid hormone and adrenocorticotropic hormone testing. Risk Manage Healthc Policy. 2016;9:271–4. https://doi.org/10.2147/RMHP.S117472.

Maher L, Gustafson D, Evans A. NHS sustainability model Institute for Innovation and Improvement. NHS Institute for Innovation and Improvement. 2010. https://www.england.nhs.uk/improvement-hub/wp-content/uploads/sites/44/2017/11/NHS-Sustainability-Model-2010.pdf

Maxwell RJ. Quality assessment in health. Br Med J (Clin Res Ed). 1984;288(6428):1470–2. http://www.ncbi.nlm.nih.gov/pubmed/6426606

Morrison C, Beauchamp T, MacDonald H, Beattie M. Implementing a non-steroidal anti-inflammatory drugs communication bundle in remote and rural pharmacies and dispensing practices. BMJ Open Qual. 2018;7(3):e000303. https://doi.org/10.1136/bmjoq-2017-000303.

NaDIA HQIP National Diabetes Inpatient Audit England and Wales 2017. 2018. https://files.digital.nhs.uk/pdf/s/7/nadia-17-rep.pdf

Ocloo J, Matthews R. From tokenism to empowerment: progressing patient and public involvement in healthcare improvement. BMJ Qual Saf. 2016;25(8):626–32. https://doi.org/10.1136/bmjqs-2015-004839.

Ogrinc G, Mooney SE, Estrada C, Foster T, Goldmann D, Hall LW, et al. The SQUIRE (Standards for QUality Improvement Reporting Excellence) guidelines for quality improvement reporting: explanation and elaboration. Qual Saf Health Care. 2008;17(Suppl 1):i13–32. https://doi.org/10.1136/qshc.2008.029058.

Øvretveit J. Does improving quality save money? A review of the evidence of which improvements to quality reduce costs to health service providers. London; 2009. https://online.manchester.ac.uk/bbcswebdav/orgs/I3075-COMMUNITY-MEDN-1/DONOTDELETE-PEPQualityandEvidence/QE-PEP-HTML5/AN-C50883C1-C877-58A4-FF18-DEBFA69D2ED3.html

Pereira ZL, Aspinwall E. Total quality management versus business process re-engineering. Total Qual Manag. 1997;8(1):33–40. https://doi.org/10.1080/09544129710422.

Reed JE, Card AJ. The problem with plan-do-study-act cycles. BMJ Qual Saf. 2016;25(3):147–52. https://doi.org/10.1136/bmjqs-2015-005076.

Rotter T, Plishka C, Lawal A, Harrison L, Sari N, Goodridge D, et al. What is lean management in health care? Development of an operational definition for a cochrane systematic review. Eval Health Prof. 2018;016327871875699:366. https://doi.org/10.1177/0163278718756992.

Seddon J. Systems thinking in the public sector : the failure of the reform regime … and a manifesto for a better way. Bridport: Triarchy Press; 2008.

Shebl NA, Franklin BD, Barber N. Failure mode and effects analysis outputs: are they valid? BMC Health Serv Res. 2012;12(1):150. https://doi.org/10.1186/1472-6963-12-150.

Shiu J, Mysak T. Pharmacist clinical process improvement: applying lean principles in a tertiary care setting. Can J Hosp Pharm. 2017;70(2):138. https://www.ncbi.nlm.nih.gov/pmc/articles/PMC5407423/

Shiyanbola OO, Mott DA, Croes KD. The structural and process aspects of pharmacy quality: older adults' perceptions. Int J Clin Pharm. 2016;38(1):96–106. https://doi.org/10.1007/s11096-015-0211-3.

Smith B. Using the lean approach to transform pharmacy services in an acute trust|news|pharmaceutical journal. Pharm J. 2009;282(457). https://www.pharmaceutical-journal.com/news-and-analysis/using-the-lean-approach-to-transform-pharmacy-services-in-an-acute-trust/10884114.article?firstPass=false

Taylor MJ, McNicholas C, Nicolay C, Darzi A, Bell D, Reed JE. Systematic review of the application of the plan-do-study-act method to improve quality in healthcare. BMJ Qual Saf. 2014;23(4):290–8. https://doi.org/10.1136/bmjqs-2013-001862.

The Health Foundation. Quality improvement made simple. 2013. http://www.health.org.uk/sites/health/files/QualityImprovementMadeSimple.pdf

The King's Fund. Reforming the NHS from within: beyond hierarchy, inspection and markets. The King's Fund. 2016. https://www.kingsfund.org.uk/sites/default/files/field/field_publication_file/reforming-the-nhs-from-within-kingsfund-jun14.pdf

Tully V, Al-Salti S, Arnold A, Botros S, Campbell I, Fane R, et al. Interprofessional, student-led intervention to improve insulin prescribing to patients in an Acute Surgical Receiving Unit. BMJ Open Qual. 2018;7(2):e000305. https://doi.org/10.1136/bmjoq-2017-000305.

Weir NM, Newham R, Corcoran ED, Ali Atallah Al-Gethami A, Mohammed Abd Alridha A, Bowie P, et al. Application of process mapping to understand integration of high risk medicine care bundles within community pharmacy practice. Res Social Adm Pharm. 2018;14(10):944–50. https://doi.org/10.1016/j.sapharm.2017.11.009.

World Health Organization. Quality of care: a process for making strategic choices in health systems. WHO Press; 2006. p. 38. https://doi.org/10.1542/peds.2010-1791

Yaduvanshi D, Sharma A. Lean six sigma in health operations. J Health Manag. 2017;19(2):203–13. https://doi.org/10.1177/0972063417699665.

Chapter 5
Covert and Overt Observations in Pharmacy Practice

Filipa Alves da Costa

Abstract Observation is a powerful method to capture the reality in pharmacy practice. It is divided into participant and non-participant observations according to the involvement of the researcher into the process being studied. Depending on the level of disclosure, observation may be classified as overt or covert, where covert observation has the advantage of minimising the Hawthorne effect while overt observation produces in depth observations, capturing a wider scope of processes. This chapter details the main features and the pros and cons of these different types of observation, mentioning useful tools to support such studies and finalising by commenting on the impact of observation in pharmacy practice.

5.1   Introduction

It is common to divide research methods according to the perspective taken, where a qualitative approach is more focused on the interpretation and the quantitative approach is mainly centred on the empirical perspective. There is a third category, named mixed methods where both perspectives are considered, and often with the aim of supplementing each other.

Once the research methodology has been chosen, data collection is planned and implemented and again various formats to collect data are available. These should be appropriate to the research perspective adopted, which in turn will depend on the research question. Perhaps the most common form for collecting data in pharmacy practice research is through self-report, often using questionnaires, but observation

F. A. da Costa (✉)
Research Institute for Medicines (iMED.ULisboa), Faculty of Pharmacy, University of Lisbon, Lisbon, Portugal

Center for Interdisciplinary Research Egas Moniz (CiiEM), Uuniversity Institute Egas Moniz, Lisbon, Portugal

© Springer Nature Singapore Pte Ltd. 2020
Z. Babar (ed.), *Pharmacy Practice Research Methods*,
https://doi.org/10.1007/978-981-15-2993-1_5

is an alternative method, increasingly used given the recognised advantages (Puspitasari et al. 2009a).

Self-report is subject to various biases, the most common being social desirability bias, which is applicable both to patients and healthcare professionals. Humans in general tend to know what is right and wrong, but that does not mean they always act well. Hence, when questioned, there seems to be a tendency to report correct behaviours, e.g. taking medicines prescribed (in the case of patients) and always advising patients how to take their medicines (in the case of pharmacists). In fact, it has been shown that investigating the same phenomenon, depending on the viewpoint, leads to different results (Puspitasari et al. 2010). Another common bias in self-report is the response bias, very common when the topic researched is satisfaction with services, where there is undoubtedly a tendency to only capture the extremes of the scale (the totally satisfied are more likely to answer as a sign of "gratitude" whereas the totally unsatisfied may use these opportunities to express their anger). Observation is able to overcome these two limitations of self-report, although not exempt from all sorts of bias.

Observation is a powerful means to obtain information about a phenomenon or behaviour, through which the researcher does not influence real-life events. Therefore, the action happens in its natural environment. In pharmacy practice research, one may resort to observation to study the functioning of the pharmacy in an organisational context, the behaviour of pharmacy staff, either focusing on technical or communication aspects or even on ethical and legal conduct, and ultimately to study patients' behaviour as consumers of care, either in the pharmacy, in the hospital, in the nursing home or even in their home. Observation can fit into qualitative or quantitative research, depending on the way it is conducted.

5.2 Participant and Non-participatory Observation

Observation can be implemented through the participation of the researcher in the processes or activities being investigated, with varying degrees of activities and disclosures of the role possible to adopt. In the context of pharmacy practice research, the researcher may, for example, work as a pharmacy locum during a given period with the purpose of covertly evaluating the performance of pharmacy staff, being part of the activity although not directly influencing it and being totally covert; he may take the role of a pharmacy customer, hence directly participating in the activity being studied and again being totally covert. Alternatively, observation can also happen without the researcher's participation in the activities being studied. In this case, normally the researcher will announce his presence, explain the aim of the observation, seek agreement and use long periods of observation. This approach is normally more appropriate if the intention is to capture details of interactions happening in pharmacy practice, like the communication terms used, the gesture, the depth of advice provided or even the consistency of performance throughout the day. The disadvantage of this approach is that individuals being researched are aware they are being observed and therefore may change their normal behaviour, a phenomenon known as Hawthorne effect. This effect is more intense in an initial phase, but there is a human tendency to revert back to normal behaviour, which is the reason why in this type of observation, long periods are used, where the initial ones are then discarded and considered the wash-out period.

5.3   Covert Observation

Covert observation, also known as pseudo-patient methodology or mystery shopping, is a technique through which a person acts as a pharmacy customer, with the aim of observing and registering aspects of service provision in pharmacy practice. This is not the only applicability of this technique to pharmacy practice research but certainly is the most common. Covert observation has the advantage of minimising the Hawthorne effect, enabling the researcher to observe real interactions as they occur. The pitfall of covert observation applied to pharmacy practice is that in general it only captures one interaction (or a few at most), which does not necessarily represent the scope of practice of the pharmacy (between subject evaluation) or even the pharmacist evaluated in that instance (within subject evaluation).

5.3.1   Applicability of Covert Observation in Pharmacy Practice

The earliest reports of the use of mystery shoppers in pharmacy practice research date from 1984, where this technique was used to explore the role of the pharmacist as medication counsellors, a public health role just emerging at that time (Mason and Svarstad 1984).

However, the most common use of covert observation is in the context of continuous professional development as audits with subsequent feedback to the pharmacy team of aspects to be improved. One of the first well-structured initiatives of using this technique in pharmacy practice to improve practice was established by the University of Sydney, through the creation of the Quality Care Pharmacy Support Centre (QCPSC) in 2002. Previous successful experience from this research group with the use of this technique as an education and training method made it clear that adaption to pharmacy practice research and upscaling nationally was possible (Almeida Neto et al. 2000). Therefore, the QCPSC was established with the aim of continuously monitoring the application of the Standards of Practice developed by the Pharmacy Guild to guide pharmacists into the process of providing the right medicine to the right patient and instructing him/her to use it in the right moment, adding value to the service. As part of a continuous development programme, since 2000 pharmacies were financially incentivised to participate and agree to periodic visits of pseudo-patients (Benrimoj et al. 2008). Although it was not mandatory, the advantages were clear, leading to an almost total adherence (over 4200 pharmacies). A total of 59 scenarios were developed to capture all the situations to be assessed against the Standards of Practice (Benrimoj et al. 2007a). Prior to national implementation, the system was tested and demonstrated its ability to significantly increase compliance with the Standards (Benrimoj et al. 2007b).

Also in other corners of the world, various research groups and pharmacy associations used the pseudo-patient methodology adapted to their settings and national priorities, and interesting data emerged also in Germany (Berger et al. 2005), Slovenia (Horvat and Kos 2015), the USA (Svarstad et al. 2003), Scotland (Watson et al. 2004, 2009), Portugal (Gomes et al. 2011) and Finland (Pohjanoksa-Mäntylä et al. 2008), to name a few.

Some of these have changed the scope of application of the technique to be able to assess new services available to answer current consumers' needs, including email or online pharmacy services (Pohjanoksa-Mäntylä et al. 2008). Adaptions of this method continue to be used in Sydney, where undergraduates act as mystery shoppers, still with the purpose of continuously improving performance (Collins et al. 2017a). However, it has been argued that this method does not include performance feedback to improve counselling skills or to encourage behaviour change as often as desired to achieve its full potential (Xu et al. 2012).

Another application of covert observation in pharmacy practice is to use it with the intent to judge if legal regulations are being obeyed. One of the first initiatives published with such aim was undertaken in New Zealand, a country where the legislation foresees various categories of medicines, including restricted medicines. Access to this class has been investigated using pseudo-patients, and wide variability has been reported, believed to be related to the proximity to medical care and also to the population served, where different patterns were suggested for pharmacists serving the Maori population (Norris 2002a, b). Later studies undertaken in the USA, where legal regulations vary across states, transformed a simple research question into a challenge. Pseudo-patients were used to measure the quality of performance in different states and to compare the effect of regulation on pharmacists' behaviour (Svarstad et al. 2004). The conclusions taken were that the frequency of information provision varied widely (from 40 to 94%) and increased proportionally to the state regulations' intensity. This same research group also suggested that chain pharmacies and those with more staff more frequently engaged in the provision of written information leaflets, also considered to be of higher quality in such pharmacies (Svarstad et al. 2003). Some years later, it has been suggested that while state legislation is a very relevant predictor of the intensity of advice given, even more powerful is having a pharmacist involved in the interaction; also of note was the availability of a private area for counselling (Kimberlin et al. 2011).

Illegal situations have also been identified in other studies, focusing on other aspects of counselling, and reported in the range of 5% of visited sites (Alte et al. 2007).

Compliance with regulations is a phenomenon very much related to the country where research is being conducted, which will be influenced by the stringency of regulations imposed, the audits in place and also the cultural background of pharmacists and of society in general. A study undertaken in Catalonia, Spain, focusing on the sale of antibiotics without a medical prescription, has shown worrisome levels of legal compliance, although varying according to the situation. In acute bronchitis, the law was transposed in 17% of the situations, raising to 35% in the case of sore throat and reaching as high as 80% in urinary tract infection (Llor and Cots 2009).

A third application of covert observation is through the involvement of consumer protector agencies. These have adopted this research method and made it more feasible and less robust, to judge various aspects of service provision which may subsequently be revealed in the wider public arena. The Portuguese Association for Consumer Protection (DECO) is one example where this research method has been often used to evaluate aspects of access and quality of advice in anecdotal samples but in relevant topics. One of these studies focused on the pattern of dispensing of orlistat in 36 pharmacies and 12 pharmacy outlets, suggesting very poor performance (Consumidor, Associação Portuguesa para a Defesa do 2010).

Another study, involving 90 sites where emergency oral contraception is available (healthcare centres, hospitals and pharmacies), highlighted pharmacies as the worst performing in terms of assessment and advice provided (*Teste Saúde* 2003).

A study focusing on behaviour adopted in situations requiring medical attention portrayed two symptom-based requests, depression and pregnancy, each of them presented to 48 sites (pharmacies, pharmacy outlets and dietetic stores). Overall, only 28% of clients received any questions, although in 47% and 40% of cases, respectively, were products not sold (*Teste Saúde* 2008).

Consumers are not that focused on pharmacists' performance but on access aspects in general, regardless of the site or healthcare professional involved. A study somehow similar to that reported by Llor was conducted by DECO, where visits were made to pharmacies and general practitioners (GPs) simulating a case of sore throat lasting for 3 days, with some discomfort when swallowing and no other symptoms. The study revealed that 55% of GPs issued an unnecessary prescription for antibiotic, most of them spontaneously and a few subsequent to a consumer request. Conversely, only 9% of pharmacies showed no resistance to the sale of an antibiotic (*Teste Saúde* 2007).

5.3.2 Evaluation of Performance

The evaluation may focus on the structure, the process, the outcome or on all of them weighed in varied formats, depending on its intended use. When mystery shopping is used outside of pharmacy practice and seen as a method to capture commercial transactions and the impact the environment may have on those, it is quite common to have evaluations focusing on the structure. In such cases, the checklists used tend to value if the premises are clean, if the surrounding sound is appropriate, the colours used (either in walls, in counters or even in outfits, as these may influence the consumer's reactions), etc. In continuous professional development, the evaluations tend to also capture these aspects, but valuing them less, in favour of process measures. In pharmacy practice, the process is generally divided into three main phases: evaluation of the situation, selection of therapy and provision of advice. In such evaluations, normally phases I and III are valued. Phase I is quite commonly judged against the WWHAM questioning method:

- Who (is it for)?
- What (are the symptoms)?
- How (long have these been present)?
- Action (taken to solve the current situation)?
- Medication (concurrently taken)?

This reasoning assumes that only once the pharmacist has consistently been able to apply the various steps of the process, he/she will be able to consciously select the most appropriate therapy. However, it may also be argued that if the entire process is well conducted but the wrong medication is selected, the outcome for the patient will be negative or at least suboptimal. This has led some research groups to put more focus on the process (Benrimoj et al. 2008), while others favour the outcome (Gomes et al. 2011) and others analyse both simultaneously (Watson et al. 2009). All approaches may be correct, depending on the intended purpose of the measurement and the phase of continuous development.

5.3.3 Scenarios

Depending on the behaviour to be assessed, the scenario needs to offer enough variability for the observed person to display varying degrees of competence. When designing a scenario, all possible behaviours need to be anticipated and all the details that may influence evaluation carefully explained. For example, in the most common structure of pharmacies in industrialised countries, there is either a long counter or various individual counters, either way in general aligned across the back of the pharmacy. It has been shown that pharmacy staff tends to work in the same positions and the way these are chosen is not incidental. Therefore, the description of the scenario needs to indicate where the pseudo-patient should go first, i.e. the right, middle or left counter, and what to do if the planned behaviour is not possible to execute (e.g. the right counter already has a customer).

When using scenarios to score the quality of advice given when dispensing non-prescription medication, there are mainly two types of scenarios: symptom-based requests (SBRs) and direct product-based requests (DPRs) (Benrimoj et al. 2007a). Consistently, symptom-based scenarios lead to higher scores, most likely to result from the pharmacist's perception of openness from the customer for greater interaction, leading inevitably to more questions being asked. However, it has also been shown that even within the same type of scenario, the medicine requested leads to variability in average performance (Kelly et al. 2009), suggesting some areas may be easier to advise on, perhaps as a result of more intense education available, or eventually that there is some variability in the difficulty attributed to varying scenarios. These aspects are particularly important to take into account when planning the observation, especially when incorporated into the continuous development process. In such context, it is more important to ensure that different measurements in time are developed either using the same scenario (therefore needing a minimum time for re-evaluation) or, if that is not possible, using scenarios within the same typology (SBRs or DPRs) and with equivalent levels of difficulty. In one of the studies conducted by Benrimoj et al., it was shown that although wide variability in performance was identified at baseline, significant increases in the quality of performance were identified after three visits, in the range of 5% after the second visit and 10% after the third visit (Benrimoj et al. 2007a).

Much work has been undertaken mostly in the areas of non-prescription medicines and minor ailments in general (Collins et al. 2017b, 2018). However, some research groups have been focusing on particular areas. Anderson et al. have investigated to a greater extent the provision of emergency oral contraception aiming to judge the adherence to a patient group direction protocol for supply of emergency hormonal contraception (Anderson and Bissell 2004). This area has more recently been researched in developing countries (Tavares and Foster 2016; Huda et al. 2018). Extensions of the technique using telephone-based assessments to judge differential access to emergency contraception with different legal status have also been conducted in the USA and in Hawaii (Shigesato et al. 2018; Bullock et al. 2016). Schneider et al. have focused on the provision of advice about correct inhaler technique, showing poor baseline performance, which after educational interventions consistently resulted in reduced supply of reliever medication without assessment and counselling and an increase in physician referral (Schneider et al. 2009, 2010). This area of research has later been expanded to the assessment of chronic cough with onward medical referral (Schneider et al. 2011). Most recent studies are focusing on the assessment of pharmacists' ability to provide appropriate paediatric advice (Wigmore et al. 2018). Also, an emerging area of interest is the use of codeine-containing analgesics (Byrne et al. 2018).

Emerging research from the Middle East and from developing countries confirms the spread of the technique as a useful research methodology in pharmacy practice, sometimes combined with other research techniques such as self-report and applied to various research questions and disease areas (Huda et al. 2018; Alaqeel and Abanmy 2015; Surur et al. 2017; Netere et al. 2018; Osman et al. 2012; Adnan et al. 2015; Belachew et al. 2017).

In industrialised countries, the tendency seems to be the use of pseudo-patients to investigate new services being developed, with a great recent example on the use of simulated smokers to investigate the UK NHS Stop Smoking Service (Jumbe et al. 2019).

But the use of mystery shoppers is not restricted to the assessment of performance when dispensing non-prescription medication, although simply easier. When used to assess advice upon dispensing of prescription-only medicines, the ethical issues of needing a "fake" prescription sometimes block the feasibility of such research. Nonetheless, research groups have developed ways to overcome such barriers and used this technique to evaluate, for instance, the quality of advice when a first prescription for antidepressant therapy is issued (Liekens et al. 2014; Chong et al. 2014).

Box 5.1 Scenario Template

IDENTIFICATION OF THE SCENARIO TYPE: *Direct product-based request OR symptom-based request*

    INFORMATION FOR THE PSEUDO-PATIENT: *Please enter the pharmacy and head towards the pharmacy staff on your right-hand side. Remember you should only give the information if you are asked for it.*

    PATIENT IDENTITY: *Identify who the product is for (self, father, spouse, child, grandmother, etc.); mention age.*

    PRIOR EXPERIENCE: *Depending on the scenario, in this section information should be made available on previous use of the product requested (in which case, if asked, the shopper should be able to indicate how he first heard about the product or who indicated it, when it was last used, what was the experience and outcome associated with its use) or previous experience with the symptoms presented (when they were last present, other associated symptoms, similarities and differences with previous episode(s), periodic recurrence, how they were treated last time, experience and outcome).*

    CURRENT SYMPTOMS: *In this section, maximum detail must be given about the symptoms the patient complains about, other associated signs or symptoms he/she may have to report if questioned, duration of symptoms, onset type, laterality (if applicable), aggravating and attenuating factors and previous exposures that could relate to the symptoms (e.g. food intake, travel).*

    TREATMENTS ALREADY USED FOR THE CURRENT SYMPTOMS: *Indicate if there were any attempts made to deal with the current situation, including non-pharmacological measures (e.g. rest for 1 day) or treatments used (which, for how long, how taken, experience and outcome so far).*

    OTHER MEDICATIONS TAKEN AND DIAGNOSED CHRONIC CONDITIONS: *When describing a scenario, it is not possible to anticipate how the questions will be asked. Therefore, it is best to provide as much information as possible, which the trained shopper will only provide according to the question made. Some pharmacy staff may ask about concurrent medications (as a proxy for identifying medical conditions), while others may simply ask directly if the patient is aware of having any chronic condition. Please note that the questions may be posed in an open manner (e.g. do you have any chronic condition?) or as closed questions (e.g. do you have diabetes?), and the patient should be instructed how to answer one or the other, with no room for improvisation. When instructed about the drugs taken, the patient should be able to know if he is expected to provide precise indications (e.g. captopril 50 mg twice a day) or general indications (e.g. I take a pill for lowering my cholesterol). In this section, indications about the presence of specific situations may also be included, e.g. pregnancy or breastfeeding and allergic reactions (again, like in previous sections, the patient should be instructed if she should offer this information when questioned about "do you have any other conditions" or only if specifically asked "are you pregnant or breastfeeding?" or "are you aware of being allergic to any substance?").*

PREVIOUS MEDICAL HISTORY: *If relevant for the scenario, the patient should be informed of any previous related event, in case he is asked. For example, if he has had a previous stroke (if so, when exactly, how it was treated and information about the recovery) and if he has had previous urinary tract infections (how many in the previous year, action taken at the time including information on any antibiotics taken, antibiotic sensibility tests made, completion of course of treatment).*

OTHER INFORMATION: *Depending on the type of research, it may be appropriate to provide information about the possible disclosures. For example, in PBRs the patient should be instructed what to do if he is not given the drug requested but is advised instead on the use of an alternative medication (Should he buy it? Regardless of the price? Should he thank the advice and note it but say he needs to think about it? Should he get angry and insist?). Another aspect worth detailing is how the patient should act when provided (or not) information on the product (what should he answer if questioned "do you need any information about the drug use?" Should he ask for it in case not offered?). The most common is to instruct pseudo-patients to be passive and wait for information to be given, but depending on the research question, that might not be always the best solution (Adapted from Benrimoj et al. (2008)).*

5.3.4 Recording the Interaction

In covert observation, interactions must occur naturally. Therefore, the pseudo-customer may not pause the interaction to take notes. However, the assessment of interactions must be very objective and not subject to recall bias or information bias. There are three main methods for recording these interactions, either through the use of tape recorders which will capture the sound, video recorders which will capture the images and sound or memory which will capture the interaction, which is immediately transcribed into a checklist upon leaving the pharmacy.

Recording transcriptions verbatim has the advantage of enabling focus on patterns and similarities in the various phases of the pharmacists' consultation, *i.e.* identification of the situation and its characterisation, selection of the most appropriate therapy and provision of advice on safe medication use including what to do when symptoms persist. On the other hand, the devices must be hidden, which may lead to difficulties in field work and potential ethical problems.

The question is really the extent of discrepancy that may exist when one or the other recording methods are used. Differences within the range of 10% in performance have been recognised, which may be seen as little in absolute terms, but when we are aiming to identify behaviour changes that fall into this range of values, it may definitely have an impact on the accuracy of findings (Benrimoj et al. 2007a).

5.3.5   Checklists

The way checklists are rated will depend on the development of a scenario which intends to judge behaviour against a standard considered to be of high quality. This implies that when the person being judged does exactly what is expected, he/she will receive a mark of 100% (or equivalent).

Factors that may affect different performance need to be captured in the checklist, which may be contextual (*e.g.* time of the day or of the week), organisational (*e.g.* ratio of staff to customers at the moment of interaction) or professional (*e.g.* professional category). For example, it has been shown that interactions where a pharmacist is involved result in significantly higher scores than those with other staff (Collins et al. 2017a; Alte et al. 2007), that larger-sized pharmacies tend to provide higher-quality advice (Alte et al. 2007) and that the location of pharmacy influences the way information is conveyed with metropolitan area pharmacies tending to adopt an oral style, whereas rural pharmacies more frequently deliver written information (Puspitasari et al. 2009b).

Box 5.2 Checklist Template

SECTION A—CHARACTERISATION OF THE PHARMACY STRUCTURE. *In this section, it may be relevant to capture aspects that may influence different behaviours. A few are given as examples*

Date and time of visit: Week day/weekend, morning/lunch time/afternoon/ evening/out of hours (night shifts)

Time waiting to be served: Record exact number of minutes

Number of pharmacy staff visible

Number of clients waiting (including yourself)

Professional identification: Pharmacist/pharmacy technician/unidentified/others

Gender:

Apparent age: Age categories may be used

Scenario tested: These may be coded if various are available

SECTION B—CHARACTERISATION OF THE EVALUATION PROCESS. *Please tick all boxes where the question was presented. Please note that some of the questions may not be applicable to the scenario (and these should be crossed out in the evaluation form)*

Who is the medication for?/Who has those symptoms?

What are the symptoms? Can you detail the symptoms (e.g. runny nose, blocked nose)?

How long have these been present?

Have you taken any action to solve/minimise the current situation?

If the question was made and the answer was yes: Was it effective? Did you experience any side effects? (Consider if these additional questions add extra marks or if they are considered as part of the previous question)

Do you take any other medication? Do you have any chronic condition? Are you pregnant or breastfeeding? Do you have any known allergy? (Consider if these additional questions add extra marks or if they are considered as part of the previous question)

SECTION C—CHARACTERISATION OF THE SELECTION PROCESS. *(Please note that according to the scenario, the scoring of these items needs to be carefully considered. Equally important is to consider how judgement will be made on the selection process)*

Was the medication supplied? Yes/no. If yes please indicate which:_____
Was a relevant precaution transmitted when supplying? Yes/no
Was an alternative product supplied?
Was the patient referred to the GP?

SECTION D—CHARACTERISATION OF THE DISPENSING PROCESS
Did you receive information on how to take?
Did you receive information on maximum tolerated dose?
Did you receive information on the duration of therapy?
Did you receive information on what to do if a dose is missed?
Did you receive information on possible side effects?
Did you receive information on interactions (drug-drug OR food-drug)?
Did you receive information on lifestyle advice?
Did you receive any written information?
Did you receive advice on what to do if the symptoms persist?
Were you asked if you had any additional questions? (Adapted from Benrimoj et al. (2008) and Gomes (2012))

When finalising the development of the checklist, additional reflection needs to put on eventual weighting of dimensions involved. In the formerly shown example, there are three main dimensions and each of them has a different number of items to be ranked. This implies that if no weighing is attributed, the last domain will be the most important because it contains more items. This may or not be the best solution depending on what the research intends to capture.

5.3.6 Ethical Aspects in Covert Observation

The need to seek ethical approval to undertake a research study using covert observation is not straightforward and will depend on the level of anonymity being used and also the legal regulations in the country/continent. In general, if it is possible to identify the individuals being audited, permission from them should be sought. Identification will be possible or not depending on the variables being collected. If the pharmacy identification, for instance, is collected, depending on the pharmacy size, not much more is needed to identify the individual. In addition, some researchers also capture gender, professional category, etc., making the identification of the subject immediate. Another aspect is the way the information gathered is used. Is it to report back to the pharmacy owner or manager? To report back to the individual? Simply to characterise the situation at a macro level? How are performance scores treated by management? Are these used to incentivise continuous development or to penalise consistently poorly performing individuals? All these aspects deal with the benefit of research, the harm of research and the autonomy of individuals involved in research and therefore will impact on the ethics around the research study and the need to collect informed consent from the individuals or for the decision to engage in a pseudo-patient study.

5.4   Overt Observation

Overt observation is another form of observation, where research intentions are openly shared, having the advantage of avoiding ethical dilemmas or lack of informed consent. In addition, because the observation period is generally quite long, it enables to capture various interactions, which leads to a greater confidence that it indeed represents reality. On the other hand, a drawback is that, depending on the topic of research, social desirability and the Hawthorne effect may occur. Overt observation originates in behavioural psychology and is more effective when observation lasts longer, leading observed ones to progressively act "normal".

The way through which data is collected and analysed also varies, where covert tends to be more quantitative and overt more qualitative, which means that the focus of the first is the nature and frequency of the event, whereas the latter focuses on details related to understanding the reasons why phenomena occur. Both techniques have their use in pharmacy practice. Overt observation may be most useful to capture details that are not properly explored in quantitative assessments, such as communication techniques.

The use of Roter's theory, for example, has been applied to detail the complex interactions in pharmacy practice that need to happen when trying to move from a product-based practice into person-centred pharmaceutical care (Cavaco and Roter 2010).

Other studies resorting to non-participatory research have also focused on communication skills but considering other standards. The Calgary-Cambridge guide was originally developed in medical practice but adapted in studies aiming to explore in depth pharmacist consultation styles (Greenhill et al. 2011). Other studies have used similar approaches but focusing on counter assistants' performance (Watson et al. 2007).

A practical aspect that needs to be considered when using overt observation in pharmacy practice is where to stand or to sit so that the researcher's presence has the minimal influence possible but is still near enough to capture all relevant aspects to be measured.

Because the nature of overt observation tends to be more qualitative and also because research is announced and allowed, the use of audio or video recording generally poses no barriers and is used as a means to capture all details of interactions. In fact, using field notes could never capture the details occurring in a complex interaction to the same extent as recordings (Murad et al. 2014).

Subsequent transcriptions of the collected material are needed and qualitative analysis, using various possible approaches (as detailed in Chap. 4), may be used for the emergence of codes and resulting search for meanings and interpretations.

When conducting the analysis, a decision needs to be made on the constructs of interest and decide if only verbal communication is of interest or if other aspects of behaviour are to be captured and analysed. Focusing on communication, the observation may encompass non-verbal behaviour, spatial behaviour (*e.g.* distance between subjects interacting), extra-linguistic behaviour (*e.g.* speed and loudness) and linguistic behaviour (*i.e.* content and structure of the message conveyed) (Kaae and Traulsen 2015).

The sampling frame to be used is also approached differently to the one sought in covert observation, again because the nature tends to be more qualitative. This implies that in covert observation, sampling frames will benefit from large samples ideally selected randomly or stratified by area (depending on the research purpose) so that they represent as much as possible the entire remit of pharmacy practice in the region or country to be characterised.

In overt observation, the focus is put on the richness of interactions; therefore, the sample may depend on the duration of the observation, when it is undertaken with concurrent analysis and constant comparison searching for saturation of themes (in which case convenient sampling frames are used, eventually exhaustive within given convenience criteria, *e.g.* all interactions during 1 week in one pharmacy); or if there are reasons to believe there are factors leading to different intensity or quality of interactions, purposive sampling may be used, eventually comparing and contrasting interactions occurring in rural and metropolitan pharmacies (as a mere example).

In both cases, the unit of analysis must be precociously identified, *i.e.* will researchers be focusing on patients or on encounters? What exactly constitutes an encounter; is it the whole experience since entering the pharmacy or is it restricted to the moment where the individual is directly interacting with the pharmacist?

The definition of the unit of analysis is extremely important when the analysis is centred on the relationship between codes and on the factors that may influence the adoption of different behaviours, such as contextual factors (time of day), recipient factors (type of patient, age, education level, occupation, socio-economic status) or host factors (professional category, previous attendance of specific courses).

5.4.1 Applicability of Overt Observation in Pharmacy Practice

There is limited research published in pharmacy practice resorting to overt observation, but is a potentially useful area for future studies, especially when interested in investigating complex situations or advanced practice. One of the first studies identified in pharmacy practice using non-participant overt observation focused on advice-giving behaviour of community pharmacy staff. Due to its nature, this study explored the reasons for customers to seek pharmacists, identifying the presence of minor ailments as key (Hassell et al. 1997). A subsequent study of this same research group further highlighted the nature of interactions and the different perspectives from both parties involved. According to the authors, consumers are more interested in information about the effectiveness of products, in contrast with pharmacy staff who concentrate on providing advice on the safety of medicines (Hassell et al. 1998).

A study, also dated from 1998, used non-participant observation in a very little researched area, the in-depth features of the essential drug programme in Burkina Faso. In this study, observation occurred in various access points, namely, healthcare centres, pharmacies and patients' homes (Krause et al. 1998).

A much more recent study has used this method to characterise dispensing practice when dealing with prescribed medicines in Swiss pharmacies and to investigate factors that may influence pharmaceutical interventions initiated. This study, based on one single day's observation in each of the 18 community pharmacies involved, was able to capture 556 prescription encounters (unit of analysis) and suggested the main factors leading to intervention were the interaction involving a pharmacist and the situation being of a new prescription, of a new customer, or of a prescription filled by carers. Although resorting to non-participant observation, the study may be classified as mainly quantitative because it was mostly empirical and focus was put on quantifying interactions using a checklist (Maes et al. 2018).

As referred in the previous section, the use of overt observation as a technique seems quite popular when desiring to explore communication aspects as it enables capturing details not possible otherwise. Communication may be researched in various settings, and certainly pharmacy practice is no exception. A Danish study focused on this aspect and used overt observation to capture 100 interactions occurring at the pharmacy counter between the staff and customers and classified each of them according to five types described by previous research. The main findings suggest the more the pharmacist or pharmacy assistant practises, the more successful he/she becomes in engaging customers in medication dialogues (Kaae et al. 2014).

Another study used this same technique but aiming to identify opportunities for improving medication reviews in Canada. This study was undertaken in four pharmacies and complemented the ethnographic observation with in-depth interviews with pharmacists and patients. In this case, the period of observation was restricted to 72 h, and the unit of analysis was the medication review process, where a total of 29 were characterised (Patton et al. 2018). The main findings highlight a wide variability in the dimensions of the service examined, which comprise the duration of the encounter, the interaction style and the location.

In fact the approach here described of combining overt observation with in-depth interviews is commonly used with the main intention to change behaviour as it enables those observed to reflect on their behaviour by exposing them to their performance, normally using video recordings.

The impact of educational interventions to improve the quality of advice in community pharmacy has also been explored using a before and after design where overt observation was one of the measures to assess performance, similar to experiences previously referred using covert observation. Pharmacy staff's performance considered the use of evidence-based supply of non-prescription medicines, using vignettes for four specific situations: athlete's foot, cough, menstrual pain and nasal congestion. The quality of performance increased significantly as a result of education. Using overt observation made it possible to classify the evidence to support recommendations made (*e.g.* international guidelines, pharmacy-based protocols, pharmaceutical society recommended practice, etc.), as opposed to recommendations based on "personal experiences" (Ngwerume et al. 2015). This aspect is much easier to capture using self-report combined with overt observation as it enables registering where information needed was sought to support the advice given. Another aspect worth highlighting in this study was the use of a long observation period (8 h in each moment) as recommended to minimise the Hawthorne effect. A great advantage of overt observation, which was well explored in this study, is the ability to observe all members of staff, so in this case interactions were recorded between 9 a.m. and 10 p.m., allowing for staff working in different shifts to be captured.

Service delivery in pharmacy practice may be considered as a broad area of interest for the application of overt observation. In fact, depending on the way it is structured, it is an interesting method to capture the duration of interactions between care provider and customer, the nature of the interaction in terms of content (*i.e.* technical *vs* lay explanations of the way medication acts), the initiator of the interaction (*i.e.* service requested by the customer, suggested by the pharmacist, referenced from elsewhere, etc.) and the particular features of the interaction (*e.g.* need for privacy). This information may be particularly useful for decision-makers in pharmacy practice to opt for a range of services to implement depending on the pharmacy's mission, vision and values. These studies are also useful ahead of implementation or in early phases, so that findings may still be incorporated to overcome barriers eventually encountered.

A study in Sweden explored the nature of interactions during generic substitution and found, during such interactions, most time was spent on non-medical aspects of counselling, including financial considerations (Olsson et al. 2017). Another study explored the New Medicine Service, soon after its initial implementation, and showed that the service was implemented with no changes made to the previously existing activities, workforce and workload, inevitably suggesting the service would have to be simplified to be delivered or it was deemed to fail, despite being commissioned (Latif et al. 2016).

Box 5.3 Examples of Aspects to be Observed and Recorded (Later Transcribed and Coded to Answer the Identified Aspects) During a Pharmacy Practice Interaction Using Overt Observation

SECTION A—CHARACTERISATION OF A PHARMACY PRACTICE INTERACTION

Please describe the service for which the identification was observed: (Medication review, New Medicine Service, Immunisation, etc.)

Date and time of interaction:

Duration of interaction (from the moment the pharmacist addressed the customer until leaving the pharmacy; if a service is offered and then booked another occasion for service delivery, please break down all of those durations):

Professional engaged in the interaction:

Number of pharmacy staff visible not engaging in the interaction:

Other staff that at some point participated in the interaction (even if remotely, e.g. hospital pharmacist, GP, etc.)

Number of clients waiting in the pharmacy premises:

When did the interaction occur (if a change in location happened during the interaction, please indicate why, when and how)?

SECTION B—IDENTIFICATION OF THE NEED FOR THE SERVICE

What was the factor(s) that triggered the need for this service?

How was the interaction initiated?

Was the service known to the customer?

If not, how was the explanation made?

Was this explanation well received?

Were the potential benefits from the service explained to the customer? And the potential risks from the service? Was there a timeline/frequency of delivered mentioned? Were there any responsibilities of the customer mentioned?

SECTION C—CHARACTERISATION OF SERVICE DELIVERY

Did the provider at some point need to consult information sources (e.g. standard operating procedures, clinical criteria databases, etc.)? Which sources were consulted? Were these easily available?

Did the provider at some point need to consult patient information (medical record, e.g. laboratory tests)? Which data were consulted? Were these easily available?

Did the provider at some point need to interact with other healthcare providers? Which healthcare providers were contacted? Were these possible to reach? Please describe the nature of the interaction (e.g. solving a drug-related problem), the duration and format (e.g. by telephone or face to face) and the type that best characterises the way the interaction was conducted (e.g. shared decision-making vs submissive enquiry)

Was any problem identified at that moment? Which? How addressed?

Was this eventual problem solved? How? Is there any follow-up measure to be adopted in the near future? How and when?

SECTION D—POTENTIAL BARRIERS OBSERVED IN SERVICE DELIVERY

During all the interactions observed, did you identify any potential barriers in any of the phases of service delivery? We are interested to know about, for instance, the communication established when the need for the service was identified and subsequently explained, the actual process of service delivery or the subsequent phases that may exist even if remotely delivered. In all these phases, we want to hear about your experience as observer of the pharmacist, of any other healthcare professional involved or of the customer. Please use expressions (verbal or physical to support your opinions whenever possible); *e.g.* the pharmacist had difficulty in finding reliable information about a drug-drug interaction after consulting source A and B (add sources you observed the pharmacist is consulting), or the customer was apparently suspicious about this new service and wanted to consult his spouse before taking a decision (add quote after transcribing the recording).

It would be interesting for future research to resort to non-participatory observation to investigate other advanced services like home medicines review or even pharmacists prescribing or working in GP practices. In fact, this technique has already been used for exploring concordance during nurses' independent prescribing interactions (Latter et al. 2007). Another area worth further investigation is the role and impact of technology on pharmacy workflow and on outcomes for patients. In this area, a published research protocol has presented the possibility to explore the impact of a paediatric prescribing system on hospital care provision (Farre and Cummins 2016). Similar approaches have been used to investigate the impact of automation on dispensing errors observed in hospital pharmacy (James et al. 2013) and the experience with electronic prescribing in a group of community pharmacies adopting the service (Harvey et al. 2014).

A slight modification of the traditionally overt observation has been recently explored in the context of social media and new ways of communicating and sharing experiences. Using non-participant observation, this study analysed themes within discussion fora of psychostimulant drug users in modern societies (Robitaille 2018). At first sight it is distant from pharmacy practice but certainly motivating to find new venues for understanding the experiences of medication users resorting to technology and perhaps using the knowledge to develop person-centred new services that are able to address the identified problems.

5.5   Impact of Observation Research Methods in Practice

During this chapter, various examples have been used to demonstrate the varied application of covert and overt observation in pharmacy practice research. In addition to discussing each of these methods' advantages and limitations, it is perhaps worth reflecting how these studies have had an impact on care provision and on medicines use. There is enough evidence to support the use of covert observation as a powerful method for continuous professional development, and personally I believe the work of QCPSC had a major impact on the performance of pharmacists and pharmacy staff in Australia, undoubtedly contributing to an improved practice (Benrimoj et al. 2007a, b, 2008). However, the system was totally focused around the pharmacy infrastructure, including service provision and a concern for ensuring quality standards were met. The extent to which these quality standards directly transfer into consumer's improved medication use is unclear.

The use of covert observation as a tool to verify legal practice may be occasionally used to unveil priority areas for action but does not change practice *per se* and merely contributes to poor performers developing dissimulated behaviours. In addition, it has absolutely no impact on medicines' use by consumers.

To contribute to improved medicines' use, probably the work developed by consumer associations, despite its low robustness in scientific terms, is the one that played a greater role into creating awareness among citizens about the importance, for example, of ensuring antibiotics are only to be used in the presence of bacterial infection. Furthermore, these small studies contributed to alert policy makers about the importance of listening to consumers (*Teste Saúde* 2007).

Thinking about the future, making use of consumers as the decision-makers to which services are needed to improve medicines' use may be the way to go into creating useful services sought by those in need. Probably overt observation will be an interesting method to explore, eventually combined with self-report to help understand success factors for service implementation.

5.6   Conclusion

Observation is a powerful technique to capture real behaviours as they occur, shown to be quite useful in pharmacy practice research. Not all studies conducted in the area have been mentioned, because the intention was to highlight various areas of applicability and not to conduct an exhaustive review of their use. It has been shown that covert observation is a technique long used in pharmacy practice, which given the advantages continues to expand worldwide. Overt observation, although equally dating from long ago, has not been so widely used in pharmacy practice but presenting promising applications in the context of emerging services and technologies.

References

Adnan M, Karim S, Khan S, Al-Wabel NA. Comparative evaluation of metered-dose inhaler technique demonstration among community pharmacists in Al Qassim and Al-Ahsa region, Saudi-Arabia. Saudi Pharm J. 2015;23(2):138–42.
Alaqeel S, Abanmy NO. Counselling practices in community pharmacies in Riyadh, Saudi Arabia: a cross-sectional study. BMC Health Serv Res. 2015;15:557.

Almeida Neto AC, Benrimoj SI, Kavanagh DJ, Boakes RA. Novel educational training program for community pharmacists. Am J Pharm Educ. 2000 64:302–7.

Alte D, Weitschies W, Ritter CA. Evaluation of consultation in community pharmacies with mystery shoppers. Ann Pharmacother. 2007;41(6):1023–30.

Anderson C, Bissell P. Using semi covert research to evaluate an emergency hormonal contraception service. Pharm World Sci. 2004;26(2):102–6.

Belachew SA, Tilahun F, Ketsela T, Achaw Ayele A, Kassie Netere A, Getnet Mersha A, Befekadu Abebe T, Melaku Gebresillassie B, Getachew Tegegn H, Asfaw Erku D. Competence in metered dose inhaler technique among community pharmacy professionals in Gondar town, Northwest Ethiopia: knowledge and skill gap analysis. PLoS One. 2017;12(11):e0188360.

Benrimoj SI, Werner JB, Raffaele C, Roberts AS, Costa FA. Monitoring quality standards in the provision of nonprescription medicines from Australian Community Pharmacies: results of a national programme. Qual Saf Health Care. 2007a;16:354–8.

Benrimoj SC, Gilbert A, Quintrell N, Neto AC. Non-prescription medicines: a process for standards development and testing in community pharmacy. Pharm World Sci. 2007b;29(4):386–94.

Benrimoj SI, Warner JB, Raffaele C, Roberts AS. A system for monitoring quality standards in the provision of non-prescription medicines from Australian community pharmacies. Pharm World Sci. 2008;30:147–53.

Berger K, Eickhoff C, Schulz M. Counselling quality in community pharmacies: implementation of the pseudo customer methodology in Germany. J Clin Pharm Ther. 2005;30(1):45–7.

Bullock H, Steele S, Kurata N, Tschann M, Elia J, Kaneshiro B, Salcedo J. Pharmacy access to ulipristal acetate in Hawaii: is a prescription enough? Contraception. 2016;93(5):452–4.

Byrne GA, Wood PJ, Spark MJ. Non-prescription supply of combination analgesics containing codeine in community pharmacy: a simulated patient study. Res Social Adm Pharm. 2018;14(1):96–105.

Cavaco A, Roter D. Pharmaceutical consultations in community pharmacies: utility of the Roter Interaction Analysis System to study pharmacist-patient communication. Int J Pharm Pract. 2010;18(3):141–8.

Chong WW, Aslani P, Chen TF. Pharmacist-patient communication on use of antidepressants: a simulated patient study in community pharmacy. Res Social Adm Pharm. 2014;10(2):419–37.

Collins JC, Schneider CR, Naughtin CL, Wilson F, de Almeida Neto AC, Moles RJ. Mystery shopping and coaching as a form of audit and feedback to improve community pharmacy management of non-prescription medicine requests: an intervention study. MBJ Open. 2017a;7(12):e019462.

Collins JC, Schneider CR, Faraj R, Wilson F, de Almeida Neto AC, Moles RJ. Management of common ailments requiring referral in the pharmacy: a mystery shopping intervention study. Int J Clin Pharm. 2017b;39(4):697–703.

Collins JC, Schneider CR, Wilson F, de Almeida Neto AC, Moles RJ. Community pharmacy modifications to non-prescription medication requests: a simulated patient study. Res Social Adm Pharm. 2018;14(5):427–33.

Consumidor, Associação Portuguesa para a Defesa do. Venda sem conselhos. Teste Saúde. 2010;84:34–5.

Farre A, Cummins C. Understanding and evaluating the effects of implementing an electronic paediatric prescribing system on care provision and hospital work in paediatric hospital ward settings: a qualitatively driven mixed-method study protocol. BMJ Open. 2016;6(2):e010444.

Gomes MAV. Feedback imediato Como metodologia de formação às farmácias comunitárias no atendimento de MNSRM. Caparica: Instituto Universitário Egas Moniz; 2012.

Gomes M, Costa FA, Cruz P, Guerreiro M, Placido G. Influência da formação no atendimento em medicamentos não sujeitos a receita médica. Rev Port Farm. 2011;LII(Suppl. 5):119.

Greenhill N, Anderson C, Avery A, Pilnick A. Analysis of pharmacist-patient communication using the Calgary-Cambridge guide. Patient Educ Couns. 2011;83(3):423–31.

Harvey J, Avery AJ, Barber N. A qualitative study of community pharmacy perceptions of the Electronic Prescriptions Service in England. Int J Pharm Pract. 2014;22(6):440–4.

Hassell K, Noyce PR, Rogers A, Harris J, Wilkinson J. A pathway to the GP: the pharmaceutical 'consultation' as a first port of call in primary health care. Fam Pract. 1997;14(6):498–502.

Hassell K, Noyce P, Rogers A, Harris J, Wilkinson J. Advice provided in British community pharmacies: what people want and what they get. J Health Serv Res Policy. 1998;3(4):219–25.

Horvat N, Kos M. Contribution of Slovenian community pharmacist counseling to patients' knowledge about their prescription medicines: a cross-sectional study. Croat Med J. 2015;56(1):41–9.

Huda FA, Mahmood HR, Alam A, Ahmmed F, Karim F, Sarker BK, Al Haque N, Ahmed A. Provision of menstrual regulation with medication among pharmacies in three municipal districts of Bangladesh: a situation analysis. Contraception. 2018;97(2):144–51.

James KL, Barlow D, Bithell A, Hiom S, Lord S, Pollard M, Roberts D, Way C, Whittlesea C. The impact of automation on workload and dispensing errors in a hospital pharmacy. Int J Pharm Pract. 2013;21(2):92–104.

Jumbe S, James WY, Madurasinghe V, Steed L, Sohanpal R, Yau TK, Taylor S, Eldridge S, Griffiths C, Walton R. Evaluating NHS Stop Smoking Service engagement in community pharmacies using simulated smokers: fidelity assessment of a theory-based intervention. BMJ Open. 2019;9(5):e026841.

Kaae S, Traulsen JM. Qualitative methods in pharmacy practice. In: [autor do livro] Zaheer-Ud-Din Babar, editor. Pharmacy practice research methods. Auckland: Springer International Publishing; 2015.

Kaae S, Saleem S, Kristiansen M. How do Danish community pharmacies vary in engaging customers in medicine dialogues at the counter—an observational study. Pharm Pract (Granada). 2014;12(3):422.

Kelly FS, Williams KA, Benrimoj SI. Does advice from pharmacy staff vary according to the non-prescription medicine requested? Ann Pharmacother. 2009;43(11):1877–86.

Kimberlin CL, Jamison AN, Linden S, Winterstein AG. Patient counseling practices in U.S. pharmacies: effects of having pharmacists hand the medication to the patient and state regulations on pharmacist counseling. J Am Pharm Assoc (2003). 2011;51(4):527–34.

Krause G, Benzler J, Heinmüller R, Borchert M, Koob E, Ouattara K, Diesfeld HJ. Performance of village pharmacies and patient compliance after implementation of essential drug programme in rural Burkina Faso. Health Policy Plan. 1998;13(2):159–66.

Latif A, Waring J, Watmough D, Barber N, Chuter A, Davies J, Salema NE, Boyd MJ, Elliott RA. Examination of England's New Medicine Service (NMS) of complex health care interventions in community pharmacy. Res Social Adm Pharm. 2016;12(6):966–89.

Latter S, Maben J, Myall M, Young A. Perceptions and practice of concordance in nurses' prescribing consultations: findings from a national questionnaire survey and case studies of practice in England. Int J Nurs Stud. 2007;44(1):9–18.

Liekens S, Vandael E, Roter D, Larson S, Smits T, Laekeman G, Foulon V. Impact of training on pharmacists' counseling of patients starting antidepressant therapy. Patient Educ Couns. 2014;94(1):110–5.

Llor C, Cots JM. The sale of antibiotics without prescription in pharmacies in Catalonia, Spain. Clin Infect Dis. 2009;48:1345–9.

Maes KA, Ruppanner JA, Imfeld-Isenegger TL, Hersberger KE, Lampert ML, Boeni F. Dispensing of prescribed medicines in Swiss community pharmacies-observed counselling activities. Pharmacy (Basel). 2018;7(1):1. https://doi.org/10.3390/pharmacy7010001.

Mason HL, Svarstad BL. Medication counseling behaviors and attitudes of rural community pharmacists. Drug Intell Clin Pharm. 1984;18(5):409–14.

Murad MS, Chatterley T, Guirguis LM. A meta-narrative review of recorded patient-pharmacist interactions: exploring biomedical or patient-centered communication? Res Social Adm Pharm. 2014;10:1–20.

Netere AK, Erku DA, Sendekie AK, Gebreyohannes EA, Muluneh NY, Belachew SA. Assessment of community pharmacy professionals' knowledge and counseling skills achievement towards headache management: a cross-sectional and simulated-client based mixed study. J Headache Pain. 2018;19(1):96.

Ngwerume K, Watson M, Bond C, Blenkinsopp A. An evaluation of an intervention designed to improve the evidence-based supply of non-prescription medicines from community pharmacies. Int J Pharm Pract. 2015;23(2):102–10.

Norris PT. Purchasing restricted medicines in New Zealand pharmacies: results from a "mystery shopper" study. Pharm World Sci. 2002a;24(4):149–53.

Norris P. Which sorts of pharmacies provide more patient counselling? J Health Serv Res Policy. 2002b;Suppl 1:S23–8.

Olsson E, Wallach-Kildemoes H, Ahmed B, Ingman P, Kaae S, Kälvemark Sporrong S. The influence of generic substitution on the content of patient-pharmacist communication in Swedish community pharmacies. Int J Pharm Pract. 2017;25(4):274–81.

Osman A, Ahmed Hassan IS, Ibrahim MI. Are Sudanese community pharmacists capable to prescribe and demonstrate asthma inhaler devices to patrons? A mystery patient study. Pharm Pract (Granada). 2012;10(2):110–5.

Patton SJ, Miller FA, Abrahamyan L, Rac VE. Expanding the clinical role of community pharmacy: a qualitative ethnographic study of medication reviews in Ontario, Canada. Health Policy. 2018;122(3):256–62.

Pohjanoksa-Mäntylä MK, Kulovaara H, Bell JS, Enäkoski M, Airaksinen MS. Email medication counseling services provided by Finnish community pharmacies. Ann Pharmacother. 2008;42(12):1782–90.

Puspitasari HP, Aslani P, Krass I. A review of counseling practices on prescription medicines in community pharmacies. Res Social Adm Pharm. 2009a;5(3):197–210.

Puspitasari HP, Aslani P, Krass I. How do Australian metropolitan and rural pharmacists counsel consumers with prescriptions? Pharm World Sci. 2009b;31(3):394–405.

Puspitasari HP, Aslani P, Krass I. Pharmacists' and consumers' viewpoints on counselling on prescription medicines in Australian community pharmacies. Int J Pharm Pract. 2010;18(4):202–8.

Robitaille C. "This drug turned me into a robot": an actor-network analysis of a web-based ethnographic study of psychostimulant use. Can J Public Health. 2018;109(5–6):653–61.

Schneider CR, Everett AW, Geelhoed E, Kendall PA, Clifford RM. Measuring the assessment and counseling provided with the supply of nonprescription asthma reliever medication: a simulated patient study. Ann Pharmacother. 2009;43(9):1512–8.

Schneider CR, Everett AW, Geelhoed E, Padgett C, Ripley S, Murray K, Kendall PA, Clifford RM. Intern pharmacists as change agents to improve the practice of nonprescription medication supply: provision of salbutamol to patients with asthma. Ann Pharmacother. 2010;44(7–8):1319–26.

Schneider CR, Everett AW, Geelhoed E, Kendall PA, Murray K, Garnett P, Salama M, Clifford RM. Provision of primary care to patients with chronic cough in the community pharmacy setting. Ann Pharmacother. 2011;45(3):402–8.

Shigesato M, Elia J, Tschann M, Bullock H, Hurwitz E, Wu YY, Salcedo J. Pharmacy access to Ulipristal acetate in major cities throughout the United States. Contraception. 2018;97(3):264–9.

Surur AS, Getachew E, Teressa E, Hailemeskel B, Getaw NS, Erku DA. Self-reported and actual involvement of community pharmacists in patient counseling: a cross-sectional and simulated patient study in Gondar, Ethiopia. Pharm Pract (Granada). 2017;15(1):890.

Svarstad BL, Bultman DC, Mount JK, Tabak ER. Evaluation of written prescription information provided in community pharmacies: a study in eight states. J Am Pharm Assoc (2003). 2003;43(3):383–93.

Svarstad BL, Bultman DC, Mount JK. Patient counseling provided in community pharmacies: effects of state regulation, pharmacist age, and busyness. J Am Pharm Assoc (2003). 2004;44(1):22–9.

Tavares MP, Foster AM. Emergency contraception in a public health emergency: exploring pharmacy availability in Brazil. Contraception. 2016;94(2):109–14.

Chumbo no atendimento. Teste Saúde. 2003;46:9–13.

Antibióticos fora de controlo. Teste Saúde. 2007;66:9–13.

Venda de produtos naturais. Teste Saúde. 2008;75:11–4.

Watson MC, Skelton JR, Bond CM, Croft P, Wiskin CM, Grimshaw JM, Mollison J. Simulated patients in the community pharmacy setting. Using simulated patients to measure practice in the community pharmacy setting. Pharm World Sci. 2004;26(1):32–7.

Watson MC, Cleland J, Inch J, Bond CM, Francis J. Theory-based communication skills training for medicine counter assistants to improve consultations for non-prescription medicines. Med Educ. 2007;41(5):450–9.

Watson MC, Cleland JA, Bond CM. Simulated patient visits with immediate feedback to improve the supply of over-the-counter medicines: a feasibility study. Fam Pract. 2009;26(6):532–42.

Wigmore BC, Collins JC, Schneider CR, Arias D, Moles RJ. Ability of pharmacy students, pharmacists and pharmacy support staff to manage childhood fever via simulation. Am J Pharm Educ. 2018;82(10):6445.

Xu T, de Almeida Neto AC, Moles RJ. A systematic review of simulated-patient methods used in community pharmacy to assess the provision of non-prescription medicines. Int J Pharm Pract. 2012;20(5):307–19.

Chapter 6
Realist Research in Pharmacy Practice

Hadar Zaman, Geoff Wong, Sally Lawson, and Ian Maidment

Abstract Research is a creative process and the topic of research methodology particularly realist methods is complex and varied. This chapter is designed to introduce beginners to the basics of realist research focussing on essential concepts rather than burdening the reader with voluminous detail. As realist research is a complex area, it may require you to read the chapter on a number of occasions to gain familiarity or understanding around the area. To make this easier for the reader, concepts have been illustrated with worked examples or case studies and links provided for further reading. It goes without saying that the best way of learning any new type of research methodology is to practically get involved and immerse yourself undertaking research using the methodology of interest and learning as you go along.

6.1   Introduction to Realist Research

There are many forms of realism (scientific, direct and critical) and this chapter sets out one of the more well-developed and commonly used form of realism pioneered by Pawson and Tilley which is scientific realism (Pawson 2006). The goal of scientific realism is to examine regular patterns that exist within reality and offer a more comprehensive understanding of these patterns by providing in-depth explanations through the exploration of causal mechanisms, which are sensitive to contextual

H. Zaman (✉)
Bradford School of Pharmacy and Medical Sciences, Faculty of Life Sciences,
University of Bradford, Bradford, UK
e-mail: H.Zaman4@bradford.ac.uk

G. Wong
Nuffield Department of Primary Care Health Sciences, University of Oxford, Oxford, UK

S. Lawson · I. Maidment
School of Health and Life Science, Aston University, Birmingham, UK

© Springer Nature Singapore Pte Ltd. 2020   115
Z. Babar (ed.), *Pharmacy Practice Research Methods*,
https://doi.org/10.1007/978-981-15-2993-1_6

and social influences. It is recognised that perfect understanding of reality is not possible; however, as knowledge is emergent, over time one might contribute to what is understood (Salter and Kothari 2014).

Very crudely, scientific realism as defined by Pawson and Tilley sits between 'positivism' ('there is a real world that exists separate to our consciousness, which we can directly observe and measure, and about which we can derive facts') and 'constructivism' ('since all our observations are shaped and filtered through human senses and the human brain, it is not possible to know for certain what the nature of reality is') (Bunniss and Kelly 2010; Illing 2014).

Pawson and Tilley's view of knowledge is that there is a real world, and through our senses, brains and culture, we process our knowledge of it. To elaborate on this interpretation further, the world comprises of solid objects and those things that are 'created by people and/or societies' (e.g. laws, regulations and social norms). However, in common with 'constructivism', Pawson and Tilley assert that our ability to fully understand the nature of the world that is external to us is imperfect as all our observations are shaped and filtered through human senses and the human brain. This assertion can be explained in a clinical context where there is a real world of patients, signs and symptoms (positivism), and these are open to a variety of interpretations which depend on the complex interaction of external influences on the clinician such as length of practice (constructivism) (Graham and McAleer 2018).

What realism adds is the idea of mechanisms which are hidden, casual forces that are context sensitive resulting in outcomes that we may or may not be able to observe. The way we think about the world we live in forms the fundamental core of Pawson and Tilley's realist research approaches and will be expanded upon in this chapter.

6.2   Causation and Complexity in Realist Research

Realist research focusses on causation which differentiates it from other forms of approaches. Causation (how interventions cause change) and attribution (whether observed changes can be attributed to the intervention or were they caused by other confounding factors) are critical questions for realist researchers. Any observable outcome of an intervention undoubtedly is a result of many interactions across and within systems and cannot be simply attributed to the intervention itself or, in other words, be regarded as cause and effect relationship. Therefore, any outcomes which have occurred are due to many mechanisms/factors and thus causation itself is not simple or linear (Pawson et al. 2004).

One of the key principles realist research embraces is the notion of complexity which it recognises as inherent in social systems, and the way individuals respond to their surroundings (contextual features) will affect the outcome. Therefore, suggesting intervention A leads to outcome B is very simplistic. In reality it is not necessarily a linear relationship, but more like a web of causal processes generating outcomes (Westhorp 2013; Shearn et al. 2017).

In realist philosophy these causal processes are referred to as 'mechanisms' and occur at a different level of the system to observable outcomes. Mechanisms operate as part of whole systems and any changes within these systems, whether elements are removed or changed, will have direct impact on the ability of an intervention to 'cause' change. This explanation of causation can be expressed in the short form as context (C) + mechanism (M) = outcome (O) (CMO configurations) (see Box 6.1). Although this may be a very simplistic representation of causation for realist researchers, it is seen as an essential building block (Pawson and Tilley 2015; Langlois et al. 2018).

Mechanisms provide an explanatory focus of how and why changes occur by exploring concepts around reasoning and resources. When an intervention is implemented, this will either provide resources to participants or take them away. This interaction of resources and how the participants interpret and act upon them (reasoning) is known as 'intervention mechanism' (see Fig. 6.1). Moreover, the activation or not of mechanisms is heavily influenced and interconnected with the context they are operating in. One of the aims of realist research is to make explicit the ways in which the various contexts interact and affect the outcomes of an intervention via the activation or inhibition of key mechanisms (Dalkin et al. 2015). For detailed discussions around the concept of mechanism, please visit the RAMESES website: http://www.ramesesproject.org/Standards_and_Training_materials.php.

Box 6.1 Example of How to Express and Write CMO Configurations
To illustrate the application of CMO configurations, take the following example of vaccination uptake rates in low- and middle-income countries through mobile outreach vaccination clinics, provided by trained healthcare professionals. We can explain this example through a realist lens where the intervention (mobile outreach clinic) has changed the context from one where no vaccinations were available in a remote village to one where trained healthcare professionals now attend the village to provide this service. This new context (locally available vaccinations) activates the mechanism of perceived convenience among the villagers and causes the outcome of a slight increase in vaccination uptake. This can be summarised by using the following CMO configuration (CMOc): when remote villages are offered vaccinations by mobile clinics (C, for context), the population perceives this to be convenient (M, for mechanism) and so people get vaccinated (O, for outcome).

Fig. 6.1 A CMO
configuration framework.
Intervention resources are
introduced in a context, in
a way that enhances a
change in reasoning. This
alters the behaviour of
participants, which leads to
outcomes (Taken from
Dalkin et al. 2015)

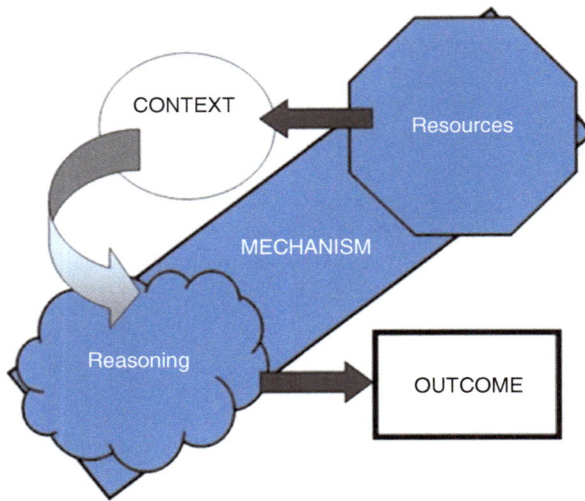

Realist approaches potentially provide a powerful strategy for addressing causal explanation (i.e. mechanisms only activate when the context is conducive). At best, realist research can make sense of the complex processes underlying interventions by formulating plausible explanations through the development of CMO configurations. It can indicate the conditions in which the intervention works (or not) and how it does so. This allows decision makers to assess whether interventions that proved successful in one setting may do so in another setting and assist policy makers in adapting interventions to suit specific contexts (Lacouture et al. 2015).

6.3   Importance of Programme Theory in Realist Research

Central to realist evaluation or review is the development of programme theory or theories which are a set of ideas about how the intervention causes the intended or observed outcomes. Programme theory or theories are the means to providing plausible explanations for certain interventions on whether they work or not in certain circumstances (Shearn et al. 2017). All interventions according to Pawson (2006) have a theoretical underpinning, and by undertaking realist research, one of the key tasks is to 'surface' (i.e. bring to the surface or develop) these theories (Pawson 2006). These theories then explain what works, for whom, under what circumstances and how, which are then 'tested' (confirmed, refuted or refined) using the best available evidence.

To develop a realist programme theory, it is important to understand 'the basic programme theory'. The most basic format for programme theories is set out in the following statement: 'If we do "x", "y" will happen, because…'. It is important to note that the 'because…' element of this structure is critical. Without it, there may be a theory of action ('we expect this to be done or that this was done'), but there will not be a theory of change (Feather 2018).

Once the basic programme theory has been developed, the second step is the generation of CMO hypothesis followed by the final step which is to refine the basic programme theory and the CMO hypothesis by answering the following realist questions:

1. For whom will this basic programme theory work and not work, and why?
2. In what contexts will this programme theory work and not work, and why?
3. What are the main mechanisms by which we expect this programme theory to work?
4. If this programme theory works, what outcomes will we see?

As programme theories are developed, it is crucial that the theories reflect the realist understanding of causation. That means that the theory should not be limited to statements about whether or not the programme will lead to outcomes, but how and why it will do so and for what kinds of settings and populations (Jagosh et al. 2015).

More information about developing realist programme theory can be found on the RAMESES website by visiting the following link: http://www.ramesesproject. org/media/RAMESES_II_Developing_realist_programme_theories.pdf.

6.4   Using Realist Approaches

Realist research has gained significant amount of attention and interest in the last few years and calls for it to become an established part of evaluative practice within the Medical Research Council framework. Examples where realist methods have been used are for evaluation of health systems, illicit drug deterrence programmes, shared care in mental health and modernisation of healthcare systems (Carnes et al. 2017). Although the uses of randomised controlled trials (RCTs) are seen as the gold standard to assess for intervention effectiveness, there are some questions and concerns around this type of study design. Issues around them are as follows: (a) 'intervention-on/intervention-off' comparisons answer some of the important questions but do not fully explore the reasons behind success or failure; (b) experimental comparisons are sometimes impractical, unethical, inappropriate or unaffordable, and (c) people behave differently when they are participating in trials (Marchal et al. 2013; Wong et al. 2012).

In contrast to RCT methods, realist research is less concerned with the effectiveness of intervention and/or effect size. The main purpose is to understand and explain how, why, for whom, in what contexts and to what extent interventions 'work' or not. The underlying assumption is that some things work for some people, some of the time, to some extent, and the goal of realist research approaches is to work out, who, when, how and why (Van Belle et al. 2016).

Developing a better understanding of how interventions 'work' allows policy makers to tailor the intervention to the needs of certain people and/or settings. Take for example the design and implementation of antimicrobial prescribing by junior doctors. Despite the wealth of antimicrobial stewardship programmes, it is often difficult to know how best to target resources to maximise intended outcomes. Most antimicrobial prescribing interventions target both junior and senior doctors as a uniform body of healthcare professionals and assume they have similar needs and operate under the same circumstances. A realist review was undertaken to shed further light on the varying contexts in which antimicrobial prescribing initiatives need to be embedded into practice, moving away from a hierarchical approach and making antimicrobial learning relevant to every healthcare professional regardless of seniority. Furthermore the realist review found that creating an environment of trust so doctors in training feel safe to ask questions and whereby they can challenge decisions made by others was also seen as an important factor that affected the success of antimicrobial prescribing interventions (Papoutsi et al. 2017).

Developing and implementing interventions like the one mentioned above can be very complex. Complex health interventions do not act as an independent agent for change, but rather operate within open systems, interacting with personal, interpersonal and environmental factors outside of the intervention. While these factors are usually controlled for within the experimental paradigm, realism seeks to explore and understand how these interactions impact on intervention success or failure. Realism looks to provide an explanation of complexity by exploring why outcomes differ in various contexts primarily due to interaction and activation of certain mechanisms (Wong et al. 2015a; Cooper et al. 2017; Wong 2013).

The next section will provide an overview of what realist reviews and evaluations are which is then followed by a step-by-step process describing how to undertake both types of realist research.

6.5   Realist Reviews

The context in which an intervention is rolled out is dynamic, complex and multifaceted, and often successful outcomes from an intervention may not be reproducible at different sites. When evaluating the success of interventions, traditional methods such as systematic reviews often provide limited answers as to whether an intervention works or not; however, they cannot answer the question of complexity (Rycroft-Malone et al. 2012).

A good illustration of when to use a realist review or a systematic review can be summarised in the following example: imagine you wanted to investigate the efficacy of drug X. It would clearly be most appropriate to undertake a systematic review (with or without a meta-analysis). However, if you wanted to gain a better understanding of why some elderly patients take their medications or not or which types of elderly patients are more likely to take their medications, then using a realist approach (be it a realist evaluation or realist review) would be more desirable.

Table 6.1 Paradigm differences between realist review and systematic review

Realist review	Systematic review (meta-analysis)
Theory driven	Method driven
Deprioritises methodology hierarchies and emphasises fallibility of all knowledge sources (constructivist lens)	Appraises papers based on a hierarchy of study design. Prioritises experimental design (i.e. randomised controlled trial) as gold standard
Uses all parts of primary research papers as evidence	Uses the results of primary studies in meta-analysis
Uses a variety of data sources, including grey literature, commentaries, etc.	Often uses primary research results only
Moves away from generalisable claims and advocates for cumulation of evidence-informed theory over the course of time	Seeks research results that can be generalised across contexts

Taken from Rycroft-Malone et al. (2012)

A realist review provides a method to understand which elderly patients decide to take their medications or not, how those decisions are made and what contextual factors affect those decisions.

Pawson and colleagues describe realist reviews in the following words:

Realist review is an approach to reviewing research evidence on complex social interventions, which provides an explanatory analysis of how and why they work (or don't work) in particular contexts or settings. It complements more established approaches to systematic review, which have been developed and used mainly for simpler interventions like clinical treatments or therapies (Pawson et al. 2004).

Realist reviews follow similar stages to a traditional systematic review but with some notable differences (see Table 6.1):

A realist review therefore applies a theoretically driven, qualitative approach to synthesising qualitative, quantitative and mixed methods research evidences that have a bearing on a single research question or set of questions. Methodologically, reviewers may begin by eliciting from the literature the main ideas that went into developing the programme theory. The programme theory as discussed earlier in the chapter sets out how and why an intervention is thought to 'work' to generate the outcome(s) of interest. The programme theory is then tested using relevant evidence (qualitative, quantitative, comparative, administrative and so on) from the primary literature relating to the intervention (Wong et al. 2013).

For each aspect of the programme theory, reviewers seek out the contextual (C) influences that are hypothesised to have triggered the relevant mechanism(s) (M) to generate the outcome(s) (O) of interest. The reviewers then look at 'how the programme was supposed to operate' comparing to the 'empirical evidence on the actuality in different situations'. The reviewers analyse the data generated from the realist review to describe and understand the many factors that affect the likelihood of such interventions generating their intended outcomes through the interplay between contextual elements and mechanisms. This approach moves away from generalisable claims and universal regularities and towards exploratory questions about how programmes are shaped by particular contexts and how programme mechanisms are activated when contexts are conducive (Jagosh 2019). This in turn provides guidance about what policy makers or practitioners might put in place to change their own contexts or provide resources in such a way as to most likely to activate the right mechanism(s) to produce the desired outcome (Wong et al. 2013).

In Box 6.2 is another brief example of a realist review which was supplemented by a traditional systematic review to help you understand the key steps involved in undertaking a realist review and show you how a systematic review can be helpful in doing your realist review. A more detailed explanation of how to do a realist review follows in the next section 'How to Do a Realist Review'.

Box 6.2 Example Application of a Realist Review

Kastner et al. wanted to understand how, for whom, under what circumstances and why effective multi-chronic disease management interventions work and influence health outcomes in older adults. They started by undertaking a systematic review investigating the effectiveness of multimorbidity interventions in older adults and supplemented this with a realist review.

Firstly, the initial programme theories were developed (i.e. what multimorbidity interventions are composed of, how and why they are expected to work and what outcomes they might generate), using team discussions and a Delphi survey. Searches for papers to include were done simultaneously for the systematic and realist review. Data extraction was undertaken to refine the programme theory through CMO configurations (i.e. could you infer an explanation for the cause [M] for a particular outcome [O] under the influence of one or more particular contexts [C]?). For example, computer-based counselling systems (intervention) targeting older adults and providers in primary care (C) are not acceptable (O) if they do not show any relative advantage over the current system (M1) and if they are inconsistent with providers' current practice workflow (M2).

The realist review contributed to the limited knowledge of underlying mechanisms of complex multi-chronic disease management interventions in older adults which can help better inform policy and practice on multimorbidity management. Care coordination was one such type of intervention that proved to be effective because of its structured and holistic approach. You can read further about this study by visiting the following link:

Kastner M, Hayden L, Wong G, et al. Underlying mechanisms of complex interventions addressing the care of older adults with multimorbidity: a realist review. *BMJ Open* 2019;9:e025009. doi: https://doi.org/10.1136/bmjopen-2018-025009

6.6   How to Perform a Realist Review?

The table below summarises the key steps involved in conducting a realist review by providing you examples of some important questions to ask yourself at the relevant stages. Using Table 6.2 we can apply this step-by-step guide to an actual realist

Table 6.2 Approach to realist review (adapted from Pawson and Greenhalgh 2004) taken from Rycroft-Malone et al. (2012)

Stage	Action	Activity
Define the scope of the review	Identify the question	What is the nature and content of the intervention? What are the circumstances or context of its use? What are the policy intentions or objectives? What are the nature and form of its outcomes or impacts? Undertake exploratory searches to inform discussion with review stakeholders
	Clarify the purpose(s) of the review	Theory integrity—does the intervention work as predicted? Theory adjudication—which theories around the intervention seem to fit best? Comparison—how does the intervention work in different settings, for different groups? Reality testing—how does the policy intent of the intervention translate into practice?
	Find and articulate the candidate programme theories	Search for relevant 'theories' in the literature Draw up list of programme theories Group, categorise or synthesise theories Design a theoretically based evaluative framework to be 'populated' with evidence Develop bespoke data extraction forms
Search for and appraise the evidence	Search for the evidence	Decide and define purposive sampling strategy Define data/information sources, search terms and methods to be used (including cited reference searching) Set the thresholds for stopping searching at saturation
	Test of relevance	Test relevance—does the research address the theory under test? Test rigour—does the research support the conclusions drawn from it by the researchers or the reviewers?
Extract and synthesise findings	Extract the results	Extract data to populate the evaluative framework with evidence
	Synthesise findings	Compare and contrast findings from different studies Use findings from studies to address purpose(s) of review Seek both confirmatory and contradictory findings Refine programme theories in the light of evidence including findings from analysis of study data
Develop narrative		Involve commissioners/decision makers in review of findings Disseminate review with findings, conclusions and recommendations

review conducted by Wong et al.—Interventions to Improve Antimicrobial Prescribing of Doctors in Training: The IMPACT (**IMP**roving **A**ntimicrobial Pres**C**ribing of Doctors in **T**raining) Realist Review. Rather than using a traditional systematic review which would have reported on the effectiveness of an intervention, the IMPACT realist review examined how doctors-in-training responded to the resources made available to them (*mechanisms*) and in which circumstances these mechanisms were triggered (*contexts*) to generate certain behaviours or *outcomes* for antimicrobial prescribing.

The full paper can be viewed by visiting the following citation:

Chrysanthi Papoutsi, Karen Mattick, Mark Pearson, Nicola Brennan, Simon Briscoe, Geoff Wong, Social and professional influences on antimicrobial prescribing for doctors-in-training: a realist review, Journal of Antimicrobial Chemotherapy, Volume 72, Issue 9, September 2017, pp. 2418–2430, https://doi.org/10.1093/jac/dkx194.

6.7   Define the Scope of the Review

The aim of this realist review was to understand how interventions aiming to change antimicrobial prescribing behaviours of doctors-in-training produce their effects. There have been a broad range of interventions to improve antimicrobial stewardship implemented within the UK, such as the TARGET toolkit and 'Start Smart Then Focus' initiatives. Although these initiatives have shown promising impact in terms of reducing antimicrobial use, these improvements are insufficient to address the scale of the problem. The literature indicates that 28% of interventions designed to change antimicrobial prescribing behaviour in new prescribers are through distribution of educational materials. The theory underlying such a practice is that poor prescribing behaviour is partly due to knowledge deficits, and the way to address this problem is through educational means.

The realist review was structured around the following areas:

- What are the mechanisms by which antimicrobial prescribing behaviour change interventions are believed to result in their intended outcomes?
- What are the important contexts which determine whether the different mechanisms produce and activate intended outcomes?
- In what circumstances are such interventions likely to be effective?

The goal of this step is to identify theories that explain how antimicrobial prescribing behaviour change interventions are supposed to work (and for whom), when they do work and when they do not achieve the desired change in clinical practice. Before any literature search was started, the research team drawing on their experiential and professional knowledge devised an initial programme theory, which was then used as a guide for refining assumptions against the data in the literature.

6.8   Search for and Appraise the Evidence

The purpose of this step is to find a relevant 'body of literature' that might contain data with which to further develop and refine the initial programme theory (IPT) which was developed in the earlier step when the review was being scoped out.

The searches were guided by the search strategy from a previous closely related systematic review on educational interventions to change the behaviour of prescribers in the hospital setting, with a particular emphasis on new prescribers. It is helpful to see if they are any previously conducted systematic reviews in the area you are researching, to help you start your realist review. Further additional searching was done to help inform programme theory development which focussed on issues emerging as significant from the main literature search. This additional search focussed on social and professional influences in clinical training and more specifically related to hierarchies, team-working and decision-making to provide an explanatory backbone for the wider contextual influences identified as important from the analysis of the literature in the main search.

Documents were selected based on relevance (whether data can contribute to theory building and/or testing) and rigour (whether the methods used to generate the relevant data are credible and trustworthy). Each document that was included in the review was relevant to the programme theory development and/or helped to develop CMO configurations.

6.9   Extract and Synthesise Findings

Data were extracted from relevant sections of texts relating to contexts, mechanisms and/or their relationships to outcomes. Data was analysed using realist 'logic of analysis' to make sense of the IPT. This process involved constantly moving from data to theory to refine explanations about why certain behaviours occurred in different settings. This included inferences about which mechanisms may be activated in specific contexts, as these often remained hidden or were not articulated adequately in the literature.

A cross-case comparison method was used to understand and explain how and why observed outcomes have occurred, for example, by comparing interventions where prescribing behavioural change has been 'successful' against those which have not, to understand how context has influenced reported findings from different studies. Particular focus was placed on identifying 'causation', looking for how different groups of doctors-in-training reasoned about and responded (by way of 'hidden' mechanisms) to contextual influences available in their environment to produce reported outcomes.

6.10 Develop a Narrative

At this stage, the final programme theory was formulated by bringing together the different CMO configurations which had been generated in the earlier stages that helped explain the data presented in the literature. The narrative was further substantiated by drawing on a range of social science and learning theories to make inferences about mechanisms, contexts, outcomes and configurations between these elements and to enhance the plausibility and coherence of the arguments.

6.11 Realist Evaluations

Realist evaluations are a relatively new approach in the field of health services research and are a helpful and constructive way of understanding and unpacking the 'black box' of many complex interventions. It was first developed by Pawson and Tilley (1997) and has subsequently been modified in different ways. It is widely acknowledged that in the real world traditional evaluative approaches provide over-simplified model of assessment and little information about the effectiveness of complex interventions within uncontrolled, context-rich settings and may be insufficient to inform future implementation efforts (Pawson and Tilley 1997).

Pawson and Tilley describe realist evaluations as 'logic of inquiry' that attempts to answer the question, 'What works, for whom, in what circumstances…and why?'. This is done through the formation of CMO configurations (see earlier in the chapter for more details) (Salter and Kothari 2014). The CMO configurations are used as the main structure for analysis for both realist evaluations and realist reviews (Berwick 2008).

Realist evaluations are particularly suited in certain circumstances and examples with citations have been provided below:

- **For evaluating new initiatives, pilot interventions and trials or programmes/interventions that seem to work but 'for whom and how' are not yet understood**; for example on the implementation of a maternal and newborn health programme in Bangladesh, see Alayne Adams, Saroj Sedalia, Shanon McNab, Malabika Sarker, Lessons Learned in Using Realist Evaluation to Assess Maternal and Newborn Health Programming in Rural Bangladesh, Health Policy and Planning, Volume 31, Issue 2, March 2016, pp. 267–275.
- **For evaluating interventions that will be scaled up, to understand how to adapt the intervention to new contexts**; for example on the scaling-up of a new integrated care network in Southeast Asia, see Nurjono, M.; Shrestha, P.; Lee, A.; Lim, X.Y.; Shiraz, F.; Tan, S.; Wong, S.H.; Foo, K.M.; Wee, T.; Toh, S.A.; and Yoong, J., 2018. Realist Evaluation of a Complex Integrated Care Programme: Protocol for a Mixed Methods Study. BMJ open, 8(3), p. e017111.
- **For evaluating interventions that have previously demonstrated mixed patterns of outcomes, to understand how and why the differences occur**; for

example on the implementation of the integrated palliative care pathway in primary care by multidisciplinary teams, see Dalkin, S. M.; Lhussier, M.; Philipson, P.; Jones, D.; and Cunningham, W. (2016). Reducing Inequalities in Care for Patients with Non-malignant Diseases: Insights from a Realist Evaluation of an Integrated Palliative Care Pathway. Palliative Medicine, 30(7), 690–697.

6.12   How to Do a Realist Evaluation?

While there is not a sequential or linear method of undertaking a realist evaluation, rather it is seen as more of an iterative process. Pawson and Tilley suggest that the process of realist evaluation itself proceeds according to a traditional cycle of hypothesis generation, testing and refinement (see Fig. 6.2) (Pawson and Tilley 2015).

1. **Formulation of initial programme theories (IPT)**: The most common method is through review of intervention-related documents (policy papers, studies, documentary analysis and protocols) including informal discussions and interviews with programme stakeholders to allow the development of potential CMO configurations, generating testable IPT hypothesis. Development of an IPT serves other functions too, such as informing evaluation design, data collection approaches and evaluation focus. More information on how to develop IPT can be found on the RAMESES project website (http://www.ramesesproject.org/Standards_and_Training_materials.php).

Fig. 6.2 Diagram showing the key steps involved in undertaking a realist evaluation

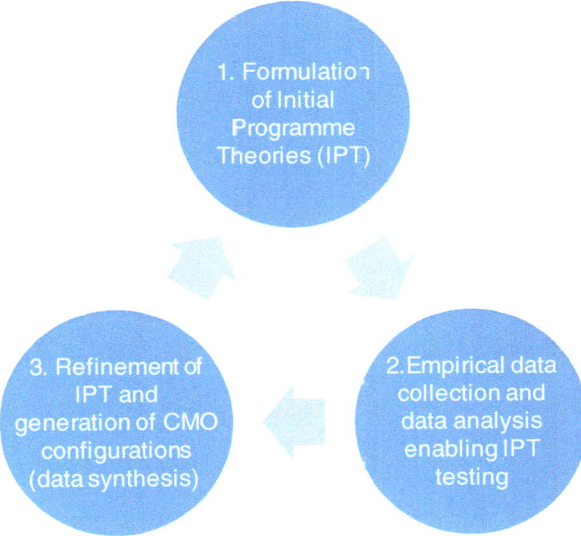

2. **Empirical data collection and data analysis enabling IPT testing**: Realist evaluations are method neutral and do not support or prefer one data collection method over the other. It is important to note that using a single method of data collection may not be appropriate as the data collected may be too narrow to test the IPT. Data collection methods can be varied (i.e. qualitative, quantitative, mixed methods, ethnographic, documentary analysis, interviews, focus groups) but should be appropriate to the hypothesised CMO configurations. Data analysis examines the outcome patterns observed from the collected data and tests the hypothesised CMO configurations and provides the realist explanation of causation for outcomes found within the IPT.

3. **Refinement of IPT and generation of CMO configurations (data synthesis)**: Data is analysed developing CMO configurations to explain outcome patterns. Building on findings in step 2, CMO configurations are developed, validated, refined or refuted, and the IPT is further refined through the collation of more data.

Finally, realist evaluations seek to better understand, identify and evaluate why complex interventions succeed or fail in order to inform spread, replicability and sustainability of effective interventions. Realist evaluations provide a way of explaining in more detail how outcomes are actually achieved. This knowledge can be used to enhance the likelihood of success when implemented in other areas. Below is a worked example of a realist evaluation applying the steps discussed above (Greenhalgh et al. 2015).

6.13 Example of a Realist Evaluation: Eliminating Medications Through Patient Ownership of End Results (EMPOWER) Study

This study conducted a realist evaluation using a mixed methods approach alongside a randomised clinical trial exploring the mechanisms and contexts for engaging patients in deprescribing of benzodiazepines that led to positive and/or negative deprescribing outcomes.

The full paper can be viewed by visiting the following citation:

Martin P, Tannenbaum C. A realist evaluation of patients' decisions to deprescribe in the EMPOWER trial, BMJ Open 2017;7:e015959. doi: https://doi.org/10.1136/bmjopen-2017-015959.

1. **Formulation of Initial Programme Theories (IPT)**

The IPT formulated was that older adults are unaware of the age-related harms of taking long-term benzodiazepines and do not understand the importance of discontinuing medications. This is a barrier to deprescribing. Using an interactive educational brochure (EMPOWER brochure) detailing the risks and safer alternatives would improve patients' motivation and capacity to initiate the deprescribing process.

2. **Empirical data collection and data analysis enabling IPT testing**

Data were collected via mixed methods to test this IPT. Questionnaires were disseminated pre- and post-intervention (EMPOWER brochure) providing quantitative data to gain a better understanding around patients' knowledge of benzodiazepine use and deprescribing, particularly focussing on the three key mechanisms of increasing motivation, capacity and opportunity. Qualitative data collection methods such as semi-structured interviews were used to ascertain a more detailed understanding around the contexts under which the deprescribing mechanism was successful or not.

The results from the qualitative analysis showed the contexts in which the EMPOWER intervention was associated with positive deprescribing outcomes. Favourable personal contexts such as 'stable health' (i.e. those who were not dealing with acute health issues) facilitated receptiveness to tapering of benzodiazepines. External influences associated with successful discontinuation of benzodiazepines were previous and ongoing support or encouragement from a healthcare provider.

The contexts in which the EMPOWER intervention failed to achieve successful outcomes to elicit motivation to deprescribe were more likely in individuals who reported poor health. Contexts that led participants to abort the deprescribing process once they showed initial motivation, capacity and opportunity included lack of support from a healthcare provider.

3. **Refinement of IPT and generation of CMO configurations (data synthesis)**

The final stage after data analysis was to refine the IPT. At the outset of this trial, it was believed that the EMPOWER brochure would trigger the motivation and capacity in patients to review and potentially stop the use of benzodiazepines by increasing their knowledge about the harms of benzodiazepine use. The assumption was that healthcare professionals would provide a supportive context, encouraging patients to stop their benzodiazepines. The initial IPT was revised in order to recognise the complexity of internal and external contexts on initiating and completing the deprescribing process. Internal influences included perceptions about one's health status, long-term health goals, fear of symptom recurrence and psychological attachment to the drug. The main external influence that was identified was the lack of support from a healthcare provider.

This realist evaluation was conducted in parallel with a clinical trial and provided important insights about deprescribing from the patient's perspective and increased current understanding about the specific mechanisms and contexts that generate positive or negative outcomes when attempting to engage patients in curbing the overuse and potentially inappropriate use of medicines.

6.14   Realist Synthesis

Finally we did not introduce the term realist synthesis as we did not want to confuse you with what a realist evaluation or review is. Some authors use the term realist synthesis interchangeably with the term realist review. However, in this context and for simplicity, we have used the term to describe when you do a realist evaluation and realist review simultaneously and bring the findings together (synthesise). The methodology remains exactly the same as mentioned above for undertaking a realist review or evaluation. The following research project is an example of realist synthesis where references have been provided in the text if you want to learn more about it.

Illustrative case study demonstrating realist methods which combined a realist evaluation and a realist review to produce a realist synthesis: MEMORABLE (**Me**dication **M**anagement in **O**lder People: **R**ealist **A**pproaches **B**ased on **L**iterature and **E**valuation—Realist Synthesis)

The MEMORABLE realist research project looked at understanding how medication management works for older people in the UK who take complex medication regimens and live in the community (Maidment et al. 2017a). The project is built on some earlier qualitative work and is one of the first projects, worldwide, to use realism to understand medication management (Maidment et al. 2017b; Aston et al. 2017).

Outcomes from interventions to optimise medication management are caused by multiple context-sensitive mechanisms; for example, if a patient trusts their doctor, they are more likely to adhere to their medication. The MEMORABLE project used realist synthesis (combining the results of a realist evaluation and realist review) to understand how, why, for whom and in what contexts interventions, to improve medication management in older people, are effective. The MEMORABLE project viewed medication management as a complex social programme involving human actions and decisions concerning medication management. It then aimed to understand how different interventions may or may not work and from this identify possible improvements.

The project had three discrete phases. The first phase involved a systematic review of the literature in the form of a realist synthesis. This focussed on developing an IPT setting out how and why outcomes within an intervention for medicines management occur. This IPT was developed by consulting stakeholders (patients and clinicians) and identifying literature with relevant explanatory theories. Iterative discussions within the project team around the various theories uncovered allowed a coherent programme theory to be formulated; this was further refined with input from the stakeholder group. At this stage the theory was mapped out to a series of outcome steps required with associated context and mechanisms.

The second phase of the project used realist interviews to generate primary data. Interviews were conducted with patients, carers and healthcare and social care providers exploring how and why an intervention such as medication management might work. The interviews tested the hypothesis contained within the programme theory (that was developed from the literature review) by gathering data to confirm, refute or refine aspects of the theory. The interview data allowed further development and refinement of the programme theory and identified aspects of the programme theory not found in the literature; for example, the issue of 'burden' was much more prominent in the interviews than the literature.

Interview data was analysed using realist logic of analysis, and then through discussion and disputation, the project team with input from the stakeholder group refined the programme theory further. Quality control processes, including regular review of the outputs by the core team, following RAMESES guidance, were implemented to ensure consistency and transparency of reporting. For further information on how to conduct a realist interview, read the following paper: http://www.ramesesproject.org/media/RAMESES_II_Realist_interviewing.pdf.

The final phase involved combining the literature and interview data to identify the most important mechanisms within the programme theory that need to be 'triggered' and the contexts related to these 'key' mechanisms. Ultimately, the project aimed to identify intervention strategies, which might be able to use to change the contexts in such a way that 'key' mechanisms are triggered to produce desired outcomes. For example, the desired outcome might be adherence to medication. One mechanism to achieve this might be patient/carer education within the context of the patient/clinician consultation. By changing the context, such as lengthening the time for the consultation, patient education is improved (the mechanism is triggered) leading to better outcomes (adherence to medication).

The results from MEMORABLE are yet to published; if you would like to be made aware of publications, follow the principal investigator (Dr. Maidment) on Twitter®: @maidment_dr.

For more information on MEMORABLE, check the project website www.aston.ac.uk/memorable, or email Dr. Maidment directly at i.maidment@aston.ac.uk.

6.15   Guidance and Resources for Undertaking Realist Research

The use of realist methodology in health services research is gaining popularity, and concerns and confusion among researchers have been expressed in relation to what constitutes high-quality or conversely substandard research. This has led to the development of reporting standards, quality standards and training materials for both realist reviews and evaluations by the RAMESES project team (Realist And Meta-narrative Evidence Syntheses: Evolving Standards) which can be accessed by visiting www.ramesesproject.org.

Publication standards, developed by the RAMESES project team, are similar to currently used standards in health services research, reporting on, for example, randomised controlled trials which use CONSORT criteria or AGREE which is used in the development of clinical guidelines or PRISMA when reporting on Cochrane-style systematic reviews. The development of RAMESES is crucial for researchers using realist methodology, not only to provide guidance and consistency in the approach used but also from a user perspective for example, so stakeholders or policy makers can be assured about the quality and rigour of subsequent research findings.

6.16   Strength and Limitations of Realist Research

Realist research involves analysis and interpretation of data from qualitative and quantitative studies or both which enhances the credibility of research findings and allows for generation of in-depth insights. Exploring and developing theories about mechanisms that mediate and moderate the relationship between action and outcome are invaluable for policy makers and add value to intervention evaluation by revealing why an intervention works. Gaining a deeper understanding of how outcomes are achieved by discerning the causal pathway is one of the real strengths of realist research. This in turn can better inform the design and evaluation of future interventions.

Realist research explanatory power allows the formation of 'generalisable knowledge' which is essential in learning from one intervention in a different context with varying mechanisms at play to produce outcomes. Realist research recognises that a 'one-size-fits-all' approach is not the way to respond to problems. Any interventions that are developed and implemented are dependent on contextual factors and how people interact with and adapt the intervention to produce outcomes. This potentially provides transferable learning from one setting to another.

Undertaking realist research can be intellectually challenging, requiring sustained thinking and imagination to work through programme theory, to define expected outcome patterns and to figure out exactly the required and essential data to test or arbitrate between theories. With the emphasis of realist research being on context and mechanisms, this can be very difficult for health economists or policy makers to interpret when assessing the effectiveness of an intervention. Furthermore, when it comes to data analysis, synthesis and interpretation, differences between research teams in respect of findings can arise. However, this can be countered by increasing transparency, so that it is clear how data has been interpreted and for which CMO configurations. Finally, realist research is an iterative process, and some researchers can find this challenging. It is important to manage the 'journey' of discovery and understanding which is inherent to realist approaches.

Acknowledgement   Thank you to Justine Tomlinson, Dr. Jon Silcock, Sarah Baig and Agostina Secchi for their helpful peer review and constructive feedback.

Definition of Common Terms Used in Realist Research (Wong et al. 2015b)

Realist methodology   A theory-driven, interpretative approach to uncovering underlying middle-range theories (or logics) driving interventions and their multiple components, as well as illuminating the contextual factors that influence mechanisms of change to produce outcomes.

Middle-range theory (MRT) A theory that is specific enough to generate hypotheses (e.g. in the form of propositions) to be tested in a particular case, or to help explain findings in a particular case, but general enough to apply across a number of cases or a number of domains.

Context-mechanism-outcome (CMO) configurations A CMO configuration is a statement, diagram or drawing that spells out the relationship between particular features of context, particular mechanisms and particular outcomes. In a sentence, they take the form of 'In "X" context, "Y" mechanism generates "Z" outcome'. A more detailed explanation of a CMO is as follows: 'CMO configuring is a heuristic used to generate causative explanations pertaining to the data. The process draws out and reflects on the relationship of context, mechanism, and outcome of interest in a particular program. A CMO configuration may pertain to either the whole program or only certain aspects. One CMO may be embedded in another or configured in a series (in which the outcome of one CMO becomes the context for the next in the chain of implementation steps). Configuring CMOs is a basis for generating and/or refining the theory that becomes the final product of the review'.

Context Often pertains to the 'backdrop' of programs and research. '… As these conditions change over time, the context may reflect aspects of those changes while the program is implemented. Examples of context include cultural norms and history of the community in which a program is implemented, the nature and scope of existing social networks, or built program infrastructure. … They can also be trust-building processes, geographic location effects, funding sources, opportunities, or constraints. Context can thus be broadly understood as any condition that triggers and/or modifies the behaviour of a mechanism'.

Mechanism There are many definitions of mechanism. What they all have in common is that mechanisms generate outcomes. Examples include the following: 'Mechanisms are the agents of change. They describe how the resources embedded in a program influence the reasoning and ultimately the behaviour of program subjects'. '…mechanisms are underlying entities, processes, or structures which operate in particular contexts to generate outcomes of interest'. There are three essential clues located in a 'realist' reading of mechanisms. These are that (1) mechanisms are usually hidden, (2) mechanisms are sensitive to variations in context and (3) mechanisms generate outcomes. Outcomes are not only intended outcomes (was the intervention successful or not?) but also all the intermediate outcomes as well as unplanned and/or unexpected impact of interventions. These are important because unplanned outcomes can sometimes have a greater influence on success of an intervention. Furthermore, unintended impacts may have 'ripple effects' in that they lead to new effects which then lead to more effects, thus changing the context of research over time.

References

Aston L, et al. Exploring the evidence base for how people with dementia and their informal carers manage their medication in the community: a mixed studies review. BMC Geriatr. 2017;17(1):242.

Berwick DM. The science of improvement. JAMA. 2008;299(10):1182–4.

Bunniss S, Kelly DR. Research paradigms in medical education research. Med Educ. 2010;44(4):358–66.

Carnes D, et al. The impact of a social prescribing service on patients in primary care: a mixed methods evaluation. BMC Health Serv Res. 2017;17(1):835.

Cooper C, et al. Protocol for a realist review of complex interventions to prevent adolescents from engaging in multiple risk behaviours. BMJ Open. 2017;7(9):e015477.

Dalkin SM, et al. What's in a mechanism? Development of a key concept in realist evaluation. Implement Sci. 2015;10(1):49.

Feather JL. Developing programme theories as part of a realist evaluation of a healthcare quality improvement programme. Int J Care Coord. 2018;21(3):68–72.

Graham AC, McAleer S. An overview of realist evaluation for simulation-based education. Adv Simul. 2018;3(1):13.

Greenhalgh T, et al. Protocol—the RAMESES II study: developing guidance and reporting standards for realist evaluation. BMJ Open. 2015;5(8):e008567.

Illing J. Thinking about research: theoretical perspectives, ethics and scholarship. Understanding medical education: evidence, theory and practice. 2nd ed. Chichester: Wiley Blackwell; 2014. p. 331–48.

Jagosh J. Realist synthesis for public health: building an ontologically deep understanding of how programs work, for whom, and in which contexts. Annu Rev Public Health. 2019;40:361–72.

Jagosh J, et al. A realist evaluation of community-based participatory research: partnership synergy, trust building and related ripple effects. BMC Public Health. 2015;15:725.

Lacouture A, et al. The concept of mechanism from a realist approach: a scoping review to facilitate its operationalization in public health program evaluation. Implement Sci. 2015;10(1):153.

Langlois EV, Daniels K, Akl EA, editors. Evidence synthesis for health policy and systems: a methods guide. Geneva: World Health Organization; 2018.

Maidment I, et al. Developing a framework for a novel multi-disciplinary, multi-agency intervention (s), to improve medication management in community-dwelling older people on complex medication regimens (MEMORABLE)—a realist synthesis. Syst Rev. 2017a;6(1):125.

Maidment ID, et al. A qualitative study exploring medication management in people with dementia living in the community and the potential role of the community pharmacist. Health Expect. 2017b;20(5):929–42.

Marchal B, et al. Realist RCTs of complex interventions—an oxymoron. Soc Sci Med. 2013;94:124–8.

Papoutsi C, et al. Social and professional influences on antimicrobial prescribing for doctors-in-training: a realist review. J Antimicrob Chemother. 2017;72(9):2418–30.

Pawson R. Evidence-based policy: a realist perspective. London: Sage; 2006.

Pawson R, Tilley N. An introduction to scientific realist evaluation. Evaluation for the 21st century: a handbook; 1997. p. 405–18.

Pawson R, Tilley N. Realist evaluation. 2004. Google Scholar. 2015.

Pawson R, et al. Realist synthesis: an introduction. Manchester: ESRC Research Methods Programme, University of Manchester; 2004.

Rycroft-Malone J, et al. Realist synthesis: illustrating the method for implementation research. Implement Sci. 2012;7(1):33.

Salter KL, Kothari A. Using realist evaluation to open the black box of knowledge translation: a state-of-the-art review. Implement Sci. 2014;9(1):115.

Shearn K, et al. Building realist program theory for large complex and messy interventions. Int J Qual Methods. 2017;16(1):1609406917741796.

Van Belle S, et al. Can "realist" randomised controlled trials be genuinely realist? Trials. 2016;17(1):313.

Westhorp G. Developing complexity-consistent theory in a realist investigation. Evaluation. 2013;19(4):364–82.

Wong G. Is complexity just too complex? J Clin Epidemiol. 2013;66(11):1199–201.

Wong G, et al. Realist methods in medical education research: what are they and what can they contribute? Med Educ. 2012;46(1):89–96.

Wong G, et al. RAMESES publication standards: realist syntheses. BMC Med. 2013;11(1):21.

Wong G, et al. Interventions to improve antimicrobial prescribing of doctors in training: the IMPACT (IMProving Antimicrobial presCribing of doctors in Training) realist review. BMJ Open. 2015a;5(10):e009059.

Wong G, et al. Realist synthesis: Rameses training materials, 2013. London: The RAMESES Project; 2015b.

Chapter 7
Importance of Mixed Methods Research in Pharmacy Practice

Cristín Ryan, Cathal Cadogan, and Carmel Hughes

Abstract Irrespective of the field of research, the underpinning methodologies used are critical in generating high-quality data and evidence. Most importantly, the method selected should answer the research question that has been posed. It is important to accept that no single method will answer all research questions, and in the field of health services and pharmacy practice research, there may be a number of questions that will form part of an overarching programme or project. In such circumstances, more than one method will be required to answer all the research questions within a single programme or project, an approach known as mixed methods.

This chapter provides an overview of the current definition of mixed methods research and the advantages and limitations of this approach. The importance of mixed methods research in pharmacy practice and the considerations required when designing and analysing a mixed methods research study or programme are outlined. The various typologies of mixed methods research are described using illustrative examples from the pharmacy practice research literature, and guidance is provided on choosing the most applicable type/typology for a given research question. Key considerations in appraising and reporting mixed methods research are also outlined.

C. Ryan
School of Pharmacy and Pharmaceutical Sciences, Trinity College Dublin, Dublin, Ireland

C. Cadogan (✉)
School of Pharmacy and Biomolecular Sciences, Royal College of Surgeons in Ireland, Dublin, Ireland
e-mail: cathalcadogan@rcsi.ie

C. Hughes
School of Pharmacy, Queen's University Belfast, Belfast, UK

© Springer Nature Singapore Pte Ltd. 2020
Z. Babar (ed.), *Pharmacy Practice Research Methods*,
https://doi.org/10.1007/978-981-15-2993-1_7

137

7.1   Introduction

Irrespective of the field of research, the underpinning methodologies used are critical in generating high-quality data and evidence. Most importantly, the method selected should answer the research question posed (Sackett 1997). Traditionally, research studies have been designed using single method research designs. However, single method research studies often report various limitations and weaknesses in their study design; for example, single study designs do not consider multiple viewpoints and perspectives (Johnson et al. 2007; Driscoll et al. 2007).

Consequently, the practice of using more than one research method, or a mixed methods approach as it is more commonly termed, to answer the research question posed has become increasingly popular. This enables expansion of the scope or breadth of research to offset the weaknesses of using any approach alone (Driscoll et al. 2007). Mixed methods research is now a recognised research paradigm in the health services and pharmacy practice research fields. This is evidenced by the publication of a dedicated journal of mixed methods research, the *Journal of Mixed Methods Research*. This journal aims to act as an impetus for creating bridges between mixed methods researchers and to provide a platform for the discussion of mixed methods research issues and the sharing of ideas across academic disciplines (Tashakkori and Creswell 2007).

Despite the relative novelty of this approach in the health services research arena, the process of using more than one research method within a single study or a research programme has been conducted for decades in other research fields. As noted above, mixed methods research adds further insights to research questions which would otherwise not be answered if a single research approach was used. Whilst this chapter focuses on mixed methods research in pharmacy practice, a mixed methods approach may not always be appropriate. It is important to refer back to the research question posed and to let the research question guide the study design. The selection of study design should be considered in tandem with the way in which the research question is asked, and in some instances, single study designs may be preferable. Sackett emphasises the importance of letting the research question guide the study design, stating that 'the question being asked determines the appropriate research architecture, strategy, and tactics to be used- not tradition, authority, experts, paradigms or schools of thought' (Sackett 1997).

A variety of terms have been used to describe the mixed methods research approach including 'integrated', 'hybrid', 'combined', 'mixed research', 'mixed methodology', 'multi-methods', 'multi-strategy' and 'mixed methodology' (Bryman 2006; Johnson et al. 2007; Driscoll et al. 2007). Throughout this chapter, we will use the term 'mixed methods' to describe research approaches which use more than one research method to answer the research question posed.

This chapter provides an overview of the current definition of mixed methods research and the advantages and limitations of this research approach. The importance of mixed methods research in pharmacy practice and the required considerations when designing and analysing a mixed methods research study or programme will be outlined. We also describe the various typologies of mixed methods research using illustrative examples from the pharmacy practice research literature and provide guidance on how to choose the most applicable typology for a given research question. Key considerations in appraising and reporting mixed methods research are also outlined.

To inform this chapter, we conducted a literature search using the following electronic databases: International Pharmaceutical Abstracts, MEDLINE and Web of Science, and using the following search terms: 'mixed-methods', 'pharmacy, 'triangulation', 'parallel design', 'embedded design' and 'sequential design'. Searches were restricted to include only full-text papers published in the English language within the last 15 years (2004–2019).

7.2   Current Definition of Mixed Methods Research

Mixed methods research can be viewed as a distinct category of multiple methods research. Multiple methods research (also referred to as multi-methods research) is an overarching term that refers to all of the various combinations of research methods involving more than one data collection procedure (Fetters and Molina-Azorin 2017). This can include combinations of exclusively qualitative and/or quantitative approaches. As the field of mixed methods research is still evolving, several researchers believe that the definition of mixed methods research should remain open to allow for its development and refinement, as the practice of mixed methods research grows across academic disciplines (Johnson et al. 2007). However, there is a general consensus that mixed methods research typically involves both a qualitative and a quantitative component embedded within a single study or research programme (Tashakkori and Creswell 2007; Creswell et al. 2004; Fetters and Molina-Azorin 2017).

Johnson et al. (2007) approached 19 experts in the field and invited them to propose a definition of mixed methods research to ensure a common and uniform understanding of the term. They subsequently summarised their findings and proposed the following definition:

> Mixed methods research is the type of research in which a researcher or team of researchers combines elements of qualitative and quantitative research approaches (e.g. use of qualitative and quantitative viewpoints, data collection, analysis, inference techniques) for the broad purpose of breadth and depth of understanding and corroboration. (Johnson et al. 2007)

In addition, they also specified that mixed methods research is a specific programme of research: 'A mixed methods study would involve mixing within a single study; a mixed method program would involve mixing within a program of research and the mixing might occur across a closely related set of studies' (Johnson et al. 2007).

Mixed methods research is therefore a synthesis that can include findings from both qualitative and quantitative research and, importantly, the integration of the findings from each research strand. Integration refers to the interaction between the different research strands (O'Cathain et al. 2010). We outline an approach to integrating findings from different strands of research at the end of this chapter.

7.2.1   Advantages of Mixed Methods Research

The use of a mixed methods approach to research is especially useful in understanding contradictions between quantitative results and qualitative findings. For example, within a large research programme on prescribing errors, junior doctors rated their level of confidence in a variety of prescribing-related tasks, e.g. selecting the most appropriate dose, as very high, overall, in a questionnaire study (Ryan et al. 2013), despite prior indication that they were responsible for a large proportion of prescribing errors identified in a related prevalence study (Ryan et al. 2014). To explore this contradiction and to examine the disparity between doctors' perceived level of confidence and the fact that prescribing errors were often made during the study period, analysis of the qualitative work revealed that doctors were not always made aware of their errors. Additionally, prescribing charts were often amended by other prescribers, without providing feedback to the original prescriber (Ross et al. 2013).

Mixed methods approaches allow participants' point of view to be reflected, provide methodological flexibility and encourage multi-disciplinary teamworking. For example, a research study conducted to evaluate the extension of prescribing rights to pharmacists consisted of a number of linked phases, which were qualitative and quantitative in nature (McCann et al. 2011, 2012, 2015). The research team consisted of pharmacists, a general practitioner (GP) and an economist. This mix of disciplines contributed to a more holistic overview of the research topic and ensured that the research objectives would be met. The study phases consisted of a cross-sectional questionnaire which was completed by qualified prescribing pharmacists (McCann et al. 2011). The questionnaire provided the quantitative baseline and background data that were explored in subsequent qualitative phases (McCann et al. 2012, 2015). Pharmacists, physicians and other healthcare professionals with a vested interest in prescribing participated in interviews which revealed the advantages and disadvantages of prescribing in greater depth than would have been gleaned from a quantitative questionnaire alone (McCann et al. 2012). However, further qualitative work with patients, who had experienced prescribing by a pharmacist, via focus groups, was even more revealing (McCann et al. 2015). Patients recognised the importance of pharmacist input, but they also cited limitations to this new model of care, particularly pharmacists' focus on one medical condition at a time. This issue had been highlighted in much of the pharmacist prescribing literature before, but never from the perspective of patients. Using these various methodologies within the one study enabled a more comprehensive and deeper understanding of how pharmacist prescribing had evolved and provided evidence for policy makers as to how this model of care could be enhanced and extended into more mainstream practice.

7.2.2   Limitations of Mixed Methods Research

Mixed methods approaches to research are labour-intensive and require a broader range of research expertise across a multidisciplinary team than those needed to conduct a single method study. Mixed methods studies are complex to plan and undertake and can pose challenges in ensuring methodological rigour of individual study components. Furthermore, the integration of data from a number of different sources can be challenging and complex as detailed below.

7.3   Mixed Methods Research in Pharmacy Practice

The use of mixed methods research in pharmacy practice research has been fuelled by a transition in the focus of health services research from a practitioner-centred approach to more of a patient-centred approach. For example, this has been highlighted by research into the development of community pharmacy-based interventions targeting alcohol use. Early work did not report any patient involvement during intervention development (Fitzgerald et al. 2008). However, a study by Krska and Mackridge (2014) describes the use of a mixed methods approach using telephone interviews with key stakeholders and survey data with patients/public to develop their intervention. Additionally, in intervention and implementation research, there is an increasing drive for theoretically derived evidence to inform the development of interventions with a growing emphasis on the science underpinning intervention development. This is illustrated by the United Kingdom's (UK) Medical Research Council's (MRC) influential guidance on the development of complex interventions (Medical Research Council 2008) which is increasingly being used in the design of pharmacy practice interventions (Hughes et al. 2016) (Fig. 7.1).

This has been adopted by pharmacy practice researchers as healthcare interventions are, in general, complex (utilising several components, rather than a single active 'ingredient') and involve a variety of healthcare professionals. Furthermore, as pharmacy practice interventions are often targeted at individual patients, effective interventions need to be tailored to these individuals accordingly.

Each phase of the MRC framework requires the application of different research methods. For example, in order to develop an intervention to improve medication adherence, researchers should firstly identify the extent of the problem of non-adherence (e.g. by quantifying the level of non-adherence) in the development

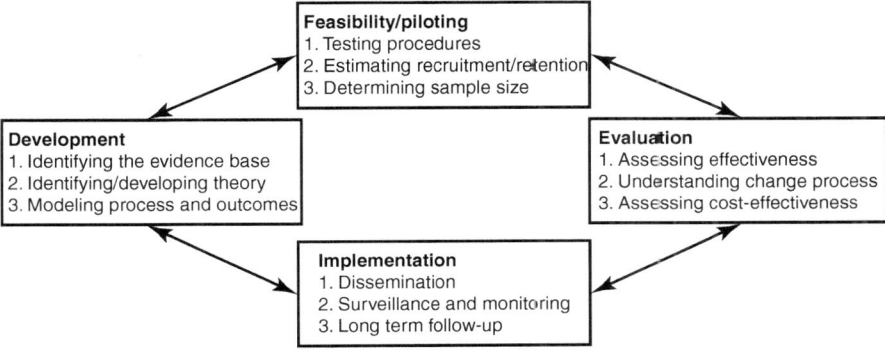

Fig. 7.1 MRC framework for the development of a complex intervention

component and then identify an appropriate theoretical basis to underpin the development of the intervention. In the feasibility/piloting component, the MRC recommends that retention, recruitment and sample size should be estimated (quantitative methods), and intervention procedures should be tested (quantitative and/or qualitative methods). This highlights the important role of mixed methods research in pharmacy practice intervention design as the research question could not be addressed using one method alone.

In order to assess the effectiveness of an intervention, specific outcome measures need to be compared before and after the intervention, e.g. the level of adherence (quantitative), as part of the evaluation component. For the change processes to be identified and understood, i.e. those mechanisms which led to changes in adherence, qualitative methods should primarily be employed to seek participants' views and experiences of the intervention. Finally, an assessment of cost-effectiveness would be quantitative in nature.

In the final component of the framework (implementation) which comprises monitoring, surveillance and long-term follow-up of the intervention, both qualitative and quantitative methods can be used either alone or in combination, but the chosen methods are largely dependent on the intervention being tested and the outcomes of interest. For example, McLeod et al. (2019) used a mixed methods study design involving both quantitative data (direct observations) and qualitative data (semi-structured interviews) to examine the implementation and impact of a hospital-based electronic prescribing and administration system. The direct observations of ward pharmacists' working practices (i.e. quantitative data) before and after implementation of the system provided data on the amount of time the pharmacists spent on different tasks, as well as information on the individuals they engaged with and where the tasks were conducted within the hospital. The interviews with the pharmacists (i.e. qualitative data) explored their perceptions of the impact of the system on ward activities and interactions with patients and other health professionals. Triangulation of the quantitative and qualitative data enabled the researchers to gain a more in-depth understanding of factors that contributed to the observed post-implementation effects of the new system such as changes in the duration of routine tasks.

As conveyed by Fig. 7.1, the various phases of the MRC framework are not necessarily constrained by a rigid sequence, but can be iterative in nature. This type of framework is ideal for the application of mixed methods.

7.4   Typologies of Mixed Methods Research

As stated previously, the choice of research methodology to adopt for a given study depends entirely on the research question. Within mixed methods research, there are a variety of categories, otherwise known as typologies, which help to formalise the approach taken and which add rigour to research projects (Bryman 2006). There are a number of classification matrices by which mixed methods research designs are described, with no one method having superiority over the other (Driscoll et al. 2007). However, each classification suggests that the factors below should be considered when deciding on the typology to use (Bryman 2006; Driscoll et al. 2007; O'Cathain et al. 2010; Hadi et al. 2013):

- Order of data collection: Are the qualitative and quantitative data collected independently or sequentially?
- Priority: Which type of data has priority, i.e. quantitative or qualitative data?
- Integration: What is the purpose of integration, e.g. triangulation?
- Number of data strands: How many constituent research components are involved?

The following section will describe four of the most common mixed methods typologies used in pharmacy practice research (*concurrent design*, *explanatory sequential design*, *exploratory sequential design and embedded design*), with examples of studies that have used these approaches. Advantages and disadvantages of each approach will also be noted.

7.4.1 *Concurrent Design*

The concurrent mixed methods design describes an approach whereby both qualitative and quantitative data are collected concurrently, in separate but related studies. This typology is also referred to as the 'convergent parallel design', 'current triangulation', 'simultaneous triangulation' and 'parallel study' (Hadi et al. 2013). Each study is given equal priority and findings are integrated only at the interpretation stage, i.e. studies are seen as separate entities during both data collection and analysis. This approach is useful for validating qualitative data with quantitative data and vice versa. This design facilitates the development of an overall understanding of the research question. For example, Ryan and colleagues used this study design type in the research programme on prescribing errors previously referred to. Whilst there were several components to this research programme, an observational prevalence study (Ryan et al. 2014) and a semi-structured interview study with junior doctors (Ross et al. 2013) were conducted concurrently. Each study was analysed separately, but data were interpreted together. The interview study offered some explanations as to why various types of errors identified in the prevalence study occurred. For example, the prevalence study revealed that errors of omission (i.e. drugs not being prescribed) at admission to hospital were one of the commonest types of errors encountered (Ryan et al. 2014). Findings from the semi-structured interviews somewhat explained these errors, in that interviewees noted difficulties in accessing prescribing information from primary care at the point of patient admission.

7.4.2   Sequential Design

Sequential design studies involve the collection of data on an iterative basis, i.e. data collected in one phase contributes to the data collection in the next phase (Driscoll et al. 2007). Subsequent phases provide more detailed data on findings from earlier phases and can help to generalise findings by verifying and augmenting study results. Sequential design studies can be either **explanatory** or **exploratory** (Hadi et al. 2013). In **explanatory** sequential design studies, the first phase consists of quantitative data collection, and this is followed by a qualitative study, the aim of which is to explain the findings from the quantitative study. The collection of quantitative data first allows application of statistical methods to determine which findings to augment in the next phase (Driscoll et al. 2007). For example, in the first phase of a study investigating prescribing errors in Scottish hospitals, the researchers defined the prevalence of prescribing errors, and in the second phase, the researchers conducted semi-structured interviews with prescribers to determine the causes and under what circumstances the prescribing errors identified in phase one occurred (Ryan et al. 2014). At study completion, i.e. at the end of the qualitative study, data were triangulated to provide a wider understanding of the occurrence of prescribing errors.

Ramsay et al. (2014) used a mixed methods approach to evaluate the effects of a ward-level medication safety scorecard to influence medication safety and the factors that influenced the use of the scorecard. A mixed methods approach was used to gain an understanding of how and why the intervention influenced staff behaviour and whether there were any unintended consequences and which factors were influential (Ramsay et al. 2014). The quantitative component (a controlled before and after study) assessed the performance of this safety scorecard, whilst the subsequent qualitative component involved interviews with hospital staff exploring governance of medication safety, experiences of scorecard feedback and implementation issues. Each component, i.e. the qualitative and quantitative aspects, was analysed separately in the first instance, and the findings were then triangulated. Using this methodological approach allowed for the evaluation of the efficacy of the scorecard, as well as considerations of contextual factors that might influence the implementation of this patient safety initiative (Ramsay et al. 2014).

Similarly, **exploratory** sequential design studies also consist of two distinct phases. The first phase consists of a qualitative study, to explore the research question in depth. Based on analysis of the qualitative data, a quantitative study is then developed to test the findings. For example, Millar et al. (2015) used semi-structured interviews to explore the views and attitudes of healthcare professionals and patients towards medicines management in intermediate care facilities. A questionnaire was subsequently developed which sought to further explore and quantify community pharmacists' views on the issues that were identified through the previous qualitative study (Millar et al. 2016). The questionnaire findings highlighted a lack of awareness and involvement amongst community pharmacists relating to intermediate care. However, community pharmacists also demonstrated willingness to being involved in intermediate care. This stepwise approach involving sequential use of qualitative and quantitative methods facilitated a logical elucidation of the main issues and challenges faced by those who work in these types of facilities. An interpretation of quantitative findings without an understanding of the contextual factors may have led to invalid or biased conclusions.

Adopting a sequential design approach allows researchers to investigate emergent and unexpected themes in more detail. However, this approach can be time-consuming.

7.4.3 The Embedded Design

The embedded design consists of both a qualitative and a quantitative phase. However, in contrast to the previously mentioned typologies, in the embedded design, one research method is designated as the key method, and the other component of the research adopts a supportive role. In essence, whilst the qualitative and quantitative components of the research study are based on the same broad topic, each research component in the embedded design answers a different research question. This design is often used in randomised controlled trials, where the quantitative component of the research study is the main focus in terms of intervention outcomes. However, the qualitative components can provide important process evaluation information in terms of issues such as implementation. The qualitative component of the research project can be incorporated into the study at any time point, e.g. at the beginning to help in the design of the intervention, during the intervention to explore participants' experiences or after the intervention to help to explain results. This is illustrated by a study which evaluated the impact of a pharmaceutical care model regarding the prescribing of psychoactive medications in older nursing home residents (Patterson et al. 2010). The original model of care (described as the Fleetwood model) had been developed in the United States (USA) by the American Society of Consultant Pharmacists for application by pharmacists in the US nursing home context (Cameron et al. 2002). However, as the model of care in US nursing homes is very different to the rest of the world, this care model required adaptation before it could be used in non-US nursing homes. Thus, a qualitative study was undertaken in Northern Ireland to allow this adaptation to take place (Patterson et al. 2007). Semi-structured interviews or focus groups were held with GPs, nursing home managers, pharmacists and advocates of older people. The American Fleetwood model was explained to all participants who were then asked for their views and opinions on how such a model could be adapted for use in the UK setting. Participants recognised that for such a model of care to work outside of the USA, consideration would need to be given as to how pharmacists would access medical records, prescribers and nursing home residents in order to implement this care model to its full potential. The resultant changes to the model enabled it to be successfully employed in 22 nursing homes as part of a randomised trial. Indeed, the adapted model of care proved to be effective and cost-effective (Patterson et al. 2010, 2011) and has since been rolled out in nursing homes across Northern Ireland.

7.5   Integrating Findings in Mixed Methods Research

As outlined in the definition given at the start of this chapter, mixed methods research does not simply involve the collection of qualitative and quantitative data; integration of findings is a central part of mixed methods research. As previously noted, integration refers to the interaction between the different research strands, and this can be achieved through the triangulation of data (O'Cathain et al. 2010).

Triangulation was initially conceptualised as a means of validating findings, but the focus has since changed and triangulation is increasingly seen as a means of enriching and completing knowledge (Flick 2009). Triangulation has been described as a process of using different methods to study a problem in order to gain a more complete picture (O'Cathain et al. 2010). This can involve the combination of multiple qualitative methods or the combination of qualitative and quantitative methods (Flick et al. 2012). Through the use of different research methods, triangulation seeks to exploit the strengths and neutralise the limitations that are inherent to each method (Jick 1979). In mixed methods research, integration can occur at different levels of the research process, e.g. study design, methods, interpretation and reporting (Fetters et al. 2013). In this chapter we focus on the integration of findings at the level of interpretation using a triangulation-based approach, once each dataset has been analysed separately, as is common practice in mixed methods healthcare studies (Östlund et al. 2011).

Triangulation looks to explore convergence, complementarity and dissonance between the findings of each method (Farmer et al. 2006). Convergence and dissonance refer to the extent to which findings from each method agree or disagree, respectively. Complementarity occurs where findings from different methods provide complementary information on the same issue. The triangulation of data from different methods offers important advantages in that it can generate richer data, uncover unexpected findings that can provide opportunity for enriching explanations and ultimately increase confidence in research findings (Jick 1979).

Triangulation has been classified into four different types (Denzin 1989): methodological triangulation (use of different research methods or data collection techniques), theory triangulation (use of different theoretical perspectives), data triangulation (use of multiple data sources or groups of research participants) and investigator triangulation (use of multiple researchers in data analysis). However, various authors have noted that little guidance has been provided to date on performing triangulation (Jick 1979; Morgan 1998; Östlund et al. 2011). Given the range of typologies in mixed methods research, as detailed earlier in this chapter, there is no single approach to triangulation that can be applied to all mixed methods research. However, as outlined in Farmer's triangulation protocol, there are a number of basic steps (i.e. sorting, convergence coding, convergence assessment, completeness assessment, researcher comparison and feedback) that can be followed in order to provide methodological transparency where triangulation is used in any given research context (Farmer et al. 2006). This triangulation protocol is considered to provide the most detailed account of how to triangulate data and is applicable to mixed methods in health research (O'Cathain et al. 2010).

The triangulation of data within mixed methods research requires decisions about the weighting given to each dataset. As noted by Jick (1979), in the absence of guidelines for systematically ordering data decisions regarding the weighting of different study components, decisions are likely to be subjective. Farmer et al. (2006) propose that decisions about weighting should be based on the contribution of the different components to the research question.

The use of a triangulation protocol can help to improve the quality and reporting of mixed methods research and to address deficiencies that have been identified in the existing mixed methods literature relating to pharmacy practice (Hadi et al. 2014), as well as the wider healthcare literature (Östlund et al. 2011). The application of Farmer's triangulation protocol is exemplified below by reference to a research project undertaken by the authors to develop an intervention to improve appropriate polypharmacy in older patients in primary care (Cadogan et al. 2015, 2016).

7.5.1   Case Study: Application of a Triangulation Protocol in a Mixed Methods Project with a Sequential Design

The triangulation protocol outlined below was adapted from the work of Farmer et al. (2006) and developed as part of an ongoing mixed methods research project seeking to develop an intervention to improve appropriate polypharmacy in older patients in primary care. The project comprised several phases, including an update of a Cochrane systematic review (Patterson et al. 2014), semi-structured interviews involving two groups of healthcare professionals (general practitioners, community pharmacists) and a feasibility study of the intervention that was subsequently developed (Cadogan et al. 2015, 2016, 2017). Triangulation was based on the completed analysis of interview data. The topic guide for the qualitative components of the project was based primarily on the Theoretical Domains Framework, an established framework which consists of 12 theoretical domains relevant to changing healthcare professionals' behaviour (Michie et al. 2005). The findings of the Cochrane review were also used to inform part of the topic guides. The main aim of the analysis was to identify the principal barriers and facilitators to changing target behaviours in healthcare professionals, namely, prescribing and dispensing, in order to achieve the desired outcome (i.e. appropriate polypharmacy) through integration of the findings from each dataset. This allowed for different perspectives on the same research question. An established taxonomy of behaviour change techniques (Michie et al. 2013) was then used to target these domains and elicit desired changes in target behaviours. Intervention delivery and related outcome assessments were informed by the findings of the updated Cochrane review.

Prior to triangulation, each qualitative dataset was independently analysed by two researchers using the framework method (Ritchie and Spencer 1994). Qualitative analysis of each dataset followed a deductive approach, and the theoretical framework (Michie et al. 2005) used to develop the topic guides served as the coding framework. The subsequent paragraphs relate to the triangulation of the findings from each dataset.

Triangulation involved multiple investigator triangulation and data source triangulation. As a single theoretical framework was used to analyse the individual datasets, theoretical triangulation was not conducted. Similarly, as a single research method was used to gather the data (i.e. semi-structured interviews), methodological triangulation was not required. Integration of the datasets focussed on the prominence of the framework domains (themes) across the datasets. Although the intervention sought to target healthcare professionals, it was also imperative that it would be beneficial to older patients who were receiving polypharmacy in primary care. Thus, the findings from each dataset (general practitioners, community pharmacists) were weighted equally as both groups of participants interacted with this patient cohort.

1. **Sorting**: Findings from each dataset were reviewed in order to identify key domains within the Theoretical Domains Framework that would need to be targeted as part of the intervention.
2. **Convergence coding**: A convergence coding matrix was developed and applied to compare the presence, frequency and examples of domains across the datasets. This allowed differences and similarities between datasets to be summarised. Convergence focussed on the prominence of domains across the datasets and the convergence of coverage (i.e. level of agreement/disagreement across the datasets).
3. **Convergence assessment**: All comparisons across the datasets were reviewed to provide a comprehensive assessment of the level of convergence. Any cases where researchers' views on convergence or dissonance differed were documented.
4. **Completeness assessment**: Findings from the datasets were compared to create an overarching summary of the findings, highlighting both unique and similar contributions to the research question. For example, both groups of healthcare professionals were aware of the potential for adverse outcomes (e.g. drug interactions, non-adherence), if actions were not taken to improve appropriate polypharmacy in older patients ('beliefs about consequences') (Cadogan et al. 2015). Despite identification of similar challenges within a number of domains that formed part of the coding framework (e.g. limited available time and work environment pressures under the 'environmental context and resource' domain), differences were identified in the groups' perceptions of other domains as barriers or facilitators to prescribing/dispensing of appropriate polypharmacy. For example, under the 'social/professional role and identity' domain, pharmacists were conscious of professional boundaries with GPs in recommending changes to older patients' existing prescriptions, whereas GPs viewed teamwork with pharmacists favourably.
5. **Researcher comparison**: Formal assessments can be used to compare the level of agreement between the researchers in terms of the degree of convergence across the datasets. For example, Farmer et al. (2006) reported that agreement between two researchers that meets or exceeds 70% can provide acceptable confidence in

the coding process. In the context of the polypharmacy research project, it was intended that any disagreements would be resolved by consensus through discussion with another researcher. However, this was not necessary as there were no disagreements.

6. **Feedback**: Triangulated results were presented to the other members of the research team for discussion. A consensus-based approach was used by the team to agree on the specific domains of the theoretical framework that should be targeted as part of the intervention. Interestingly, based on the research team's review of the summary findings from each dataset, all but one of the domains from the coding framework were considered to be relevant to both the prescribing and dispensing of appropriate polypharmacy to older patients. The importance of the same key domains for both groups highlighted commonalities in the perceived barriers to, and facilitators of, behaviour change within each group. The selected key domains were then mapped to behaviour change techniques from an established taxonomy (Michie et al. 2013) that formed the components of the final intervention.

This thorough and painstaking process yielded rich and informative results which highlighted multiple perspectives on an important issue within primary care, i.e. polypharmacy. A GP-targeted intervention has been developed and undergone feasibility testing (Cadogan et al. 2017). A single focus on a single constituency, e.g. GPs, would have provided a narrow and limited view. Any subsequent intervention development would have considered only this single view, and the resultant intervention may not have identified relevant barriers and facilitators to the prescribing of appropriate polypharmacy for older people in primary care. Researchers should be aware that adopting this kind of triangulation protocol will be time-consuming, but the findings in subsequent types of phases of research should be much more meaningful.

7.6 Enhancing Rigour and Reporting in Mixed Methods Research

Ensuring methodological rigour in mixed methods research is critical in order to maximise its potential to advance the evidence base relating to pharmacy practice and inform relevant policy/practice. Previous reviews have identified deficiencies with the conduct and reporting of mixed methods research (Brown et al. 2015; Wisdom et al. 2012; O'Cathain et al. 2008; Fàbregues and Molina-Azorín 2017; Kaur et al. 2019). For example, a systematic review of health services research involving mixed methods designs identified issues with the rigour of the included studies in terms of a lack of adequate description of study design and justification for a mixed methods approach, as well as a lack of information regarding integration of data from different study components (O'Cathain et al. 2008).

In addition to adhering to existing standards for each of the component methods, researchers must also consider how they will integrate the two components and ensure that they describe this adequately in their final published report (Hadi and Closs 2016).

Work has been undertaken to develop tools and criteria for appraising the methodological rigour of mixed methods research (Sale and Brazil 2004; Heyvaert et al. 2013; Hong et al. 2018). For example, the Mixed Methods Appraisal Tool (MMAT) has been developed to appraise the methodological quality of empirical studies as part of mixed methods systematic reviews (Hong et al. 2018). The MMAT comprises study-specific questions for appraising five different categories of study designs: quantitative randomised controlled trials, quantitative non-randomised studies, quantitative descriptive studies, qualitative studies and mixed methods studies. Responses to each question can be documented as 'yes', 'no' or 'unclear'. In applying this tool to appraise study quality, it is intended that a combination of question categories should be applied relating to each study component (i.e. qualitative and quantitative), as well as the overall mixed methods design. Assessment questions specific to appraising the quality of mixed methods study designs are listed in Table 7.1.

In order for tools such as the MMAT to be applied, studies must be adequately reported. In contrast to other research designs for which established reporting guidelines exist (e.g. 'Consolidated Standards of Reporting Trials' (Schulz et al. 2010) for randomised controlled trials), there are no universally accepted reporting guidelines for mixed methods research. In seeking to address this, the 'Good Reporting of A Mixed Methods Study' (GRAMMS) recommendations have been proposed (O'Cathain et al. 2008). These recommendations cover key considerations when designing a mixed methods study, including the integration of data sources. The GRAMMS recommendations are intended for guidance purposes as opposed to being used as a formal reporting checklist. The recommendations have been adapted for pharmacy practice research (Table 7.2) (Hadi et al. 2014).

As mixed methods research continues to evolve and grow as a paradigm in pharmacy practice research, it is important that researchers make use of available quality appraisal and reporting tools. This will ultimately help to enhance rigour and reporting in mixed methods pharmacy practice research.

Table 7.1 Sample questions from Mixed Methods Appraisal Tool (Hong et al. 2018)

Methodological quality criteria for mixed methods study designs
1. Is there an adequate rationale for using a mixed methods design to address the research question?
2. Are the different components of the study effectively integrated to answer the research question?
3. Are the outputs of the integration of qualitative and quantitative components adequately interpreted?
4. Are divergences and inconsistencies between quantitative and qualitative results adequately addressed?
5. Do the different components of the study adhere to the quality criteria of each tradition of the methods involved?

Table 7.2 Recommendations to improve mixed methods reporting in pharmacy practice research

1. Research objectives should be described in a way that clarifies the need for using a mixed methods approach
2. Rationale and justification should be provided for the choice of mixed methods approach in relation to the research question
3. Key elements of the research design (i.e. purpose, priority and timing) should be described using common mixed methods terminology
4. Research methods for each of the component qualitative and quantitative approaches should be described in sufficient detail to enable reproducibility
5. Information should be provided on how and where integration has occurred
6. Any relevant limitations for each of the component qualitative and quantitative methods should be outlined
7. An explanation should be provided of the benefits of using a mixed methods approach to answer the research question
8. An explanation should be provided of the potential implications of the research findings on pharmacy policy, practice and/or education

Adapted from Hadi et al. (2014)

7.7 Conclusion

Using a variety of methods to answer a research question can add further context and explanations to findings and interpretations. We have outlined a variety of mixed methods typologies that are used in pharmacy practice research. It is important to note there is no preferred typology that pharmacy practice researchers should adopt. Instead, researchers should ensure that the methodological approach chosen in a study is suitable for the research question posed. The growing recognition of the contribution of mixed methods to pharmacy practice research should ensure that studies are addressing key research questions in a comprehensive and meaningful way.

References

Brown KM, Elliott SJ, Leatherdale ST, Robertson-Wilson J. Searching for rigour in the reporting of mixed methods population health research: a methodological review. Health Educ Res. 2015;30(6):811–39.

Bryman A. Integrating quantitative and qualitative research: how is it done? Qual Res. 2006;6(1):97–113.

Cadogan CA, Ryan C, Francis JJ, Gormley GJ, Passmore P, Kerse N, Hughes CM. Improving appropriate polypharmacy for older people in primary care: selecting components of an evidence-based intervention to target prescribing and dispensing. Implement Sci. 2015;10:161.

Cadogan CA, Ryan C, Francis J, Gormley GJ, Passmore AP, Kerse N, Hughes C. Development of an intervention to improve appropriate polypharmacy in older people in primary care using a theory-based method. BMC Health Serv Res. 2016;16(1):661.

Cadogan CA, Ryan C, Gormley GJ, Francis JJ, Passmore P, Kerse N, Hughes CM. A feasibility study of a theory-based intervention to improve appropriate polypharmacy for older people in primary care. Pilot Feasibility Stud. 2017;20(4):23.

Cameron K, Feinberg JL, Lapane KL. Fleetwood project Phase III moves forward. Consult Pharm. 2002;17:181–98.

Creswell JW, Fetters MD, Ivankova NV. Designing a mixed methods study in primary care. Ann Fam Med. 2004;2(1):7–11.

Denzin N. The research act: a theoretical introduction to sociological methods, transaction publishers. 3rd ed. New York: McGraw-Hill; 1989.

Driscoll DL, Appiah-Yeboah A, Salib P, Rupter DJ. Merging qualitative and quantitative data in mixed methods research: how to and why not. Ecol Environ Anthropol. 2007;3(1):19–27.

Fàbregues S, Molina-Azorín JF. Addressing quality in mixed methods research: a review and recommendations for a future agenda. Qual Quant. 2017;51(6):2847–63.

Farmer T, Robinson K, Elliott SJ, Eyles J. Developing and implementing a triangulation protocol for qualitative health research. Qual Health Res. 2006;16(3):377–94.

Fetters MD, Curry LA, Creswell JW. Achieving integration in mixed methods designs—principles and practices. Health Serv Res. 2013;48(6):2134–56.

Fetters MD, Molina-Azorin JF. The journal of mixed methods research starts a new decade: principles for bringing in the new and divesting of the old language of the field. J Mixed Methods Res. 2017;11(1):3–10.

Fitzgerald N, McCaig DJ, Watson H, Thomson D, Stewart DC. Development, implementation and evaluation of a pilot project to deliver interventions on alcohol issues in community pharmacies. Int J Pharm Pract. 2008;16:17–22.

Flick U. Qualitative research at work II: triangulation. In: Flick U, editor. An introduction to qualitative research. 4th ed. London: SAGE; 2009.

Flick U, Garms-Homolova V, Herrmann WJ, Kuck J, Rohnsch G. "I can't prescribe something just because someone asks for it...": using mixed methods in the framework of triangulation. J Mixed Methods Res. 2012;6(2):97–110.

Hadi MA, Alldred DP, Closs SJ, Briggs M. Mixed-methods research in pharmacy practice: basics and beyond (part 1). Int J Pharm Pract. 2013;21(5):341–5.

Hadi MA, Alldred DP, Closs SJ, Briggs M. Mixed-methods research in pharmacy practice: recommendations for quality reporting (part 2). Int J Pharm Pract. 2014;22(1):96–100.

Hadi MA, Closs SJ. Applications of mixed-methods methodology in clinical pharmacy research. Int J Clin Pharm. 2016;38(3):635–40.

Heyvaert M, Hannes K, Maes B, Onghena P. Critical appraisal of mixed methods studies. J Mixed Methods Res. 2013;7(4):302–27.

Hong QN, Pluye P, Fàbregues S, Bartlett G, Boardman F, Cargo M, Dagenais P, Gagnon M-P, Griffiths F, Nicolau B, O'Cathain A, Rousseau M-C, Vedel I. Mixed Methods Appraisal Tool (MMAT), version 2018. Registration of copyright (#1148552). Canada: Canadian Intellectual Property Office, Industry Canada; 2018.

Hughes CM, Cadogan CA, Ryan CA. Development of a pharmacy practice intervention: lessons from the literature. Int J Clin Pharm. 2016;38(3):601–6.

Jick TD. Mixing qualitative and quantitative methods: triangulation in action. Adm Sci Q. 1979;24(4):602–11.

Johnson RB, Onwuegbuzie AJ, Turner LA. Towards a definition of mixed methods research. J Mixed Methods Res. 2007;1(2):112–33.

Kaur N, Vedel I, El Sherif R, Pluye P. Practical mixed methods strategies used to integrate qualitative and quantitative methods in community-based primary health care research. Fam Pract. 2019;36:666. https://doi.org/10.1093/fampra/cmz010.

Krska J, Mackridge AJ. Involving the public and other stakeholders in development and evaluation of a community pharmacy alcohol screening and brief advice service. Public Health. 2014;128(4):309–16.

McCann L, Haughey S, Parsons C, Lloyd F, Crealey G, Gormley G, Hughes CM. Pharmacist prescribing in Northern Ireland-a quantitative assessment. Int J Clin Pharm. 2011;33(5):824–31.

McCann L, Haughey S, Parsons C, Lloyd F, Crealey G, Gormley G, Hughes CM. "They come with multiple morbidities" – a qualitative assessment of pharmacist prescribing. J Interprof Care. 2012;26(2):127–33.

McCann L, Haughey S, Parsons C, Lloyd F, Crealey G, Gormley G, Hughes C. A patient perspective of pharmacist prescribing: "crossing the specialisms -crossing the illnesses". Health Expect. 2015;18(1):58–68.

McLeod M, Karampatakis GD, Heyligen L, McGinley A, Franklin BD. The impact of implementing a hospital electronic prescribing and administration system on clinical pharmacists' activities – a mixed methods study. BMC Health Serv Res. 2019;19(1):156.

Medical Research Council. Developing and evaluating complex interventions: new guidance. 2008.

Michie S, Johnston M, Abraham C, Lawton R, Parker D, Walker A. Making psychological theory useful for implementing evidence based practice: a consensus approach. Qual Saf Health Care. 2005;14:26–33.

Michie S, Richardson M, Johnston M, Abraham C, Francis J, Hardeman W, Wood C. The behaviorchange technique taxonomy (v1) of 93 hierarchically clustered techniques: building an international consensus for the reporting of behavior change interventions. Ann Behav Med. 2013;46(1):81–95.

Millar A, Hughes C, Devlin M, Ryan C. A cross-sectional evaluation of community pharmacists' perceptions of intermediate care and medicines management across the healthcare interface. Int J Clin Pharm. 2016;38(6):1380–9.

Millar AN, Hughes CM, Ryan C. "It's very complicated": a qualitative study of medicines management in intermediate care facilities in Northern Ireland. BMC Health Serv Res. 2015;15:216.

Morgan DL. Practical strategies for combining qualitative and quantitative methods: applications to health research. Qual Health Res. 1998;8(3):362–76.

O'Cathain A, Murphy E, Nicholl J. The quality of mixed methods studies in health services research. J Health Serv Res Policy. 2008;13(2):92–8.

O'Cathain A, Murphy E, Nicholl J. Three techniques for integrating data in mixed methods studies. Br Med J. 2010;341:1147–50.

Östlund U, Kidd L, Wengström Y, Rowa-Dewar N. Combining qualitative and quantitative research within mixed method research designs: a methodological review. Int J Nurs Stud. 2011;48(3):369–83.

Patterson SM, Cadogan CA, Kerse N, Cardwell CR, Bradley MC, Ryan C, Hughes C. Interventions to improve the appropriate use of polypharmacy for older people. Cochrane Database Syst Rev. 2014;(10):CD008165.

Patterson SM, Hughes CM, Cardwell C, Lapane K, Murray AM, Crealey GE. A cluster randomized controlled trial of an adapted U.S. model of pharmaceutical care for nursing home residents in Northern Ireland (Fleetwood Northern Ireland study): a cost-effectiveness analysis. J Am Geriatr Soc. 2011;59(4):586–93.

Patterson SM, Hughes CM, Crealey G, Cardwell C, Lapane K. An evaluation of an adapted United States model of pharmaceutical care to improve psychoactive prescribing for nursing home residents in Northern Ireland (Fleetwood NI Study). J Am Geriatr Soc. 2010;58(1):44–53.

Patterson SM, Hughes CM, Lapane KL. Assessment of a United States pharmaceutical care model for nursing homes in the United Kingdom. Pharm World Sci. 2007;29(5):517–25.

Ramsay AIG, Turner S, Cavell G, Oborne CA, Thomas RW, Cooksor G, Fulop NJ. Governing patient safety: lessons learned from a mixed methods evaluation of implementing a ward level medication safety scorecard in two English NHS hospitals. BMJ Qual Saf. 2014;23:136–46.

Ritchie J, Spencer L. Qualitative data analysis for applied policy research. In: Bryman A, Burgess TG, editors. Analyzing qualitative data. London: Routledge; 1994.

Ross S, Ryan C, Duncan EM, Francis JJ, Johnston M, Ker JS, Lee AJ, Macleod MJ, Maxwell S, McKay G, Mclay J, Webb D. Perceived causes of prescribing errors by junior doctors in hospital inpatients: a study from the PROTECT programme. BMJ Qual Saf. 2013;22:97–102.

Ryan C, Ross S, Davey P, Duncan E, Fielding S, Francis JJ, Johnston M, Ker J, Lee AJ, MacLeod MJ, Maxwell S, McKay G, McLay J, Webb D, Bond C. Junior doctors' perceptions of prescribing errors: rates, causes and self-efficacy. Br J Clin Pharmacol. 2013;76(6):980–7.

Ryan C, Ross S, Davey P, Duncan EM, Francis JJ, Fielding S, Johnston M, Ker J, Lee AJ, MacLeod MY, Maxwell S, McKay G, McLay JS, Webb DJ, Bond C. Prevalence and causes of prescribing errors: the prescribing outcomes for trainee doctors engaged in clinical training (PROTECT) study. PLoS One. 2014;9(1):e79802.

Sackett DL, Wennberg JE. Choosing the best research design for each question. BMJ. 1997;315:1636.

Sale JE, Brazil K. A strategy to identify critical appraisal criteria for primary mixed-method studies. Qual Quant. 2004;38(4):351–65.

Schulz KF, Altman DG, Moher D, CONSORT Group. CONSORT 2010 statement: updated guidelines for reporting parallel group randomised trials. BMJ. 2010;340:c332.

Tashakkori A, Creswell JW. Editorial: The new era of mixed methods. J Mix Methods Res. 2007;1(1):3–7.

Wisdom JP, Cavaleri MA, Onwuegbuzie AJ, Green CA. Methodological reporting in qualitative, quantitative, and mixed methods health services research articles. Health Serv Res. 2012;47(2):721–45.

Chapter 8
Grounded Theory in Pharmacy Practice Research

Radi Haloub and Zaheer-Ud-Din Babar

Abstract This chapter aims to provide an overview of the use of Grounded Theory methodology in pharmacy practice research. Grounded Theory does not only provide clearer insights into thoughts and feelings that determine the behaviour of individuals, but it also assists in discovering relationships and concepts that have not been previously defined or explained from the perspective of symbolic interactionism. This will consequently support the development of hypotheses and construction of new theories. Moreover, this chapter explains how the use of Grounded Theory can facilitate theoretical development through continuous comparison with the literature during the process of data collection in pharmacy practice research.

8.1 Introduction

Grounded Theory is a constructive methodology used by qualitative researchers to guide them in the theory development process in social sciences research (Pettigrew 2000). It is a comprehensive approach that produces explanations for uniformity of social action, social organisation and social change (Merton 1968). In addition to the ability of Grounded Theory to generate explanatory models of human social processes (Morse and Field 1995), it can also provide modification to existing theories and models (Strauss and Corbin 1990).

As will be discussed later, the process of data collection in Grounded Theory starts without prior knowledge about the subject to create new theory from the new data. According to Glaser and Strauss (1967), it represents a mirror reflection test for established abstract theories that fit between the theory and the reality of empirical data.

R. Haloub (✉)
Department of Management, Business School, University of Huddersfield, Huddersfield, UK
e-mail: r.haloub@hud.ac.uk

Z. Babar
Department of Pharmacy, School of Applied Sciences, University of Huddersfield, Huddersfield, UK

© Springer Nature Singapore Pte Ltd. 2020
Z. Babar (ed.), *Pharmacy Practice Research Methods*,
https://doi.org/10.1007/978-981-15-2993-1_8

They argued that Grounded Theory encapsulates "the discovery of theory from data" (p. 7) in ways that:

> …can be used as a fuller test of a logico-deductive theory pertaining to the same area by comparison of both theories than an accurate description used to verify a few propositions would provide. Whether or not there is a previous speculative theory, discovery gives us a theory that 'fits' or 'works' in a substantive or formal area – though further testing, clarification, or reformulation is still necessary since the theory has been derived from data, not deduced from logical assumptions. (p. 29)

In Grounded Theory the emphasis is on theory development. Although data is collected through the usual interview method (Morse and Field 1995), theoretical development is based on comparative analyses (or constant comparison) between or among groups of persons within a particular area of interest. It is this central feature of Grounded Theory (Strauss and Corbin 1994; Glaser and Strauss 1967) that permits researchers to recognise patterns and relationships between patterns.

In terms of pharmacy practice, the pharmacy role has been redefined recently from being a role solely of supplier of medicines to being a provider of healthcare and health services (El-Dahiyat et al. 2018). For example, the increasing number of medicines, the increased pressure to constrain healthcare costs (Thompson and Nissen 2013) and the rise of patient counselling (Palaian et al. 2006) are some of the evolving aspects to consider in the pharmacy practice.

Grounded Theory is derived from the symbolic interactionist theoretical perspective and the researchers' perspectives that are explicitly and exclusively "Grounded" as they appear in the collected data (Crotty 1998). The use of Grounded Theory allows a systematic identification of contemporary variables in pharmacy practices that could be adopted in diverse environments. The Grounded Theory also allows researchers to validate the results after reaching the saturation, which is the stage where the answers are repeated and no further questions or interviews are needed.

Despite the increase in the amount of research in social sciences and published articles using both qualitative and Grounded Theory methods (Eaves 2001), Grounded Theory is one of the most misunderstood methodologies (Shah and Corley 2006; Suddaby 2006). This chapter provides a structured approach in developing and implementing Grounded Theory with a special focus on pharmacy practice research. It is divided into six sections—Development of Grounded Theory, Building the Grounded Theory Research, The Interpretation and Development of the Story Line, Grounded Theory in Pharmacy Practice Research as well as a summary of the chapter.

8.2   The Development of Grounded Theory: Debates Between the Authors

It is important for pharmacy practice researchers to select the right approach in Grounded Theory. There are mainly three approaches, Glaser and Strauss (1967), Strauss and Corbin (1990) as well as Charmaz (2006), and these will be discussed in this section.

Grounded Theory was originally developed by Anselm Strauss and Barney Glaser in 1967 (Baker et al. 1992) and considered in the nursing doctoral programme at the University of California, where Glaser and Strauss were appointed (Stern 1985). That is why the initial studies using the Grounded Theory were in nursing (Baker et al. 1992). Glaser and Strauss (1967) emphasised the inductive approach in Grounded Theory and stated that the researchers must remain open in their approach to data collection and analysis, so that they will be able to make abstract connections in "thinking multivariately" (Glaser 2003, p. 62).

In 1990, Strauss and Corbin clarified the use of Grounded Theory in becoming more programmatic and over-formulaic (Melia 1996), which means that researchers can define the direction of research at the beginning of data collection. After Strauss and Corbin's publication, Glaser and Strauss's version of Grounded Theory became obsolete. Strauss and Corbin preferred a dimensional approach that influences behaviour, and they describe Grounded Theory as "a combination of hypothesis generation and verification" (Strauss and Corbin 1990), whereas Glaser (1992) adhered to the initial approach and argued the Grounded Theory should exist independently of the researcher. He said:

> …when the theory seems sufficiently Grounded in a core variable and in an emerging integration of categories and properties, then the researcher may begin to review the literature in the substantive field and relate the literature to his own work in many ways. Thus scholarship in the same area starts after the emerging theory is sufficiently developed. (p. 32)

Eaves (2001) supported the view that differences between approaches can be justified based on the type and aim of the research. Alammar et al. (2019) summarised the differences between the Straussian and Glaserian approaches in the following way:

> The Straussian approach allows researchers to hypothesize, contextualize, and relate certain categories and their properties together to create a theory. However, the Glaserian approach encourages the natural emergence of a theory without purposefully and directly linking categories or concepts. (p. 240)

In 2006, Charmaz established the constructivist approach of Grounded Theory as methods in theorising "social actions that researchers construct in concert with others in particular places and times" (p. 129). The process of interaction with data and creation of theory is through the shared experience and relationships with participants and other sources of data. Charmaz said that "constructivists study how—and sometimes why—participants construct meanings and actions in specific situations… so different researchers might come up with similar idea but how they render them theoretically may differ" (p. 133). Figure 8.1 shows the chronological development of Grounded Theory since 1967.

Based on the above-mentioned, there are three approaches in Grounded Theory: (a) the original (or Glaserian) approach, (b) Strauss and Corbin's (or Straussian) approach and (c) Charmaz's (or constructivist) approach (Denzin and Lincoln 2008).

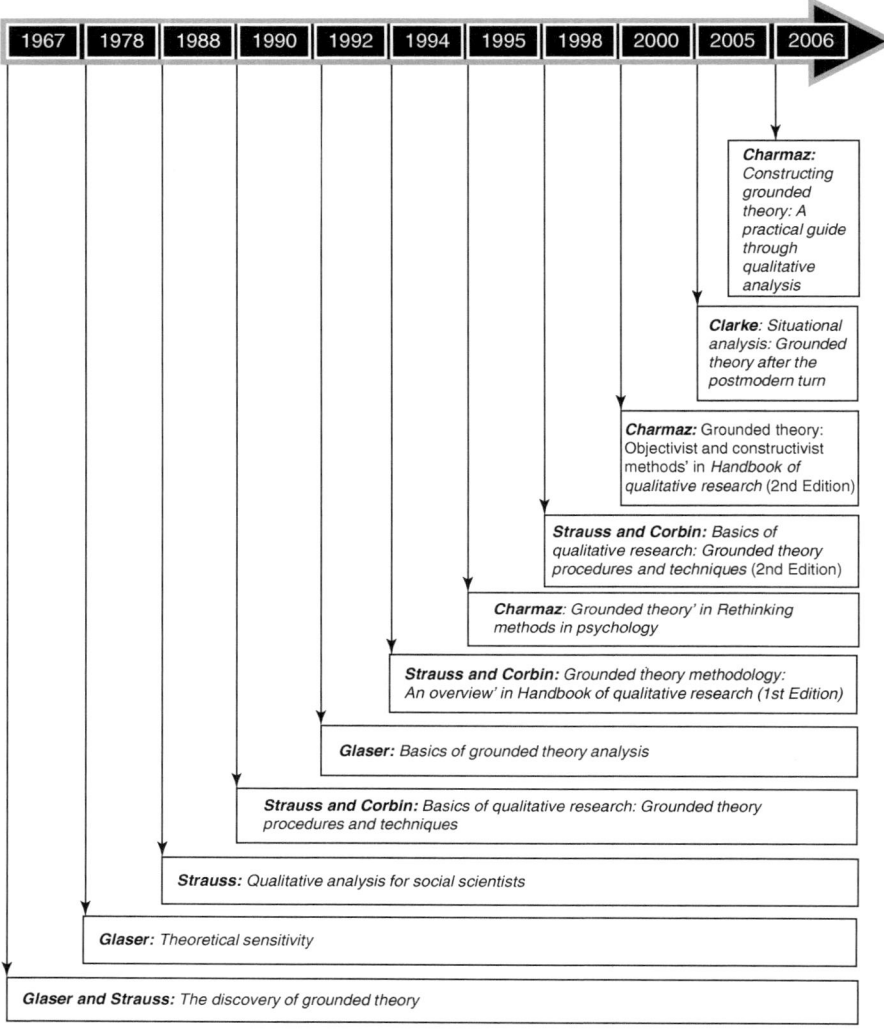

Fig. 8.1 The chronological development of Grounded Theory since 1967 (Birks and Mills 2011)

8.3   Building the Grounded Theory

With reference to Pandit (1996), there are five phases in building the Grounded Theory as shown in Fig. 8.2. These phases are not strictly sequential, and each phase contains different procedures that will be used to judge the quality of the Grounded Theory methodology. The first phase is the research design phase, which includes reviewing technical literature and selecting cases. The second phase is the data collection phase, which involves developing rigorous data collection protocol and

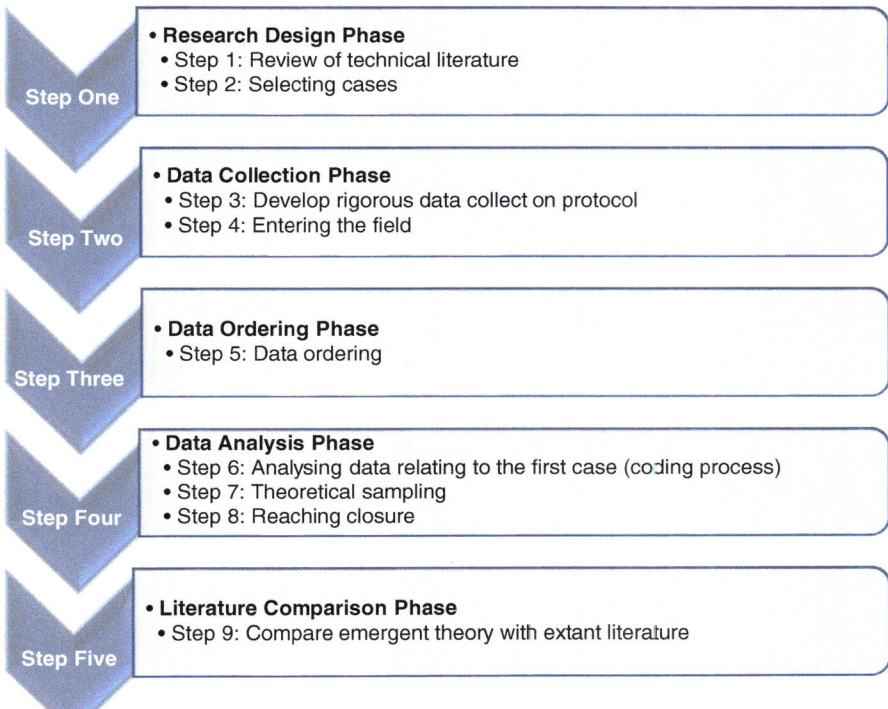

Fig. 8.2 The general five phases in building the Grounded Theory research (Pandit 1996)

entering the field. The third phase is the data ordering, which involves arranging the data in sequence. The fourth phase is the data analysis, which involves analysing data relating to the first case (coding process), theoretical sampling and reaching closure. The fifth and final phase is the literature comparison phase, which involves comparing emergent theory with literature.

8.3.1   Phase One: Research Design and Philosophies in Using Grounded Theory

The selection of Grounded Theory as an appropriate method is related to the research philosophy that stems from the review of technical literature and selecting cases. As explained by Birks and Mills (2011), these components of research design describe the relationship between the knowledge and the process by which it is developed (or emerged in the Grounded Theory research). The research methodology describes the set of principles to be linked with the research philosophy, methods and procedures that will be used in the research to analyse data. This is shown in Fig. 8.3.

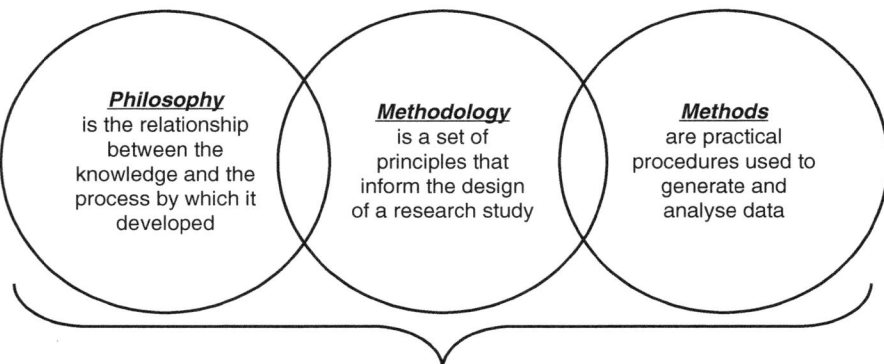

Fig. 8.3 The components of the research design. (Adapted from Birks and Mills (2011))

Choosing the target sample is very critical as respondents need to match with the phenomenon that is under investigation. This is in order to support the generalisability of the results. In Grounded Theory, the research sample cannot be planned, but sampling decisions evolve during the research process (Strauss and Corbin 1990).

8.3.2   Phase Two: Data Collection Phase

In using the Grounded Theory approach, the interview questions should evolve depending on the stage of the data collection (Strauss and Corbin 1990). The first interview should be unstructured and focused on asking general questions to test the understanding of respondents about the subject. Then each interview should be analysed separately through finding codes to be used in the following interview(s). The research questions will evolve at each step in the data collection process. The researchers can then stop conducting further interviews after reaching the saturation stage, which is the stage where the answers are repeated and nothing is added.

8.3.3   Phase Three and Four: Data Ordering and the Analytical Elements of Grounded Theory

Grounded Theory is "discovered, developed, and provisionally verified through systematic data collection and analysis of data pertaining to that phenomenon. Therefore, data collection, analysis, and theory should stand in reciprocal relationship with each other. One does not begin with a theory, then prove it. Rather, one begins with an area of study and what is relevant to that area is allowed to emerge" (Strauss and Corbin 1990: 23).

There are three fundamental elements of the data ordering in Grounded Theory including concepts, categories and propositions **Concepts** are derived from the conceptualisation of data collected, which are considered as the basic units of analysis to develop theory. **Categories** are "higher in level and more abstract than the concepts they represent. They are generated through the same analytic process of making comparisons to highlight similarities and differences that is used to produce lower level concepts. Categories are the cornerstones of developing theory; they provide the means by which the theory can be integrated" (Corbin and Strauss 1990: 7).

The third element of data ordering is the generation of **propositions** which involve conceptual relationships (Whetten 1989; Pandit 1996) that can be hypothesised and measured quantitatively in future research (Glaser and Strauss 1967).

During the data collection, the research codes and categories emerge, and this is based on full and deeper understanding of the data. Theoretical sample requires the researchers to use data in explaining the categories and in developing propositions until reaching the "theoretical saturation". This was explained by Glaser and Strauss (1967):

> ... no additional data are being found whereby the (researcher) can develop properties of the category. As he sees similar instances over and over again, the researcher becomes empirically confident that a category is saturated ... when one category is saturated, nothing remains but to go on to new groups for data on other categories, and attempt to saturate these categories also. (p. 65)

8.3.4 Phase Five: Data Analysis and Literature Comparison

The method of data analysis is identified by Strauss and Corbin (1990) as "the touchstone of your own experience may be more valuable an indicator for you of a potentially successful research endeavour" (Strauss and Corbin 1990, pp. 35–36). According to Pandit (1996), the data analysis stage is considered the central point in building the Grounded Theory research. In order to generate a Grounded Theory, the researcher should be engaged in a rigorous and iterative process of data collection and constant comparative analysis until theory is generated. This method of theory generation has to be very well defined and it should clearly use articulated techniques.

The first stage of data analysis is **"Coding"** which "represents the operations by which data is broken down, conceptualised, and [then] put back together in new ways" (Strauss and Corbin 1990: 57). According to Creswell (1994), meaningful data can be extracted through miscellaneous processes, in different directions, and then deciding the direction of data analysis and then perhaps themes emerged which are influenced by the research objectives.

Because of the nature of qualitative data and interviews, some data are not relevant to the research and can be considered as extra data which is not needed (Silverman 2000). However, despite this, researchers should not ignore irrelevant data, and it should be coded to make clear differences that are important for the research findings and contribution (Knight 2002). It is also critical to prevent short-sightedness during the process of developing codes and to have them arranged all together (Huberman and Miles 1998; Knight 2002). The generated codes that are not related to the research literature are continuously tested and checked against the categories to ensure they are fitted within them. Consequently, conditions and dimensions are developed, and finally, through an interpretive process (or selective coding), theory starts to emerge (Glaser 1978; Glaser and Strauss 1967; Strauss and Corbin 1990). Nevertheless, the data generated are not all handled at the same time, and inconsistencies or irregularities in setting codes can be identified by researchers. The coded transcripts should be double-checked at different times to evaluate their relevancy and suitability of the codes assigned.

The coding process is divided into three analytic types including open, axial and selective coding, and it is not strictly necessary to move sequentially from the open through axial to selective coding. **Open coding** is the initial stage of the Grounded Theory analysis (Glaser and Strauss 1967; Strauss and Corbin 1990), and it is related to identifying, naming, categorising and describing phenomena found in the text, where each line and sentence is read and coded, through the *constant comparative method* (Scott and Howell 2008). This method enables the researchers to derive general descriptors and understand the interrelationships between the open codes to be used as building blocks in the construction of Grounded Theory. The open codes will go through the process of elaboration and refining of the results. Similar data will be grouped together and labelled under the same conceptual label and this process is called *categorising*. These concepts were put into categories to be linked through finding the relationship in a process called **axial coding**. These connections will be in the form of hypothesised propositions specifying conditions, and the **selective coding** is the process of *integration* of the categories to create the **core categories** which are the initial theoretical framework. As explained by Strauss and Corbin (1990), "Core categories is the sun, standing in orderly systematic relationships to its planets" (p. 59). These categories are the central ideas or phenomena and are the first story line in the generation of theory.

Writing memos is an important activity during the open coding process, and it was recommended by Corbin and Strauss (1990) who mentioned that "writing theoretical memos is an integral part of doing Grounded Theory. Since the analyst cannot readily keep track of all the categories, properties, hypotheses, and generative questions that evolve from the analytical process, there must be a system for doing so. The use of memos constitutes such a system. Memos are not simply ideas; they are involved in the formulation and revision of theory during the research process" (p. 10).

There are three different types of memos including code memos, theoretical memos and operational memos. Code memos are needed to explain the links between open codes and decide the conceptual labelling, whereas theoretical memos link the axial and selective coding. Operational memos contain directions that represent the evolving research design. The categories are linked to the core category through the *core categorical relationship* or *conditional relationship guide*. Strauss and Corbin (1998) mentioned that researchers who are using Grounded Theory to analyse will "uncover relationships among categories . . . by answering the questions of who, when, why, how, and with what consequences . . . to relate structure with process" (Strauss and Corbin 1998:127). The relationship between the categories can contextualise a central phenomenon. Using the **conditional relationship guide** or a **conditional matrix** helps the researcher in constructing theory (Scott and Howell 2008; McCaslin and Scott 2003; Strauss and Corbin 1998). According to Scott (2004), the conditional relationship guide can be conducted by asking the following questions:

- What is [the category]? (Using a participant's words helps avoid bias)
- When does [the category] occur? (Using "during. .." helps form the answer)
- Where does [the category] occur? (Using "in. ." helps form the answer)
- Why does [the category] occur? (Using "because. .." helps form the answer)
- How does [the category] occur? (Using "by. .." helps form the answer)
- With what consequence does [the category] occur or is [the category] understood? (Scott 2004: 205, cited in Scott and Howell 2008: 6).

The conditional relationship guide fills the gaps in understanding the full picture after reaching the saturation stage. The consequence categories (in the last column in Table 8.1) that emerge are very useful in the **reflective coding matrix** to explain the dimensions and conditions of the story line (Glaser and Strauss 1967; Strauss and Corbin 1998). **The reflective coding matrix** is based on "the properties, processes, dimensions, contexts, and modes for understanding the consequences of the central phenomenon of interest" (Scott and Howell 2008, p. 6). It is also crucial in constructing the relational hierarchy, contextualising the core category and linking the major and minor sub-categories (Strauss and Corbin 1998). The reflective coding matrix is described in Table 8.2.

According to Richardson (2000), the subjectivity of data is the main motive for the crystallised verification in the relationships between the data collected in different

Table 8.1 The conditional relationship guide (Scott and Howell 2008)

Conditional relationship guide						
Categories	What	When	Where	Why	How	What are the consequences
Category 1	Answers from respondents' transcripts	Answers from respondents' transcripts	Answers from respondents' transcripts	Answers from respondents' transcripts	Answers from respondents' transcripts	Answers from respondents' transcripts
Category 2	Answers from respondents' transcripts	Answers from respondents' transcripts	Answers from respondents' transcripts	Answers from respondents' transcripts	Answers from respondents' transcripts	Answers from respondents' transcripts
Category 3	Answers from respondents' transcripts	Answers from respondents' transcripts	Answers from respondents' transcripts	Answers from respondents' transcripts	Answers from respondents' transcripts	Answers from respondents' transcripts

Table 8.2 The reflective coding matrix (Scott and Howell 2008)

Reflective coding matrix						
Central phenomenon	Core category name					
Processes *(actions/interactions)*						
Properties *(characteristics of category)*						
Dimensions *(property location on continuum)*						
Contexts						
Modes of understanding the consequences *(process outcome)*						
	Story one	Story two	Story three	Story four	Story five

directions, and this is why memos are a very important step in the analysis of data (Glaser and Strauss 1967; Glaser 1978).

Researchers should consider whether the continuous interactions between the participants and realities change during the time of conducting research. The use of a reflective coding matrix and conditional relationship guide can identify the changes during the time of conducting research.

8.4   The Interpretation and Development of the Story Line

The story has a descriptive nature in relation to specific phenomena of the research. As mentioned earlier, and according to Strauss and Corbin (1998), the core categories are used to integrate all the interpretive work of analysis which will explain the story line. At this stage, researchers should be ready to develop the cohesion and trustworthy story line. Reading the reflective coding matrix from left to right should describe the participants' story of the central phenomenon, and each process of the analysis is described and supported in participants' words. "Each researcher constructed a conditional matrix based on his or her study's reflective coding matrix that serves as a model representing the emergent theory" (Scott and Howell 2008: 14).

Figure 8.4 summarises Grounded Theory method until the emergence of theory. The unstructured interviews at the starting point will direct the researcher to the research problem. As mentioned earlier in this chapter, starting with totally unstructured interviews or having some direction is the main difference between the two main philosophies of Grounded Theory, between Strauss and Corbin (1990) and Glaser and Strauss (1967) at this stage. Transcribing each interview before starting the next and carrying out the analysis based on the analysis of the previous one(s) allow the emergence of knowledge about the research subject. This is done based on the principles of conducting analysis in Grounded Theory, as stated by Glaser and Strauss (1967):

> The process of data collection for generating theory whereby the analyst jointly collects, codes, and analyses his data and decides what data to collect next and where to find them, in order to develop his theory as it emerges. (Glaser and Strauss 1967: 45)

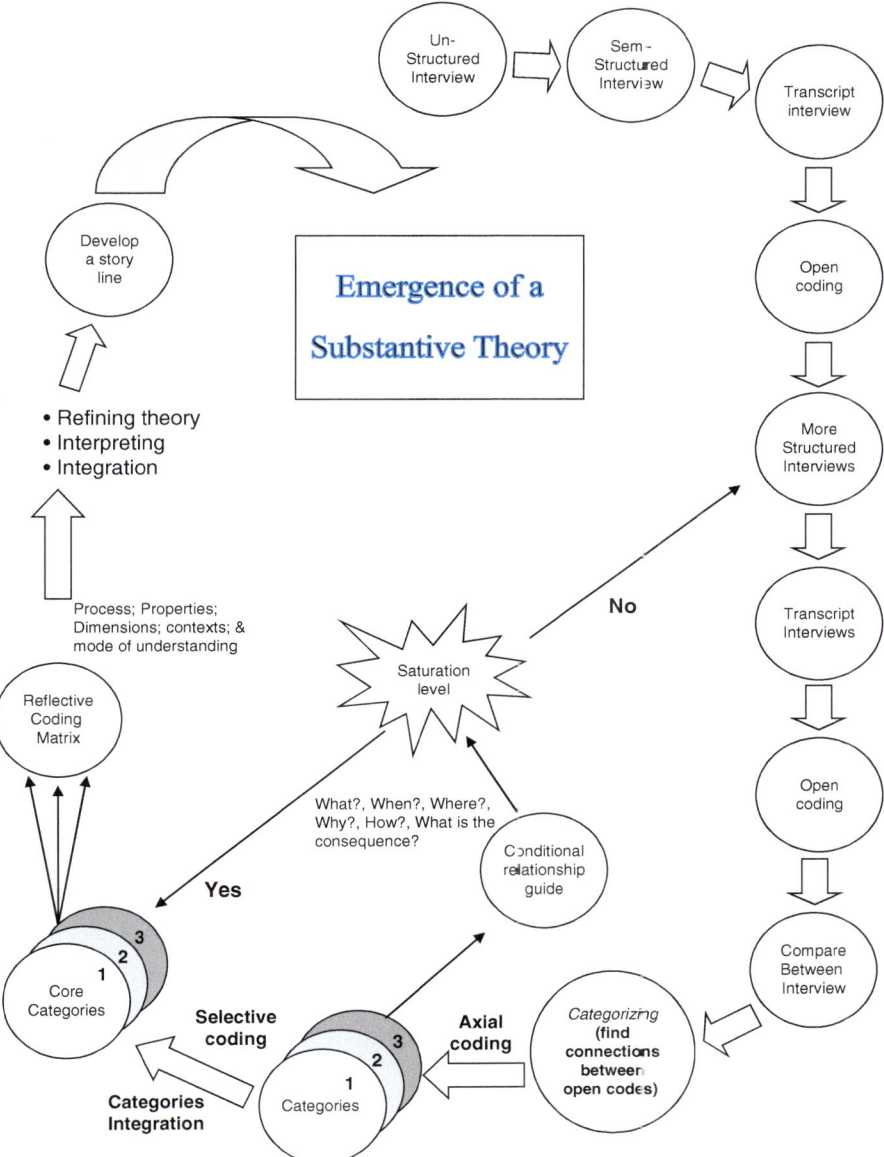

Fig. 8.4 The process of collecting data and analysis using Grounded Theory method and methodology (Haloub 2013)

The initial interviews are considered as part of building experience in the process of interviewing respondents and exploring the open codes that will be used in the analysis. After each interview, researchers should analyse it to break down the data collected into open codes, then the emerged codes should be linked to previous interviews to help the researcher identify common and conflicting points of view between respondents, and future interview questions should be designed based on this continuous comparison between responses and literature accordingly. Any uncertainties in the data should be clarified by modifying and developing new interview questions. The interviews and analysis continue until reaching the saturation level, where the same codes and information are largely repeated (Glaser and Strauss 1967). Strauss and Corbin (1990) identified the saturation level when categories identified in the research will connect to each other, and further interviews do not provide new inputs, but will rather repeat the same information in the date.

8.5   Grounded Theory in Pharmacy Practice Research

There is an increase in the amount of qualitative research undertaken by pharmacy practice researchers (Smith 1998).This is because qualitative research methods have the potential to explore emotions and behaviour from the perspectives of users (Auta et al. 2017).

However, a review of literature has identified that in pharmacy practice research only a very few articles have employed the principles of Grounded Theory. Some of these researches used Grounded Theory alone or mixed with other methods, such as quantitative methods, depending on their aim and objectives. For example, Adigwe et al. (2013) used Grounded Theory to argue the barriers and facilitators to implement changes in the UK health policy indicating nurses and pharmacists can prescribe medicines for chronic pain patients. The choice of Grounded Theory is suitable for this type of research. The authors used multilevel iterative approach based on the works of Charmaz (2006). Similarly, Patton et al. (2018) used the constructivist approach (Charmaz 2006) in evaluating the expanded clinical role of community pharmacy in Ontario, Canada. The authors used four pharmacies as cases to investigate. In addition to interviews, the authors used non-participant observation of provider, client activities and interactions with specific attention to medication reviews.

Some pharmacy practice researches also used Straussian approach. For examples, Benson et al. (2009) used Straussian approach that aims to understand pharmacists' values and include ethical dilemmas in the UK pharmacy practice. Moreover, Almutairia et al. (2013) investigated why antipsychotics continue to be prescribed in psychological symptoms of dementia (BPSD) despite guidelines calling for a reduction in their use. They justified the use of Grounded Theory as no existing theory adequately explains the continued prescribing of antipsychotics in BPSD. Due to the nature of the research, the researchers used Straussian approach, as they started with observation of the use of antipsychotics in certain conditions. Straussian approach was used by Cunningham et al. (2016) as they interviewed GPs and pharmacists in the UK (NHS); the aim of the study was to assess the perceptions and experiences of inter-professional learning and inter-professional relationships and the team-working.

Similarly, Cicelie and de Guzman (2017) used Straussian approach of Grounded Theory in their research which aimed to enhance the pharmacy curriculum and expanded the literature describing pharmacy students' experiences. Another example of Straussian approach was the work used by Daher et al. (2015) which investigated the impact of patients' religious and spiritual beliefs on pharmacy practice in Australia. The authors used semi-structured interviews and reached the saturation after 21 interviews. The use of Straussian approach in this research is because there is very little research regarding social aspect of pharmacy practice in multicultural and diverse population.

Tavakol et al. (2006) suggested the use of the Glaserian approach in medical education in hospital and ambulatory settings. Another example is a research conducted by O'Sullivan et al. (2014) as they gathered pharmacy students' opinions of the current pharmacy curriculum and what they would expect from a competency-based curriculum. By collecting the data using focus groups, Grounded Theory provided themes and trends emerging from the opinions and views of pharmacy students.

Another research conducted by Irwin et al. (2012) used Grounded Theory in analysing data, as they investigated the perceived impact of methadone[1] patient aggression on pharmacy practice in the UK. Their research suggested actions to reduce the impact of that aggression on pharmacy practice. Using the qualitative analysis, the authors reached saturation stage after conducting 16 interviews. Moreover, Sorensen and Bernard (2012) investigated the process for developing a change in package for the Health Resources and Services Administration (HRSA) by introducing measurable action items in Patient Safety and Clinical Pharmacy Services. The authors used both Grounded Theory and inductive data analysis techniques to allow systematic identification of indicators of patient safety and clinical pharmacy. Their research provided evidence of change concepts and actionable items that might be possible using different methodology.

Verweel et al. (2017) used the Grounded Theory in data collection to explore community pharmacists' perspectives of a decision aid for managing type 2 diabetes in Ontario; however, they used thematic analysis to analyse the data instead of using codes and categories. Another example of using Grounded Theory is by Katoue and Ker (2018) who used mixed methods in data collection (qualitative and quantitative), and Grounded Theory was the method used in analysis to explore the implementation of medicines reconciliation tool in practice in Kuwait. The triangulation of results provided the basis for removing barriers for implementing medicines reconciliation in Kuwait.

As seen in the examples above, all approaches of Grounded Theory were used earlier in pharmacy practice research, either alone or together with the other mixed methods research. The following part is the chapter summary.

---

[1] Methadone is a synthetic opiate used as an alternative to heroin as a painkiller.

8.6   Chapter Summary: Challenges and Future Opportunities in Using Grounded Theory in Pharmacy Practice Research

Grounded Theory is a very suitable method in evaluating complex social sciences questions; this helps to form a substantive theory from the data. This is widely used in business research (Ng 2005; Ng and Hase 2008). In order for researchers to develop a theory, they are required to understand the problem through the words of the respondents and how the respondents deal with such situations. The results of the Grounded Theory methodology are contextual explanations rather descriptions. This provides the "theoretical lens" for researchers and practitioners to share the research results in practical life (Creswell 1998; Partington 2000; Locke 2001; Dick 2002).

In the debate between the Straussian and Glaserian approaches, the main difference is the extent to which researchers use relevant material prior to the analysis of the data. Perhaps this is the point of conflict among Grounded theorists. Strauss and Corbin (1990) allow some flexibility for in-depth reading of the literature in the early stages; however, Glaser (1992) did not allow reading of literature until the identification of core categories that are formed from the collected data (Goulding 1998; Melia 1996).

Locke (2001) said that Grounded Theory is "particularly appropriate to researching managerial behaviour" as it provides explanations for the complexity of the managerial process, which further adds to its appropriateness in pharmacy practice research. Many researchers called for the use of Grounded Theory in pharmacy practice, including Austin and Sutton (2014), Smith (1998) and Norgaard et al. (2000). This method is best suited in research that involves social experiences and/or interactions in order to develop a theory or to explain a process. All examples mentioned in Sect. 8.5 provided an overview of using Grounded Theory in pharmacy practice research.

One of the main challenges in choosing Grounded Theory is the ability of researchers to choose between the historical approaches—Glaserian and Straussian—as the differences between the two approaches confuse new researchers. This sometimes leads to the flawed use of this theory in organisational and management sciences research (Alammar et al. 2019).

References

Adigwe OP, Strickland-Hodge P, Briggs M, Closs SJ. Developing a grounded theory to understand non-medical prescribing for chronic pain. Int J Pharm Pract. 2013;21(S1):1–26. Presented at the health services research & pharmacy practice conference, 9–10 May 2013, University of Central Lancashire, Preston, UK.
Alammar FM, Intezari A, Cardow A, Pauleen DJ. Grounded theory in practice: novice researchers' choice between Straussian and Glaserian. J Manag Inq. 2019;28(2):228–45.

Almutairia S, Mastersb K, Donyai P. Why are antipsychotics still being prescribed in dementia? Int J Pharm Pract. 2013;21(S1):9–10. Presented at the health services research & pharmacy practice conference, 9–10 May 2013, University of Central Lancashire, Preston, UK.

Austin Z, Sutton J. Qualitative research: getting started. Can J Hosp Pharm. 2014;67(6):436–40.

Auta A, Strickland-Hodge B, Maz J. There is still a case for a generic qualitative approach in some pharmacy practice research. Res Soc Adm Pharm. 2017;13(1):266–8.

Baker C, Wuest J, Stern P. Method slurring: the grounded theory/phenomenology example. J Adv Nurs. 1992;17:1355–60.

Benson A, Cribb A, Barber N. Understanding pharmacists' values: a qualitative study of ideals and dilemmas in UK pharmacy practice. Soc Sci Med. 2009;68:2223–30.

Birks M, Mills J. Grounded theory: a practical guide. London: SAGE Publication; 2011.

Charmaz K. Constructing grounded theory: a practical guide through qualitative analysis. London: SAGE Publications, Inc.; 2006.

Cicelie M, de Guzman A. Liminal adjustment experiences of pharmacy students: a grounded theory analysis. Pharm Educ. 2017;17(1):125–35.

Corbin J, Strauss A. Grounded theory research: procedures, canons, and evaluative criteria. Qual Sociol. 1990;13(1):3–21.

Creswell J. Research design: qualitative and quantitative approaches. USA: SAGE Publications; 1994.

Creswell J. Qualitative inquiry and research design: choosing among five traditions. Thousand Oaks, CA: SAGE; 1998.

Crotty M. The foundations of social research: meaning and perspective in the research process. London: SAGE; 1998.

Cunningham DE, Ferguson J, Wakeling J, Zlotos L, Power A. GP and pharmacist inter-professional learning – a grounded theory study. Educ Prim Care. 2016;27(3):188–95.

Daher M, Chaar B, Saini B. Impact of patients' religious and spiritual beliefs in pharmacy: from the perspective of the pharmacist. Res Soc Adm Pharm. 2015;11:e31–41.

Denzin NK, Lincoln YS. The discipline and practice of qualitative research. In: Denzin NK, Lincoln YS, editors. Strategies of qualitative inquiry. Los Angeles: SAGE Publications; 2008.

Dick B. Postgraduate programs using action research. Learn Organ. 2002;9(4):159–70.

Eaves YD. A synthesis technique for grounded theory data analysis. J Adv Nurs. 2001;35(5):654–63.

El-Dahiyat F, Curley LE, Babar Z. A survey study to measure the practice of patient counselling and other community pharmacy services in Jordan. J Pharm Health Serv Res. 2018;10:133–9.

Glaser B. Theoretical sensitivity advances in the methodology of grounded theory. Mill Valley, CA: The Sociology Press; 1978.

Glaser B. Basics of grounded theory analysis: emergence vs. forcing. Mill Valley, CA: Sociology Press; 1992.

Glaser B. Conceptualization contrasted with description. Mill Valley, CA: Sociology Press; 2003.

Glaser B, Strauss A. The discovery of grounded theory: strategies for qualitative research. Chicago: Aldine Publishing Company; 1967.

Goulding C. Grounded theory: the missing methodology on the interpretivist agenda. Qual Mark Res Int J. 1998;1(1):50–7.

Haloub, R. Assessment of forecasting management in international pharmaceutical firms. PhD thesis, University of Huddersfield. 2013.

Huberman M, Miles M. Data management and analysis methods. In: Denzin N, Lincoln Y, editors. Collecting and interpreting qualitative materials. London: SAGE Publications; 1998.

Irwin A, Laing C, Mearns K. Dealing with aggressive methadone patients in community pharmacy: a critical incident study. Res Social Adm Pharm. 2012;8:542–51.

Katoue MG, Ker J. Implementing the medicines reconciliation tool in practice: challenges and opportunities for pharmacists in Kuwait. Health Policy. 2018;122(4):404–11.

Knight P. Small scale research. London: SAGE Publications; 2002.

Locke K. Grounded theory in management research. London: SAGE; 2001.

McCaslin M, Scott K. Method for studying a human ecology: an adaptation of the grounded theory tradition. Qual Res. 2003;17(1):26–32.

Melia KM. Rediscovering glaser. Qual Health Res. 1996;6(3):368–78.

Merton R. Social structure and social theory. USA: Collier-Macmillan; 1968.

Morse J, Field P. Qualitative research methods for health professionals. 2nd ed. Thousand Oaks, CA: SAGE; 1995.

Ng Y. Managing collaborative synergy. Grounded Theory Rev. 2005;4(3):81–103.

Ng K, Hase S. Grounded suggestions for doing a grounded theory business research. Electron J Bus Res Methods. 2008;6:155–70.

Norgaard LS, Morgall JM, Bissell P. Arguments for theory-based pharmacy practice research. Int J Pharm Pract. 2000;8:77–81.

O'Sullivan TA, Danielson J, Weber SS. Qualitative analysis of common definitions for core advanced pharmacy practice experiences. Am J Pharm Educ. 2014;78(5): article 91(1–9).

Palaian S, Prabhu M, Shankar PR. Patient counseling by pharmacist – a focus on chronic illness. Pak J Pharm Sci. 2006;19(1):65–72.

Pandit N. The creation of theory: a recent application of the grounded theory method. Qual Rep. 1996;2(4):1–20.

Partington D. Building grounded theories of management action. Br J Manag Stud. 2000;11:91–102.

Patton SJ, Miller FA, Abrahamyan L, Rac VE. Expanding the clinical role of community pharmacy: a qualitative ethnographic study of medication reviews in Ontario, Canada. Health Policy. 2018;122:256–62.

Pettigrew S. Ethnography and grounded theory: a happy marriage? Adv Consum Res. 2000;27:256–60.

Richardson L. Writing: a method of inquiry. In: Denzin N, Lincoln NK, editors. Handbook of qualitative research. 2nd ed. Thousand Oaks, CA: SAGE; 2000. p. 923–48.

Scott K. Relating categories in grounded theory analysis: using a conditional relationship guide and reflective coding matrix. Qual Rep. 2004;9(1):113–26.

Scott K, Howell D. Clarifying analysis and interpretation in grounded theory: using a conditional relationship guide and reflective coding matrix. Int J Qual Methods. 2008;7(2):1–15.

Shah S, Corley K. Building better theory by bridging the quantitative-qualitative divide. J Manag Stud. 2006;43(8):1825–35.

Silverman D. Doing qualitative research: a practical handbook. London: SAGE Publications; 2000.

Smith F. Health services research methods in pharmacy: qualitative interviews. Int J Pharm Pract. 1998;6(2):97–108.

Sorensen AV, Bernard SL. Accelerating what works: using qualitative research methods in developing a change package for a learning collaborative. Jt Comm J Qual Patient Saf. 2012;38(2):89–95.

Stern P. Using grounded theory in nursing research. In: Leininger M, editor. Qualitative research methods in nursing. Orlando: Grune and Stratton; 1985. p. 140–60.

Strauss A, Corbin J. Basics of qualitative research: grounded theory procedures and techniques. Newbury Park: SAGE Publications; 1990.

Strauss A, Corbin J. Basics of qualitative research: techniques and procedures for developing grounded theory. Thousand Oaks, CA: SAGE Publications, Inc.; 1998.

Strauss A, Corbin J. Grounded theory methodology: an overview. In: Denzin NK, Lincoln YS, editors. Handbook of Qualitative Research. London: SAGE; 1994. p. 273–85.

Suddaby R. From the editors: what grounded theory is not. Acad Manag J. 2006;49(4):633–42.

Tavakol M, Torabi S, Akbar Zeinaloo A. Grounded theory in medical education research. Med Educ Online. 2006;11(1):4607, (1–6).

Thompson W, Nissen LM. Australian Pharmacists' understanding of their continuing professional development obligations. J Pharm Pract Res. 2013;43(3):213–7.

Verweel L, Gionfriddo MR, MacCallum L, Dolovich L, Rosenberg-Yunger ZRS. Community pharmacists' perspectives of a decision aid for managing type 2 diabetes in Ontario. Can J Diabetes. 2017;41:587–95.

Whetten D. What constitutes a theoretical contribution? Acad Manag Rev. 1989;14:490–5.

Chapter 9
Pharmacoepidemiological Approaches in Health Care

Xiaojuan Li and Christine Y. Lu

Abstract Pharmacoepidemiology studies the utilization patterns of medicines—also known as drug utilization research—which is an important component of pharmacy practice research. Pharmacoepidemiology also studies the relationship between medicines or other medical treatments and outcomes in large populations under nonexperimental situations. Providing an introduction to pharmacoepidemiology, this chapter describes frequently used metrics to understand drug utilization and medication adherence. This chapter also covers the key concepts involved in studying the association between medical or surgical treatments and outcomes. These concepts include forming a research question, selecting sources of data, defining the study population, and defining drug exposures, covariates, and outcomes. The chapter also discusses a range of study designs used in pharmacoepidemiologic research, including, but not limited to, cohort studies, case-control studies, within-subject studies, cross-sectional studies, ecological studies, and quasi-experimental designs. Finally, the chapter draws on key challenges such as confounding bias as well as commonly used analytical techniques to overcome these challenges.

9.1 Pharmacoepidemiology and the Need for Pharmacoepidemiological Research

Pharmacologic treatments are a major component of modern medicine. Pharmacoepidemiology is a discipline that uses similar methods in epidemiologic studies to study pharmacologic treatments but focuses on the area of clinical pharmacology. The birth of pharmacoepidemiology may be dated to the early 1960s (Wettermark 2013). Initially pharmacoepidemiologic investigations focused on adverse drug reactions but in recent decades also include studies of the beneficial

X. Li · C. Y. Lu (✉)
Department of Population Medicine, Harvard Medical School and Harvard Pilgrim Health Care Institute, Boston, MA, USA
e-mail: christine_lu@hphci.harvard.edu

© Springer Nature Singapore Pte Ltd. 2020
Z. Babar (ed.), *Pharmacy Practice Research Methods*,
https://doi.org/10.1007/978-981-15-2993-1_9

Fig. 9.1 Cause-effect
relationship between an
exposure and an outcome

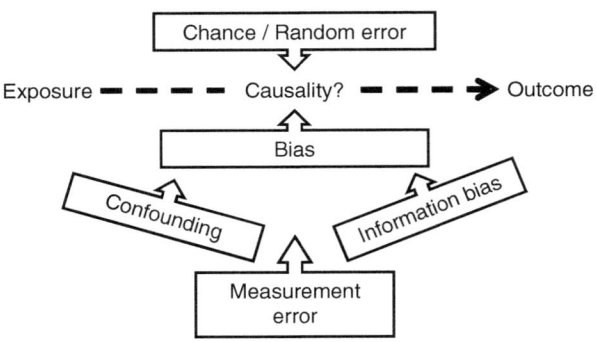

effects of medicines. In general, pharmacoepidemiology studies the utilization patterns of medicines, and the relationship between medical treatment and outcomes (good and bad)—see Fig. 9.1—in large, often diverse populations under nonexperimental settings over time (Avorn 2004). The driving forces behind the development of pharmacoepidemiology are the increasing attention on the safety and effectiveness of medicines and the growing awareness that health outcomes of medicine use in the rigorous setting of randomized controlled trials (RCTs) are not necessarily the same as health outcomes of medicine use in real-world clinical practice.

Randomized trials are regarded as the gold standard for assessing the efficacy and safety of an intervention. Randomization is the most important feature of this study design in determining causality (see Fig. 9.1), which ensures that the groups formed are similar at time of randomization, except for chance difference, in all aspects. This method maximizes the internal validity by minimizing confounding biases at time of randomization. The internal validity of a study is the extent to which the observed difference in outcomes between the study groups can be attributed to the intervention rather than other factors. However, RCTs have several important limitations. They are resource intensive and focus on effects of an intervention among a small population of carefully selected patients, who are treated and followed up for a relatively short period of time under strictly controlled conditions. Trials typically have strict inclusion and exclusion criteria that underrepresent vulnerable patient groups (e.g., children, pregnant women, the elderly, individuals with multimorbidity). Because of these limitations, the external validity of RCTs is often limited. External validity, also known as generalizability or transportability, refers to whether the causal relationship holds beyond the individuals included in the study (e.g., other settings or populations). Because RCTs only provide results of average patients in a controlled environment, they do not provide a true reflection of how medication use will impact health outcomes in patients seen in the real-world setting. In addition, RCTs are not feasible to answer many questions of importance such as rare outcomes. Therefore, clinicians, patients, and policymakers must turn to pharmacoepidemiologic studies for best available evidence.

Pharmacoepidemiologic research has an important role in supporting the rational and cost-effective use of drugs in the real world, thereby improving health outcomes.

Specifically, pharmacoepidemiologic investigations can contribute in several ways (Avorn 2004; Lu 2009). We will discuss these main research questions that pharmacoepidemiologic research can help answer in the next section.

9.2 Major Research Questions in Pharmacoepidemiology

Pharmacoepidemiologic research can define medication needs by measuring the prevalence and burden of a particular clinical problem to identify the clinical place for the new therapeutic agent. Pharmacoepidemiologic research can assess utilization patterns of medicines (also referred to as drug utilization research) and issues such as medication adherence (sometimes noted as compliance). Importantly, pharmacoepidemiologic research can examine the safety and *effectiveness* of medicines in large, diverse populations; effectiveness describes how well a medication performs in the real-world setting, that is, when it is used by clinicians treating typical patients over a prolonged period of time and in comparison with other available therapeutic alternatives. Pharmacoepidemiologic research can be used for drug safety surveillance by quantifying the frequency and severity of adverse effects of a drug or drug class.

9.2.1 Drug Utilization Research

Drug utilization research is an essential part of pharmacoepidemiology and pharmacy practice as it describes the extent, nature, and determinants of drug exposure (Introduction to Drug Utilization Research 2019). Drug utilization research provides insights into the following aspects of drug prescribing and use. It can estimate the number of patients exposed to a drug or drug class within a given time period. We can estimate all drug users, regardless of when they started to use the drug (prevalence), or patients who started to use the drug within a given time period (incidence). Drug utilization research also describes the extent and profiles of medicines use at a certain time point and/or in a certain region (e.g., country, state, hospital) and trends and costs of medicines use over time. On the basis of epidemiologic data on a disease, drug utilization research also estimates the extent of appropriate use, overuse, or underuse of medicines. It describes the utilization pattern of a group of medicines and their relative market share for a certain disease. Examining utilization patterns by patient or prescriber characteristics (e.g., sociodemographic factors, provider specialty) can help identify the target population for educational interventions to improve medicines use. Drug utilization research also compares observed patterns of medicines use with clinical recommendations or guidelines for the treatment of a certain disease or local drug formularies. Such comparison can help generate hypotheses whether discrepancies represent less than optimal clinical practice, determine whether educational or other types of interventions are required, or identify if the guidelines need to be reviewed in the light of actual practice. In addition, drug utilization research compares utilization patterns and costs of medicines between different regions and time periods. Such comparisons can generate hypotheses to further investigate reasons for and health implications of the differences found. Geographical variations and changes over time in medicines use may have medical, social, and/or economic implications both for the individual patient and for society and are thus important to identify, explain, and intervene, if necessary.

Drug utilization research often uses cross-sectional (see Sect. 9.4.3.5) or longitudinal study designs. Cross-sectional studies provide a snapshot of medicines use at a certain time (e.g., year 2019). Such studies may use similar data to compare medicines use between countries, different regions in a country, or different hospitals. Longitudinal data are often used to describe trends in medicines use (Vitry et al. 2011; Kelly et al. 2015; Chung et al. 2008; Lu et al. 2007a, b). Longitudinal data for drug utilization research can be obtained through administrative healthcare claims databases, based on a statistically valid sample of pharmacies or medical practices, or obtained from repeated cross-sectional surveys. Data collection in repeated cross-sectional surveys is continuous, but the patients or providers surveyed are continually changing. Thus, such data can reflect overall trends but cannot provide information about prescribing trends for individual practitioners or practices.

9.2.2 Drug Safety and Effectiveness Research

As indicated by its name, pharmacoepidemiology uses the study designs, methods, and techniques of epidemiology to study the uses and effects of medicines. In addition to characterize the use of medicines in drug utilization research, pharmacoepidemiology can study the effects of medicines in large numbers of people. One specific application is in the context of post-marketing drug surveillance, which has been broadened to include more areas in recent years, including effectiveness (Strom et al. 2012). As safety issues of medicines lead to major public concerns and both their effectiveness and safety affect evidence-based prescribing, studies discerning the effectiveness and safety of medicines have increasingly become a major emphasis.

Randomized trials are a great way to test the safety and efficacy of a new drug. The baseline randomization of the interventions, the careful collection and adjudication of the outcomes, and the execution of a rigorous, pre-specified protocol enable RCTs greater power to infer causal effects. However, RCTs are expensive, time- and resources-intensive, and sometimes unethical. RCTs also tend to have limited generalizability due to their strict eligibility criteria and other reasons mentioned in Sect. 9.1. In addition, some RCTs are powered for testing efficacy but are too small for studying adverse events (Evans 2012).

Pharmacoepidemiologic research, with large, diverse populations, can be used to examine the safety and effectiveness of medicines. In contrast to the well-"controlled" environment of RCTs, pharmacoepidemiologic studies can study the effects of medicines in the "real-world" setting where patients are treated in routine clinical care. Due to the large number of individuals included in the studies, pharmacoepidemiologic studies can potentially detect the adverse effects, for which RCTs mainly targeted for efficacy are generally underpowered. In addition, pharmacoepidemiologic research can study long-term effects of treatments over a long period of time and in comparison with other available therapeutic alternatives, which would be too costly for RCTs.

While data from RCTs remain the cornerstone of regulatory decisions, there is growing interest in utilizing robust real-world evidence generated from high-quality pharmacoepidemiologic research with real-world data to support regulatory decision-making. Following the twenty-first Century Cures Act (Bonamici 2016), the US Food and Drug Administration (FDA) has determined real-world evidence one of the most important topics to be funded under the Prescription Drug User Fee Act VI (PDUFA VI 2019) and committed to facilitating the use of real-world evidence and considering its use in regulatory approval decisions.

9.2.3 Importance of a Well-Defined Research Question

In pharmacoepidemiology, a prior specification of the research question (and study population, study design, and data analysis plan) in the format of a study protocol is recommended to minimize the risk of "cherry-picking" interesting findings and a related issue of observing spurious findings because of multiple hypothesis testing (Austin et al. 2006). The rationale for the study should be explicitly stated, along with what a new study can add to existing knowledge. The research question should be concise and clearly articulate the exposure and outcome(s) of interest when the effects of medicines are of interest. The research question should be formulated considering the strengths and limitations of the available data

9.3 Sources of Data in Pharmacoepidemiology

The research question should dictate the choice of data sources and whether the question can be appropriately addressed with a particular database. Knowing the relative strengths and limitations of the available data sources shall aim the selection of the appropriate data source for a particular research question.

9.3.1 Main Computer-Based Data Sources

Pharmacoepidemiology has grown rapidly as large-scale, computer-based databases have become increasingly available over the last two decades. There are three main types of large computer-based data sources frequently used for pharmacoepidemiologic research: administrative healthcare claims databases, electronic medical records (EMR) databases, and patient registries. Administrative claims databases contain information about the delivery of services or a record of events, collected primarily for payment purposes. EMR data are recorded during the process of clinical care. While administrative claims and EMR databases are valuable resources, they are not designed for research (Motheral and Fairman 1997; Schneeweiss 2007). In contrast, patient registries, disease-based or drug-based, are established for the specific reporting of clinical information and management of certain diseases and procedures. A more comprehensive description of data sources used in pharmacoepidemiologic research, including the three main types, can be found elsewhere (Strom et al. 2012).

Administrative claims databases (Lu 2009) with millions of observations on the use of drugs, biologics, devices, and medical procedures along with health outcomes are valuable sources for drug safety and effectiveness studies (Gram et al. 2000). Rigorous longitudinal observational studies using large healthcare claims databases can complement results from RCTs by assessing treatment effectiveness in patients encountered in routine clinical practice. Comparisons of results from observational studies with RCTs have shown that these studies often produce similar results and that well-designed observational studies do not systematically overestimate the magnitude of treatment effects and do provide valid additional information (Benson and Hartz 2000; Concato et al. 2000). Furthermore, observational studies overcome the limitations found with current pharmacovigilance systems, many of which rely on voluntary reporting.

There has been an enormous growth in the use of large administrative healthcare claims databases for pharmacoepidemiology, including outcomes research, drug safety surveillance, and healthcare quality improvement programs. Table 9.1 lists a few examples of healthcare claims databases used in pharmacoepidemiology.

Table 9.1 Examples of large electronic healthcare databases

Country	Name	Website
United States	HMO Research Network	http://www.hmoresearchnetwork.org/
	Healthcare Cost and Utilization Project (HCUP)	http://www.hcup-us.ahrq.gov/databases.jsp
	SEER-Medicare Linked Database	http://appliedresearch.cancer.gov/seermedicare/
	Medicare and Medicaid Databases	https://www.resdac.org/
	Veterans Administration Databases	http://www.virec.research.va.gov/
Canada	Population Health Research Unit	http://metadata.phru.dal.ca/
	Population Data BC	https://www.popdata.bc.ca/researchers
United Kingdom	The Clinical Practice Research Datalink	http://www.cprd.com/intro.asp
The Netherlands	PHARMO Record Linkage System	http://www.pharmo.nl/
Australia	Medicare Benefits Scheme Data, Pharmaceutical Benefits Scheme Data	http://www.humanservices.gov.au/corporate/statistical-information-and-data/?utm_id=9

Administrative healthcare claims databases have several strengths (Lu 2009). There is a good level of compliance with reporting, and the accuracy of data submitted is usually high, because the data are collected for administrative purposes and often closely audited due to the importance of correct filling for reimbursement reason. These databases contain information on patient demography, some clinical diagnoses, use of medical services and drugs, and detailed information on charges. Data can be used to answer a variety of research questions at a low cost in a relatively short time span. In addition, routine healthcare data reflect drug effectiveness and safety in patients encountered in real-world practice. Moreover, large populations of patients can be followed over long time periods, making these databases a good source to identify clinically important, rare adverse events as compared with RCTs.

One concern about administrative healthcare claims databases is about the data incompleteness. The use of prescription medicines may not be captured in the claims in some situations; examples include when patients use medicines during hospital stay, use their partner's pharmacy benefit (Schneeweiss and Avorn 2005), use of free samples (Li et al. 2014), or pay out of pocket fully for prescription medicines (Choudhry and Shrank 2010). Therefore, caution must be exercised when determining the start date for drug exposure using the pharmacy-dispensing data from healthcare claims databases.

Electronic medical records (EMR) databases contain rich clinical information on patients that are often lacking in administrative databases (e.g., smoking status, body mass index, vital signs, laboratory data). EMR data can provide data for better confounding adjustment, particularly for studies that may be susceptible to confounding bias. However, while EMR data capture records of physician prescribing, they do not record all prescribed medications taken by patients and are generally not considered as a valid source for identifying drug exposure. Another major challenge is the variation in available data fields and data standards across EMR databases (Kush et al. 2008), which may limit data linkage and, subsequently, study sample sizes.

Patient registries are also valuable sources for tracking relevant clinical, economic, and humanistic (e.g., patient health-related quality of life, patient satisfaction) outcomes of therapeutic treatments, including medicines. Registries are prospective observational studies of patients with certain shared characteristics that collect ongoing and supporting data on well-defined outcomes of interest over time. Given patient registries are designed specifically for a purpose, they may not have data to answer a wide range of questions other than what has been pre-specified.

Merging administrative and EMR datasets or data from patient registries can provide the opportunity to leverage the strengths of each type of data. However, such practice must consider privacy issues, data quality and transferability, and feasibility of merging datasets. Data linkage is discussed in the next section. Ultimately, the choice of data sources depends on the research question and whether the question can be appropriately addressed with a particular database. It is important to note that databases do not have all the answers researchers seek in measuring drug exposure and outcomes. In selecting a data source, one must at least consider the breadth and depth of the data in the database, quality of the database itself, the patient population that contributes data, and duration of information contained in the database.

For drug utilization research, household surveys are another data source to examine drug utilization and related issues such as adherence and access to medicines (Paniz et al. 2010; Bertoldi et al. 2008). Medicines available in households have been either prescribed or dispensed at health facilities or purchased at a pharmacy (with or without a prescription) or are over-the-counter medications. The medicines may be for the treatment of a current illness or leftover from a previous illness. Thus, dispensing data and utilization data are not necessarily equivalent because they have not been corrected for nonadherence, which is a common issue in real-world pharmacoepidemiologic studies. Drug utilization can be assessed by performing household surveys, counting leftover pills, or using special devices that allow electronic counting of the number of times a particular drug is administered.

9.3.2 Data Linkage

A pharmacoepidemiologic study may require data from more than one source either to enhance data available through linkage of disparate sources or to expand the size of the study population through combination of similar data sources. Person-level linkage of disparate databases can allow a more robust evaluation by providing a more complete picture of patient care and characteristics (Lu 2009). Such linkage can improve validity of a study (e.g., mitigating missing data, improving confounding control) or generalizability (e.g., increasing sample size).

Common linkages include the combination of inpatient, outpatient, and pharmacy data or linking cancer or death registries to medical records and may be within or across institutions. In the best scenario, each dataset will include several common relevant patient descriptors to allow a high-probability match (e.g., based on medical record number or other standardized person-level identifier, date of birth and residence); the more linkage variables are available the better. For common information across sources, rules for handling potentially duplicate information must also be specified (e.g., which record to be kept). In countries like the United States where no unified patient identifier is available, linking data from different sources typically require a probabilistic or deterministic linkage algorithm to account for ambiguity, for instance, slightly different spelling of names or addresses. The choice of linking method should be based on expertise in the approach used, previous linkage of the databases (if any), and the acceptable balance of false positives and false negatives, recognizing that some linkages will be incorrect and some will be missed. Furthermore, it is important to assess the overlap in populations because low linkage will affect sample size. Sensitivity analyses should be considered to evaluate potential linkage errors. Patient privacy is a concern when conducting linkages. Approaches have been developed for anonymous linkage (e.g., secure hashing algorithms) (Dusetzina et al. 2014), which are beyond the scope of this chapter. In recent years, more electronic healthcare databases linking data from different sources are becoming available, offering a more complete picture of a patient's journey through time. The examples include SEER-Medicare Linked Database (National Cancer Institute Division of Cancer Control and Population Sciences 2019), linking data from the Surveillance, Epidemiology, and End Results (SEER) program and Medicare, and OptumLabs Data Warehouse (OptumLabs Health Care Collaboration and Innovation 2019) linking claims and EHR data for over 200 million individuals covered by a health plan.

Linkage of data sources containing similar information on different patients aims to expand the size of the study population (Brown et al. 2010). Many pharmacoepidemiologic studies require very large populations. Examples include research questions targeted on small population of interest (e.g., hypereosinophilic syndrome or chronic eosinophilic leukemia), uncommon exposures (e.g., safety surveillance of new treatments), and/or rare outcomes (e.g., rhabdomyolysis). Multiple sources, for instance, data from multiple health insurance plans, will be valuable and needed to identify an adequate size of study population when no single database is large enough to address such research questions in a timely and adequate way. Examples include FDA-funded Sentinel System (Sentinel Initiative 2019) and the Vaccine Safety Datalink Project (Vaccine Safety Datalink (VSD) 2019)

Assessment of comparability of data sources is needed before data linkage. Comparability of data sources refers to the way in which the data are captured and recorded so that the data can be reasonably combined with respect to data capture and terminology. Comparability should be assessed qualitatively through detailed understanding of the data source and quantitatively across all relevant variables to ensure that information from the different sources can be combined. For example, claims databases of different health insurers may be comparable, the data may be captured via a standardized reimbursement system, and the information is recorded using standardized coding schema. For multi-institutional studies through a distributed model (Brown et al. 2010, 2013), data partners maintain physical control of their data in adherence to their privacy and security rules instead of all data partners transferring data to a single site for analysis in a centralized model, thereby giving up control. Comprehensive analysis to characterize data should be conducted to evaluate variability across data partners with respect to overall cohort metrics (e.g., age and sex distribution) and study-specific metrics (e.g., exposure and outcome rates by age, sex, and year).

9.4 Study Designs and Methods in Pharmacoepidemiology

As mentioned in Sect. 9.2.3, having a well-pre-specified study question is of great importance in a pharmacoepidemiologic study. A detailed study protocol should explicitly state the study question, the exposure and outcomes of interest, the study population, the measurement of study variables, the study design, and the analytic plans. In this section, we will describe the specific considerations for each of these elements.

9.4.1 Selecting the Study Population

The selection/creation of study populations in pharmacoepidemiologic studies is critically important because confounding bias is a particular concern in nonexperimental research. For pharmacoepidemiologic studies interested in assessing effects of medicines, study cohorts typically include a study group of patients who have had the drug exposure and a comparison group of patients who have *not* had the same drug exposure (but may be exposed to a comparison drug). To increase comparability of the study groups, study cohorts should be restricted to patients who are homogeneous regarding their indication for the study drug exposure, which will lead to more balance of patient characteristics that predict the outcome (Perrio et al. 2007; Schneeweiss et al. 2007). This approach will reduce but not completely eliminate confounding because it is likely that some factors that influenced prescribing decisions may not be available in the data.

There are two major exclusion criteria to consider in pharmacoepidemiologic studies to maximize internal validity by reducing confounding. First, if the objective is to examine the incidence, rather than reoccurrence, of an outcome of interest, make sure to exclude patients with a history of the outcome of interest; these patients may be at an increased baseline risk for the outcome and at the same time may be more likely to take a study medication. It is often better to exclude these patients in the cohort creation/design stage instead of adjustment in the later analysis stage, particularly if the condition is a strong risk factor for future events (and thus a confounder). Second, studies may restrict to incident users of the study medications. Incident users are those starting on a study medication without prior dispensings of study drugs (i.e., no drug exposure) during a predefined time interval (also known as washout period—see Fig. 9.2). An often-used washout period is 6 months. However, this period might not be long enough for some patients who might have taken the drug 9 months ago. Thus, a longer washout period can increase the certainty that patients are truly incident users. Unfortunately, using a longer washout period reduces the number of patients eligible for the study, thus reducing precision of the effect estimates (i.e., study results). Prevalent users are individuals who have been taking a study medication for some time. Prevalent users are likely to be those

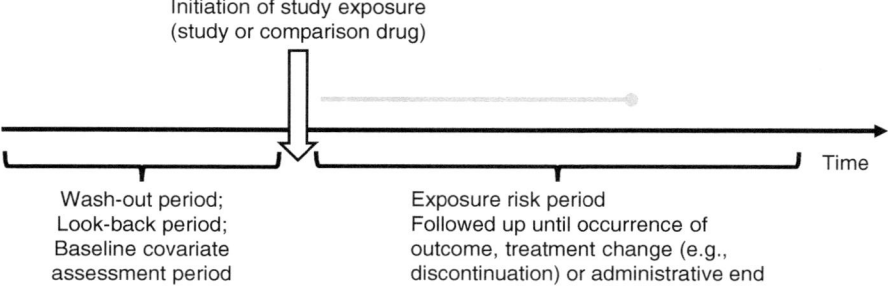

Fig. 9.2 Basic design of a pharmacoepidemiologic study

who tolerate the drug well, perceive some therapeutic benefits, and may lead to healthy user bias (Glynn et al. 2001). Restricting study cohorts to all patients in a defined population who start a course of treatment with the study medication ("new-user design") may reduce confounding (Johnson et al. 2013). The new-user design ensures the appropriate temporal ordering of baseline confounders, exposures, and outcomes, avoiding adjustment for intermediate variables that may be on the causal pathway between exposure and outcome. When used in combination with an active-comparator design (Schneeweiss et al. 2007) that compares the new users of the study drug to new users of a therapeutic alternative or comparator drug, the new-user design approach can help reduce the potential for immortal time bias (Suissa 2003) and also confounding by indication (Walker 1996) (see Sect. 9.6).

9.4.2 Defining Exposures and Outcomes

Drug exposures and outcomes in pharmacoepidemiologic studies must be operationally defined considering the formulated research question and the data source to be used. Because administrative claims data are recorded for billing purposes and not for research, both systematic and random errors can occur in the identification of exposure and outcome. Importantly, data are only captured for individuals who seek care and whose care is obtained through the insurance payment system. Claims for prescription drugs are generally considered a valid measure of drug exposure (Strom et al. 1991), although they may miss capturing some medication information, e.g., free drug samples, prescriptions paid in full by patients, etc. (see Sect. 9.3.1). Claims for medical procedures and services have been found to have a high level of specificity, but substantial variability in sensitivity exists across diagnoses when compared against the gold standard of medical records (Wilchesky et al. 2004)

Prescription claims data provide a wealth of information on drug exposure including dispensing date, pharmacy identifier, and drug information (generic and brand names, dose, duration in the format of days' supply). Drugs may be coded by established classification systems such as World Health Organization's Anatomical Therapeutic Chemical system. Using details like date of dispensing and days' supply, one can construct measures to assess medication adherence (discussed below). In comparison, while EMR data capture whether the physician prescribed medication for the patient, the dose, and intended regimen, they do not record whether the patient actually obtained the medication from the pharmacy. This nonadherence to initial treatment decision has been known as "primary nonadherence" or "primary noncompliance" and has been found to be substantial in real-world practices (Beardon et al. 1993; Fischer et al. 2010). This imperfect reflection of all dispensed medications taken by patients is a key limitation of the EMR data.

Medical claims data provide information on final end points such as fractures, stroke, myocardial infarction, or death but are limited for outcomes that involve intermediate biomarkers, self-reported symptom scales, or measures of patient functioning. Researchers may use a combination of diagnostic, procedures, and facility codes to develop proxy measures of intermediate outcomes. For instance, a study that used diagnostic and inpatient hospital stays to classify severity of chronic obstructive pulmonary disease found moderate accuracy to medical charts (McKnight et al. 2005). Recent years have seen an increasing use of laboratory result data linked to administrative claims data, but these data are not available on a large scale across the globe.

To assess the occurrence of outcomes, study cohorts are typically observed (followed) for a certain period of time after the start of treatment—see Fig. 9.2. This is known as the exposure risk window (or period). The exposure risk window is the time period during which the medication puts individuals at risk for outcome(s) of interest. The choice of exposure risk period considers the duration of medicines use and the onset and persistence of drug toxicity. Typically, there is an extension after the drug is discontinued to account for the period when a drug is still biologically active in the body. The choice of exposure risk windows can influence the estimate of outcome risks. Risk windows should be carefully evaluated, or sensitivity analysis should be conducted on the varying length of exposure risk window.

9.4.3   Study Designs

Pharmacoepidemiologic research typically uses epidemiological study designs and methods. This section introduces a range of study designs often used in pharmacoepidemiologic studies; they are also summarized in Table 9.2. It is important to consider all potential study design options before choosing the most appropriate one for the study question of interest.

9.4.3.1   Cohort Studies

A cohort study typically follows a group of individuals in which some have had or continuing to have an exposure of interest in order to determine the occurrence of outcome(s). In pharmacoepidemiologic research, the exposure is typically a drug or a medical intervention. Usually a comparison group of individuals who have not been exposed to the same medication, unexposed or exposed to a comparator drug, is also included in the cohort study. The probability of developing the outcome in one group is compared with that in the other group; this is called the relative risk. Cohort design can be prospective or retrospective and has a number of applications, including the study of incidence, causes, and prognosis (Goldacre 2001; Gurwitz et al. 2005). In a prospective cohort study, individuals are enrolled into the study before none of them has developed outcomes of interest. In a retrospective cohort study, both the exposure and the outcome of interest have already occurred, but the investigators will go back in time and assemble a cohort at a point before the occurrence of outcome of interest. As a result, no matter whether a prospective or retrospective design is used, a cohort study enrolls individuals into the study based on their exposure status and measures subsequent outcome occurrence. In other words,

Table 9.2 Study designs for pharmacoepidemiology

- **Cohort studies** follow one group that is exposed to a drug or medical intervention and another group that is exposed to a comparison drug or unexposed to determine the occurrence of the outcome (estimating the relative risk). Cohort studies can examine multiple outcomes of a single exposure

- **Case-control studies** compare the proportion of cases with a specific exposure to the proportion of controls with the same exposure (estimating the odds ratio). Case-control studies can examine multiple factors that may be associated with the presence or absence of the outcome

Within-subject methods:
- *The self-controlled case series method* assesses the association between a transient exposure and an outcome by estimating the relative incidence of specified events in a defined time period after the exposure
- *Case-crossover design* estimates the odds of an outcome by comparing the probability of exposure between the at-risk and control periods
- *Case-time-control design* is case-crossover design with the addition of a traditional control group without occurrence of outcome

- **Cross-sectional studies** are used to determine prevalence, that is, the number of cases in a population at a certain time or time period and to examine the association between an exposure and an outcome

- **Ecological studies** focus on the comparison of groups. They can be used to identify associations by comparing aggregate data on risk factors and disease prevalence from different population groups

Quasi-experimental designs:
- *Interrupted time series design* involves a time series (repeated observations of a particular outcome collected before and after the implementation of an intervention to evaluation its effects). It can be conducted without or with a time series from a comparison group (interrupted time series with comparison series)
- *Pre-post with/without comparison group design* involves one measurement of a particular outcome before and another measurement after the implementation of an intervention to evaluate its effects. Intervention effect is estimated by a difference-in-differences approach when there are also pre-post measurements from a comparison group
- *Post-only with/without comparison group design* involves only measurements of a particular outcome after the implementation of an intervention to evaluate its effects

cohort studies measure exposure and outcome in temporal sequence, thereby avoiding the debate as to which comes first and making it possible to demonstrate causal relationships. Another advantage of the cohort design compared with the case-control approach, discussed in the next section, is that one can examine a wide range of possible outcomes from the same exposure in one cohort study. A cohort study is usually cheaper and easier than a RCT.

Cohort design is inefficient for studying the incidence of a latent or rare outcome (e.g., cancer) because individuals would need to be followed for a long time. The major challenges include (1) selection bias caused by potential systematic differences between the study groups in factors related to the outcome, (2) the inability to control for *all* extraneous factors (confounders) that might be associated with the outcome and might differ between the study groups, and (3) bias caused by differential loss to follow up due to migration, death, or dropouts (Gurwitz et al. 2005). Bias and confounding are discussed later in the chapter.

9.4.3.2 Case-Control Studies

In comparison to cohort studies, case-control studies enroll individuals into study based on their status of outcome and then ascertain their prior exposure status. Thus, case-control studies are usually retrospective. One group would include individuals who have the outcome of interest (i.e., cases), and they are matched with a control group who do not (i.e., controls or non-cases). Same information on prior exposure is collected from both groups (Breslow 1982). The key measure of association in case-control study report is the odds ratio, comparing the proportion of cases with a specific exposure to the proportion of controls with the same exposure, that determines the relative importance of the exposure with respect to the presence or absence of the outcome. Due to the lack of the denominators for the two exposure groups, case-control studies cannot directly report the incidence rates or incidence ratios of the outcomes. In cases of rare diseases, the odds ratio approximates the relative risk.

As some of the individuals have been deliberately chosen because they have the outcome, case-control studies are more cost-efficient than cohort studies—that is, a smaller sample size is sufficient to generate adequate information because of a higher percentage of cases per study. Further, a large number of variables can be examined at one time while the outcome being studied is limited (i.e., presence or absence of the outcome). Case-control studies are commonly used for initial, inexpensive evaluation of risk factors and are particularly useful when there is a long time period between an exposure and the occurrence of the outcome or when the outcome is rare. The main problems with the case-control design are confounding, selection bias, and recall bias because people with the outcome are more likely to remember certain antecedents or exaggerate or minimize what they consider to be risk factors.

9.4.3.3 Nested Case-Control Studies

A nested case-control study is comprised of individuals sampled from a well-defined cohort study. The case-control study is thus "nested" inside the cohort study (Etminan 2004). Analytical methods appropriate for case-control studies are applicable to nested case-control studies with computation of an odds ratio. The nested case-control design is flexible in that it allows examination of an exposure not planned in advance if records of a specific exposure of the cases and a subset of non-cases are available. This design also reduces selection bias because case and controls are sampled from the same source population. In some settings, a nested case-control design may involve less complex analysis compared to a standard cohort design because confounding is controlled for through matching and thus avoids sophisticated statistical techniques such as propensity scores (Etminan 2004).

Traditionally, case-control and nested case-control designs are favored due to its improved efficiency relative to the cohort design in that they reduce the costs and burden of data collection. In contemporary era of pharmacoepidemiology where electronic healthcare databases are the main data sources, all exposure, covariate, and outcome data for the entire cohort are already available, so the cost of data collection for a single study approximates zero. Another feature that previously makes nested case-control studies attractive was its computational efficiency in the setting of time-dependent exposures (Essebag et al. 2005). Recent advances in computational sciences and technology make this advantage less relevant. Increasingly, researchers argue that these designs should no longer be used in secondary databases where data are already available (Schuemie et al. 2019) and suitable for a cohort design.

9.4.3.4 Within-Subject Methods (Case-Only Designs)

Cohort and case-control studies are useful for examining cumulative effects of chronic exposures. In situations where suitable comparison groups or controls are difficult to identify, within-subject methods that use self-controls offer a good alternative. The within-subject methods, also referred to as case-only designs, have the advantages that they don't require a separate comparison group and that all fixed confounders, unmeasured or unmeasured, are well controlled for (Petersen et al. 2016). These methods include self-controlled case series method, case-crossover design, and case-time-control design (Maclure et al. 2012).

In contrast to the case-crossover design discussed below, the self-controlled case series design derives from the cohort (fixed exposure, random event) rather than case-control (fixed event, random exposure) logic (Farrington 2004). The self-controlled case series method was originally published by Farrington et al (1995) to investigate the association between vaccination and acute potential adverse events and has also been used to examine effects of chronic exposures such as antidepressants (Hubbard et al. 2003). Using data on cases only, it is an alternative to cohort or case-control methods for assessing the association between a transient exposure and an outcome by estimating the relative incidence of specified events in a defined period after the exposure. This design retrieves the entire exposure history inside a given time window. Time within the observation period is classified as at-risk period or as control period in relation to the exposure. The key advantages are that the design controls for individual-level confounders (measured and unmeasured) that are stable over time and allows for changes in exposure with time (i.e., exposure trends) (Whitaker et al. 2006). Therefore, it provides valid inference about the incidence of events in at-risk periods relative to the control period and is suitable for studying recurrent outcomes.

Case-crossover studies can also eliminate within-person confounding that is stable over time because the exposure history of each case is used as his/her own control thus (Maclure 1991). They are useful for examining effects of transient exposures (e.g., use of benzodiazepine) on acute events (e.g., car accidents) and the time relationship of immediate effects to the exposure. It estimates the odds of an outcome by comparing the probability of exposure between the at-risk and control periods. However, the underlying probability of exposure must be constant (i.e., no exposure trends) so that the at-risk and control periods are comparable. Therefore, changes in prescribing over time or within-person confounding, including transient indication or changes in disease severity, may be problematic because they can influence the probability of exposure, that is, the case-crossover design may have time trend bias (Schneeweiss et al. 1997).

Case-time-control design is an elaboration of the case-crossover design (Suissa 1995). This design uses data from a traditional control group (without occurrence of outcomes) to estimate and adjust for time trend bias and control-time selection bias (Schneeweiss et al. 1997). The trend-adjusted measure of association is obtained by dividing the observed odds ratio in cases by the observed odds ratio in controls.

9.4.3.5 Cross-Sectional Studies

Cross-sectional studies are primarily used to determine prevalence, that is, the number of cases in a population at a certain time or time period. This method is also used to examine the association between an exposure and an outcome, rather than establishing causation. The subjects are assessed at one point in time to determine whether they are exposed to a medication and whether they have the outcome. A difference between cross-sectional studies and cohort and case-control designs is that some of the individuals in the study sample will not have been exposed nor have the outcome of interest. The major advantage of cross-sectional studies is that they are generally quick to conduct and inexpensive because there is no follow up. However, this method cannot differentiate between cause and effect due to the inability to discern the sequence of events and is inefficient when the outcome is rare.

9.4.3.6 Ecological Studies

Ecological or correlational studies focus on the comparison of groups rather than individuals and are typically based on aggregate secondary data. The unit of analysis in an ecological study is an aggregate of individuals, and variables are often aggregate measures collected on this group. One can use ecological studies to identify associations by comparing aggregate data on risk factors and disease prevalence from different population groups. Because all data are aggregate at the group level, relationships between exposure and outcome at the individual level cannot be empirically determined. An error of reasoning—"ecological fallacy"—occurs when conclusions are drawn about individuals on the basis of group-level data, as relationships between variables observed for groups may not necessarily hold for individuals (Wilchesky et al. 2004). Ecological studies provide relatively cheap and efficient source for generating or testing the plausibility of hypotheses for further investigation by other study designs (e.g., case-control, cohort, or experimental studies) to test whether the observations made on populations as a whole can be confirmed in individuals. Despite these practical advantages, there are major methodological problems that limit causal inference, including ecologic and cross-level bias, problems of confounder control, within-group misclassification, temporal ambiguity, collinearity, and migration across groups (Morgenstern 1995). Therefore, ecological studies should only be conducted when individual-level data are unavailable.

9.4.3.7 Quasi-Experimental Study Designs

Similar to RCTs, quasi-experimental studies aim to estimate causal effect of an intervention on an outcome, but quasi-experimental studies do not use randomization. For such studies, interventions of interest are often educational interventions, quality improvement initiatives, and health policies, rather than drug exposure in typical pharmacoepidemiologic studies. The intervention often cannot be randomized; reasons include (1) ethical considerations, (2) infeasibility to randomize patients, (3) infeasibility to randomize locations, and (4) a need to intervene quickly.

An interrupted time series design is a strong quasi-experimental design that evaluates the longitudinal effects of interventions through regression modelling (Wagner et al. 2002). It consists of repeated measures of an outcome taken at regular intervals of time (e.g., monthly or quarterly) both before and after an intervention that occurs at a defined point in time. For example, studies may aim to assess the impact of a policy or regulatory actions on drug utilization and immediate outcomes (Lu et al. 2010, 2011, 2012, 2014; Adams et al. 2009). This method can control for most threats to internal validity (e.g., secular changes in prescribing, aging of the population) because it adjusts for baseline trends in study outcomes that are unrelated to the intervention. In an interrupted time series study, the post-intervention outcomes that might have occurred in the absence of the intervention are predicted based on patterns of historical data before the intervention of interest, so it is possible to get more valid and accurate measures of intervention effects. A challenge for interrupted time series design is the typical need for relatively large effect sizes.

In an interrupted time series study, it might be challenging to conclude the observed effect was not due to co-intervention or some other events occurring around the time of intervention of interest. One useful design to minimize such confounding is the interrupted time series with comparison series design that includes a comparison time series from another region or group of providers or patients.

Pre-post with non-randomized comparison group design is another commonly used quasi-experimental study design. This design examines a single measurement before and a single measurement after an intervention in the intervention group as well as in a comparison group. The inclusion of an observation before the intervention provides some information about what rates might have been had the intervention not occurred. In most cases, if the intervention achieves its expected impacts, the differences in effects observed between the groups should come from changes in the study group. It is therefore important to show that the intervention and comparison groups were similar on a variety of factors before the intervention takes place. Statistical methods (e.g., propensity scores) are sometimes used to adjust for differences in baseline characteristics between the groups. However, studies that depend on statistical adjustment alone without strong study designs provide less convincing results.

Quasi-experimental studies can also use "pre-post without comparison group" or "post-only" designs. Pre-post without comparison group designs examine a single measurement before and a single measurement after an intervention in a single group. In contrast, post-only designs examine only measurements collected after an intervention has occurred. A pre-post study is a weak design; we cannot be confident that observed changes would have occurred anyway without the intervention due to previous trends or to external changes. A post-only study is also a weak design because of the lack of knowledge of previous levels and trends of the measured effect; thus, we cannot be certain that observed effects are due to the intervention and not to some other factors. Even if the study includes a comparison group ("post-only with comparison group"), there is no way to know whether observed effects in study and comparison groups would have been different anyway without the intervention.

9.5   Common Measures for Medication Use

This section introduces frequently used metrics to understand drug utilization and medication adherence, key study outcomes in pharmacoepidemiologic and pharmacy practice research.

9.5.1 Drug Utilization Metrics

The World Health Organization has recommended a number of quality indicators of medicines use (WHO 2018) that can be constructed from prescription or dispensing data. These include but are not limited to:

- Average number of drugs per prescription (per encounter or per patient).
- Percentage of drugs prescribed by generic name.
- Percentage of encounters with an antibiotic prescribed.
- Percentage of encounters with an injection prescribed.
- Percentage of drugs prescribed from essential drugs list or formulary.
- Proportion of treatment according to standard treatment guidelines.
- Average drug cost per encounter.

Data on drug costs are important for policy design and development to manage drug supply, pricing, and use. Costs may be determined at government, health facility, hospital, health insurance plan, or other levels within the health sector. Costs are often broken down according to drug group or therapeutic area to determine, for example, the reason for an increase in drug costs. For instance, the introduction of new, expensive oncology therapies may be found to be driving the increases in drug costs in a hospital. Changes in drug costs can result from changes in prescription volumes, quantity per prescription, or the average cost per prescription. Common cost metrics include total drug costs; cost per prescription; cost per treatment day, month, or year; cost as a proportion of total health costs; and cost as a proportion of average income (Introduction to Drug Utilization Research 2019).

A commonly used measure of drug utilization is defined daily doses (DDDs) per 1000 inhabitants per day, the standard unit recommended by the World Health Organization (WHOCC 2019). This measure allows comparisons of medication use independent of the country's population, the pack size, and dosage of the medication dispensed. The DDD is the assumed average maintenance dose per day for a drug used for its main indication in adults. Based on available information about doses (e.g., sales, prescription, or dispensing data), DDD/1000 inhabitants/day provides a crude estimate of the proportion of the study population that may be treated daily with certain medicines. For example, 10 DDDs/1000 inhabitants/day indicates that 1% of the population on average might get a certain drug or group of drugs every day. This estimate is most useful for chronically used drugs when there is good agreement between the average prescribed daily dose and the DDD. This method facilitates comparisons between drugs in the same therapeutic class and between different settings or geographic areas.

The DDD should be interpreted with caution. First, this metric is a technical unit of comparison and not a recommended dose and so does not reflect the actual prescribed dose. Second, the DDD describes the medication use in adults and needs to be adjusted first if pediatric use needs to be included. Finally, the DDD method does not consider variations in medication adherence.

9.5.2 Medication Adherence Metrics

Medication adherence generally refers to whether a patient takes a medication as prescribed, while persistence generally indicates how long a patient continues with the therapy regimen. The definitions and methods to determine adherence and persistence differ substantially in the published literature. Studies of medication adherence and persistence in large populations are important to understand factors related to low adherence (which will allow development of necessary interventions to improve adherence) and to assess clinical and economic outcomes related to low adherence and persistence. Medication adherence can be assessed by biochemical measures (e.g., levels of the drug or its metabolites in the blood or urine), patient interviews, medication diaries, pill counts, electronic drug monitors, and clinician assessments. However, these approaches are generally not practical to perform on large populations.

Administrative pharmacy claims databases are valuable sources for assessing medication adherence and persistence efficiently One major limitation worth noting is that actual utilization is likely to differ from observed utilization, and based on utilization data only, we cannot determine if the patient actually consumed the dispensed medication. Here we discuss some common measures of medication adherence using the pharmacy claims data (Andrade et al. 2006).

Two most common methods are medication possession ratio (MPR), which estimates the proportion (or percentage) of days medication was supplied during a specified time period, and proportion of days covered (PDC), which estimates the number of days covered over a time interval. Other related measures of medication availability include adherence ratio, refill adherence, compliance rate, continuous multiple-refill-interval measure of medication availability, adherence index, compliance ratio, or total number of days' supply dispensed during a specified time interval. The adherence measure is often dichotomized or categorized so that patients are considered adherent if a specified threshold was attained. A value of 80% or higher is generally considered adherent (Michael Ho et al. 2009).

In measurement of medication adherence, switching between drugs within a therapeutic class is defined as the dispensing of a different drug within the same class at some point during the study period (following the dispensing of the initial drug). Medication gap-related measures (e.g., continuous measure of medication gaps, cumulative gap ratio) are based on the number of days a patient is without medication. They can be determined for each refill interval using days' supply information in claims and the duration between refills. This allows calculation of proportion of days without medication during a specified time interval.

Metrics including discontinuation and continuation rates, often known as persistence, or the frequency of patients discontinuing/continuing medications are indicators of the acceptability of that medication. Discontinuation is generally defined by gaps between one dispensing of a drug and a subsequent dispensing, with continuous use based on the days' supply of medication dispensed or a specified time period after each dispensing (e.g., days' supply dispensed plus a grace period in days).

9.6   Challenges of Pharmacoepidemiologic Studies

It is critical to minimize the effects of chance, confounding, and other biases in pharmacoepidemiologic studies in order to provide results that are credible and convincing. Chance, confounding, and other biases are major threats to internal validity of a study and should always be considered as alternative explanations when interpreting the relationship between an exposure and the outcome. This section introduces major challenges in pharmacoepidemiologic research: misclassification, selection bias, and confounding, which are also summarized in Table 9.3.

Table 9.3 Major challenges in pharmacoepidemiologic studies

- **Selection bias**: Systematic error in creating comparison groups, such that they differ with respect to prognosis. That is, the groups differ in measured or unmeasured baseline characteristics because of the way participants were selected or assigned. This also used to mean that the participants are not representative of the population of all possible participants

- **Confounding**: A situation in which the seeming association or lack of association is due to another factor that determines the occurrence of the outcome of interest but that is also associated with the exposure, such as baseline characteristics, prognostic factors, or concomitant medications. For a factor to be a confounder, it must differ between the comparison groups and predict the outcome of interest

- **Information bias**: This occurs when systematic differences in the completeness or the accuracy of data lead to differential misclassification of individuals regarding exposures or outcomes

Definitions derived from the STROBE statement (Vandenbroucke et al. 2007)

9.6.1 Misclassification

A major challenge using claims data for defining exposure, covariates, and outcome is misclassification (information bias) (Vandenbroucke et al. 2007), that is, subjects may be classified as being exposed to a drug when they are not or as being unexposed when they are, similarly for the classification of covariate and outcome events. The likelihood of misclassification may differ between the exposure and nonexposed groups, often noted as differential misclassification. In general, the exposed group may have a lower likelihood of outcome misclassification because they have encounters with the healthcare system, which increases the likelihood of recording a diagnosis for the outcome event. In contrast, the nonexposed group is more likely to be misclassified as not having the outcome, which is an artifact of not entering the healthcare system.

With respect to drug exposure, the main data sources are prescribing or dispensing data. Research using these data sources need to be aware that drugs that are prescribed are not necessarily dispensed (primary nonadherence) and drugs that are dispensed are not necessarily taken (secondary nonadherence) (Beardon et al. 1993; Fischer et al. 2010), contributing to exposure misclassification. Misclassification can also occur when subjects receive their medications outside of the reimbursement system through multiple channels, including medication samples, patient assistance programs, paying out of pocket, taking medications belonging to someone else, secondary insurance coverage, and low-cost generic programs offered by retail pharmacies. Misclassification of drug exposure can impact outcome measurement because the risk of outcome is assessed during the time window when patients are considered "exposed" (exposure risk window—see Fig. 9.2). Misclassification of drug exposure can also affect the interpretation of the study results (Li et al. 2018).

With respect to outcomes, they are normally identified using a list of diagnostic or procedure codes. Misclassification of diagnostic or procedure codes can occur due to payment arrangements. For instance, clinicians are less incentivized to submit claims documenting care under capitated payment systems. Coding practices also vary under fee-for-service systems (e.g., upcoding—billings deliberately exaggerated to obtain higher payments, or undercoding—to avoid penalty). Ideally, researchers should consult clinicians who are familiar with the coding practice within the field under study or use definitions that have been validated against medical chart reviews in a similar setting. When several approaches are available to define the outcome, sensitivity analysis should be conducted to understand the implications of the various definitions on the results.

Correct classification of covariates is also essential for the validity of a research study. As patient characteristics and covariate status may vary with time, the assessment window of covariates is important. A common approach is to assess covariates in a fixed time window prior to start of exposure (i.e., fixed look-back period). Another approach is doing the assessment using all available historical data (Brunelli et al. 2013) and has shown to result in estimates with less bias but that requires more data assessment.

Misclassification of follow-up time in the exposure risk window can result in time-related bias, including immortal time bias (Suissa 2008), and produce delusive results. They can generally be avoided using appropriate study design and correct classification of follow-up time and exposure status in the analyses.

9.6.2   Selection Bias

Selection bias is a systematic error due to design and execution errors in sampling, selection, or classification methods that cause a distortion in the measure of association such that it does not accurately reflect the target population (Gurwitz et al. 2005). Selection bias will occur in cohort studies if the rates of enrollment into the study or the rates of loss to follow up differ by both the exposure and outcome status. Selection bias can also occur in case-control studies when the controls are not truly representative of the source population that produced the cases. One example is Berkson's bias (Berkson 1946), also known as hospital patient bias, that may occur when hospital controls are used in a case-control study.

In pharmacoepidemiologic studies, efforts should be made to avoid biased selection of study groups. Careful selection and clear identification of study population at the design stage are an important first step. Study groups need to be selected without knowing the outcome. Analytical methods including inverse probability of censoring weights can adjust for selection bias arising from the follow-up stage, such as differential loss to follow up (Robins and Finkelstein 2000).

9.6.3   Confounding

Confounding occurs when the study groups differ with respect to other factors that influence the outcome (Mamdani et al. 2005). For a variable to confound an association, it must be associated with both the exposure and the outcome, and its relation to the outcome should be independent of its association with the exposure. Confounding can cause over- or underestimation of the true exposure-outcome relationship and may even change the direction of the observed effect. Left unadjusted, results of nonexperimental studies may lead to invalid inference regarding the effects of the exposure.

Confounding by indication (also known as channeling bias) occurs when treatments are preferentially prescribed to groups of patients based on their underlying risk profile (Psaty et al. 1999). Patients with more severe disease are more likely to be treated (with higher doses) but also have higher risk of adverse outcomes. This confounding tends to make the study drug look worse when compared with nonexposed individuals. Confounding by indication is one of the most important, frequent problems encountered in pharmacoepidemiologic studies due to the natural presence of incomparability of prognosis between subjects receiving the drug and those who do not.

Confounding by frailty occurs when individuals close to death (or frailer) are more likely to receive certain drug classes or palliative treatments and are less likely to receive preventive treatments due to more focus on the main medical problem (Glynn et al. 2001; Redelmeier et al. 1998). This confounding tends to make the study drug look better when compared with nonexposed individuals.

The next section will introduce a few appropriate study designs and analytic methods that can help mitigate the potential confounding and selection bias.

9.7 Common Design Options and Analytical Techniques

Pharmacoepidemiologic studies typically use data that were originally collected for other purposes, so not all the relevant information may have been available for analysis, resulting in unknown and/or unmeasured potential confounders. This section discusses approaches that have been developed and adopted to improve the comparability between groups while limiting confounding and selection bias. Table 9.4 summarizes these strategies.

Table 9.4 Strategies to reduce confounding

Design phase

- *New-user design* restricts the study sample to individuals who are new users of a drug and follows them from the initiation of the treatment
- *Active comparator, new-user design* compares a cohort of new users for the study drug of interest to a cohort of new users of a therapeutic alternative or comparator drug, rather than a nonuser group
- *Restriction*: inclusion to the study is restricted to a certain category of a confounder (e.g., male)
- *Matching* of controls to cases (in case-control studies) to enhance equal representation of subjects with certain confounders among study groups

Analytical phase

- *Stratification*: the sample is divided into subgroups or strata on the basis of characteristics that are potentially confounding the analysis (e.g., age)
- *Statistical adjustment* estimates the association of each independent variable with the dependent variable (the outcome) after adjusting for the effects of other variables

Confounder summary scores

- **Propensity score**: the conditional probability of exposure to an intervention given a set of observed variables that may influence the likelihood of exposure

- **Disease risk score**: the conditional probability or hazard of having the study outcome conditional on their baseline characteristics
- Both scores can be used to control for confounding via matching, stratification, weighting (except for disease risk score), and regression

G-methods, including parametric g-formula, inverse probability weighting of marginal structural models, and g-estimation, have been developed to adjust for time-varying confounding affected by past treatment

Instrumental variables: a pseudo-randomization method that divides patients according to levels of a covariate that is associated with the exposure but not directly associated with the outcome unless through exposure

9.7.1 Study Design Options

The new-user design (Ray 2003), widely used in pharmacoepidemiology, restricts the study sample to individuals who are new users of a drug and follows them from the initiation of the treatment. This design avoids biases associated with prevalent users and adjusts for covariates at study entry that have been impacted by the drug already, also known as mediators.

The active comparator, new-user design is one option of new-user design that compares a cohort of new users for the study drug of interest to a cohort of new users of a therapeutic alternative or comparator drug, rather than an unexposed group. Coupled with an active-comparator design, the new-user design can help mitigate many of the biases discussed in the last section. This study design is regarded as the standard for comparative research in pharmacoepidemiology (Johnson et al. 2013).

There are additional methods to control for confounding in the design phase. First, restriction–inclusion to the study is restricted to a certain category of a confounder (e.g., male). However, strict inclusion criteria can limit generalizability of results to other segments of the population. In addition, in a case-control study, researchers can match controls to cases on certain confounders via frequency matching or one-to-one matching. However, the effect of the variable used for restriction or matching cannot be assessed and is a disadvantage of these approaches.

9.7.2 Analytic Options

In the analysis phase, stratifying the study sample into subgroups or strata on the basis of characteristics that are potentially confounders (e.g., age) can reduce confounding. The effects of the treatment are measured within each subgroup and can be summarized using the Mantel-Haenszel method (Mantel and Haenszel 1959). This approach may result in reduced power to detect effects because the number of participants in each stratum is smaller than the total study population. Subgroups may not be balanced with respect to other characteristics after stratification. It might not be appropriate to summarize the stratum-specific effects. Significant heterogeneity between stratum-specific effects suggests the presence of treatment effect modification, which is a characteristic of the effect under study rather than a source of bias that needs to be eliminated. In this case, stratum-specific estimates should be reported rather than a summarized estimate.

Statistical adjustment for dissimilarities in characteristics between study groups by including them in the regression model is a commonly used method to control for confounding (Normand et al. 2005). Regression analyses estimate the association of each independent variable (i.e., the treatment and certain characteristics of interest) with the dependent variable (the outcome) after adjusting for the effects of all the other variables.

Regardless of the approach used to control for confounding, the first important step is to capture and assess all potential confounders for the exposure-outcome relationship under study. A thorough literature review should be conducted to identify variables that can influence treatment selection or the risk of outcome. Complete adjustment for confounding would require detailed information on these variables that sometimes include clinical parameters and lifestyle changes, which are not well captured in electronic healthcare databases. Residual confounding bias due to unmeasured confounders would occur. The impact of residual confounding should be systematically evaluated in sensitivity analyses or mitigated via external adjustment if such data are available (Schneeweiss 2006).

9.7.3 Confounder Summary Scores

The rich information contained in electronic healthcare databases enable the study to control for an extensive list of potential confounders, but its sheer volume can pose challenges for statistical analyses. To adjust for the large number of confounders, confounder summary scores—the propensity score and the disease risk score—can condense the information contained in individual confounders into a single variable.

Propensity score, proposed by Rubin and Rosenbaum (1984), is the conditional probability of having the drug exposure given patients' characteristics that may influence the likelihood of exposure. Disease risk score is the conditional probability or hazard of having the study outcome conditional on their baseline characteristics (Arbogast and Ray 2011). The propensity score can be estimated from a multivariable logistic regression model, while the disease risk score can be estimated using a logistic or Cox regression model. The most critical issue of the confounder summary score techniques is the appropriate selection of covariates to include in the model to generate the score. For propensity scores, all factors that are related to the treatment selection and/or outcome should be carefully considered for inclusion (Brookhart et al. 2006). Instrumental variables, discussed below, should be excluded from the propensity score model.

Both confounder summary scores can be incorporated in the analysis via matching, stratification, weighting (except for disease risk score), and regression. When correctly estimated, matching, stratifying, or weighting treated and comparison individuals on estimated scores tend to balance the observed characteristics across groups (McWilliams et al. 2007). However, balance between unmeasured variables cannot be assumed across groups when these scores are used for confounding control.

9.7.4 Instrumental Variable

In recent years, the instrumental variable method, a technique that originates from the field of econometrics, has been used more commonly in pharmacoepidemiologic studies to overcome the potential lack of balance on unobserved prognostic factors (e.g., health behavior) (Greenland 2018). In brief, this pseudo-randomization method divides patients according to levels of a covariate that is associated with the exposure but not directly associated with the outcome unless through the exposure. The method may lead to equal distribution of characteristics in both exposed and nonexposed people and thus reduce potential confounding. For example, Brookhart et al (2006) used the prescribing physician's preference to cyclooxygenase-2 inhibitors or nonselective, nonsteroidal anti-inflammatory drugs as an instrumental variable to compare the risk of gastrointestinal complications associated with the use of these medicines. However, finding good instrumental variables has demonstrated to be remarkably difficult. Researchers should focus efforts on reducing the sources of bias (e.g., measurement error, omitted variables) instead of wishing for a "magic bullet" from instrumental variables.

9.7.5   Time-Varying Confounding

In real-world clinical practice, the treatment for a condition, in particular chronic conditions, often changes across time. To estimate the effect of the treatment, a study needs to appropriately control for time-varying confounding in the regression model. In situations where time-varying confounders are themselves affected by past treatment, standard regression methods for confounding control will be biased even when all relevant confounders are included and correctly specified in the regression model. An example is myocardial infarction in the estimation of effect of aspirin on the risk of cardiac death (Cook et al. 2002). Prior myocardial infarction affects subsequent aspirin use and the risk of subsequent cardiac death; it itself is also affected by previous aspirin use. Prior myocardial infarction is thus a time-dependent confounder between aspirin and cardiac death that is also affected by previous treatment.

Several approaches have been proposed to estimate effects of treatment in the presence of time-varying confounding affected by past treatment. Collectively referred to as "g-methods," these approaches include the parametric g-formula (Robins 1986), inverse probability weighting of marginal structural models (Robins et al. 2000; Hernán et al. 2000), and g-estimation. Few applications of these approaches exist in pharmacoepidemiology due to lack of sufficient information on time-varying confounders in administrative healthcare databases and limited availability of or familiarity with analytical tools to implement the relatively complex algorithms (Li et al. 2017). Fortunately, the increasing availability of data sources that contain more complete longitudinal information and better understanding of the g-methods begins to facilitate the use of these methods to estimate effects of complex time-varying treatment and treatment strategies.

9.8   The Future of Pharmacoepidemiology

We have been fortunate to live in an era where large amounts of data are available for research, including genetic information. Genetic information in the field of medical care includes a person's genetic predisposition to disease (e.g., results of specific genetic tests), diagnosis of heritable medical conditions, or family history of disease with a known pattern of inheritance. Genetic testing may help identify DNA variants that predict an individual's response to a drug or course of therapy, resulting in identifying groups that may benefit most in terms of treatment effectiveness while avoiding adverse effects.

The public, patients, and consumers have a lot of concerns about confidentiality and the inappropriate use of the sensitive genetic information that may affect employment or health insurance rights. Higher privacy standards may be required than those for other medical information. To address these concerns, the International Declaration on Human Genetic Data was adopted in October 2003; this and the Universal Declaration on the Human Genome and Human Rights are the only international points of reference in the field of bioethics (International Declaration on Human Genetic Data: UNESCO 2019). Furthermore, in May 2007, member countries of Organization for Economic Cooperation and Development (OECD) adopted the Guidelines for Quality Assurance in Molecular Genetic Testing, which provides principles and best practice for the quality assurance of molecular genetic testing (OECD Guidelines for Quality Assurance in Genetic Testing—OECD 2019). Based on OECD Privacy Guidelines, the protection of patient privacy has generally been safeguarded by laws in some countries including OECD member countries. Pharmacoepidemiology has begun to see increasing research questions involving genetic information and will see more in the future. Researchers in the field should pay attention to legislations, policies, and guidelines for use of genetic information for research.

The availability of electronic healthcare databases and advances in pharmacoepidemiologic methods enable researchers to identify products in which effectiveness in the real world does not match efficacy shown in the trials. This will challenge the actions of all concerned—industry, regulators, payers, healthcare providers, and patients. In recent years, the European Medicines Agency and the US FDA have required risk management plans or risk evaluation and mitigation strategies as part of the drug approval process to help ensure that the benefits of a particular medicine outweigh its risks in the real-world setting. Observational studies are also increasingly requested by payers and other agencies to assess the value of medicines. Patients may also demand better systems to monitor effectiveness and safety of medicines. In fact, it is best practice to establish a systematic, comprehensive approach to monitor all marketed drugs postlaunch, and abundant electronic healthcare databases present a unique opportunity. Such monitoring may range from descriptive utilization statistics to sophisticated comparative effectiveness research, depending on the budget impact and level of uncertainty about the risk-benefit of the medicine at the time of marketing.

The data explosion in modern society will surely continue As presented in this chapter, the nature of drug monitoring activities will be determined by the availability of data, advances in research methods and biostatistics, and competent pharmacoepidemiologists. Pharmacoepidemiology will also continue to be an area for collaboration between multiple stakeholders, including physicians, regulators, payers, manufacturers, patients, and the general public. Given the important contribution of pharmacoepidemiologic studies, collaboration should also involve decision-makers for drug formularies, health economists, and health policy researchers. Pharmacoepidemiology will likely continue to be one of the most dynamic and challenging research areas for the coming decades.

Acknowledgement We thank Caitlin Lupton, M.Sc., of Harvard Pilgrim Health Care Institute for research assistance and administrative support.

References

Adams AS, Zhang F, LeCates RF, et al. Prior authorization for antidepressants in Medicaid: effects among disabled dual enrollees. Arch Intern Med. 2009;169(8):750–6. https://doi.org/10.1001/archinternmed.2009.39.

Andrade SE, Kahler KH, Frech F, Chan KA. Methods for evaluation of medication adherence and persistence using automated databases. Pharmacoepidemiol Drug Saf. 2006;15(8):565–74. https://doi.org/10.1002/pds.1230.

Arbogast PG, Ray WA. Performance of disease risk scores, propensity scores, and traditional multivariable outcome regression in the presence of multiple confounders. Am J Epidemiol. 2011;174(5):613–20. https://doi.org/10.1093/aje/kwr143.

Austin PC, Mamdani MM, Juurlink DN, Hux JE. Testing multiple statistical hypotheses resulted in spurious associations: a study of astrological signs and health. J Clin Epidemiol. 2006;59(9):964–9. https://doi.org/10.1016/j.jclinepi.2006.01.012.

Avorn J. The role of pharmacoepidemiology and pharmacoeconomics in promoting access and stimulating innovation. Pharmacoeconomics. 2004;22(2):81–6. https://doi.org/10.2165/00019053-200422002-00009.

Beardon PH, McGilchrist MM, McKendrick AD, McDevitt DG, MacDonald TM. Primary non-compliance with prescribed medication in primary care. BMJ. 1993;307(6908):846–8.

Benson K, Hartz AJ. A comparison of observational studies and randomized, controlled trials. N Engl J Med. 2000;342:1878–86.

Berkson J. Limitations of the application of fourfold table analysis to hospital data. Biometrics. 1946;2(3):47–53.

Bertoldi AD, Barros AJ, Wagner A, Ross-Degnan D, Hallal PC. A descriptive review of the methodologies used in household surveys on medicine utilization. BMC Health Serv Res. 2008;8(1):222. https://doi.org/10.1186/1472-6963-8-222.

Bonamici S. Text—H.R.34—114th congress (2015–2016): 21st century cures act. https://www.congress.gov/bill/114th-congress/house-bill/34/text. Published 13 Dec 2016. Accessed 15 Oct 2019.

Breslow N. Design and analysis of case-control studies. Annu Rev Public Health. 1982;3(1):29–54. https://doi.org/10.1146/annurev.pu.03.050182.000333.

Brookhart MA, Schneeweiss S, Rothman KJ, Glynn RJ, Avorn J, Stürmer T. Variable selection for propensity score models. Am J Epidemiol. 2006;163(12):1149–56. https://doi.org/10.1093/aje/kwj149.

Brookhart MA, Wang P, Solomon DH, Schneeweiss S. Evaluating short-term drug effects using a physician-specific prescribing preference as an instrumental variable. Epidemiology. 2006;17(3):268–75. https://doi.org/10.1097/01.ede.0000193606.58671.c5.

Brown J, Holmes J, Shah K, Hall K, Lazarus R, Platt R. Distributed health data networks: a practical and preferred approach to multi-institutional evaluations of comparative effectiveness, safety, and quality of care. Med Care. 2010;48(6):S45. https://doi.org/10.1097/MLR.0b013e3181d9919f.

Brown J, Kahn M, Toh S. Data quality assessment for comparative effectiveness research in distributed data networks. Med Care. 2013;51:S22. https://doi.org/10.1097/MLR.0b013e31829b1e2c.

Brunelli SM, Gagne JJ, Huybrechts KF, et al. Estimation using all available covariate information versus a fixed look-back window for dichotomous covariates. Pharmacoepidemiol Drug Saf. 2013;22(5):542–50. https://doi.org/10.1002/pds.3434.

Choudhry NK, Shrank WH. Four-dollar generics—increased accessibility, impaired quality assurance. N Engl J Med. 2010;363(20):1885–7. https://doi.org/10.1056/NEJMp1006189.

Chung Y, Lu CY, Graham GG, Mant A, Day RO. Utilization of allopurinol in the Australian community. Intern Med J. 2008;38(6a):388–95. https://doi.org/10.1111/j.1445-5994.2008.01641.x.

Concato J, Shah N, Horwitz RI. Randomized, controlled trials, observational studies, and the hierarchy of research designs. N Engl J Med. 2000;342(25):1887–92.

Cook NR, Cole SR, Hennekens CH. Use of a marginal structural model to determine the effect of aspirin on cardiovascular mortality in the physicians' health study. Am J Epidemiol. 2002;155(11):1045–53. https://doi.org/10.1093/aje/155.11.1045.

Dusetzina SB, Tyree S, Meyer A-M, Meyer A, Green L, Carpenter WR. Linking data for health services research: a framework and instructional guide. Rockville, MD: Agency for Healthcare Research and Quality (US); 2014. http://www.ncbi.nlm.nih.gov/books/NBK253313/. Accessed 15 Oct 2019.

Essebag V, Platt RW, Abrahamowicz M, Pilote L. Comparison of nested case-control and survival analysis methodologies for analysis of time-dependent exposure. BMC Med Res Methodol. 2005;5(1):5. https://doi.org/10.1186/1471-2288-5-5.

Etminan M. Pharmacoepidemiology II: The nested case-control study—a novel approach in pharmacoepidemiologic research. Pharmacotherapy. 2004;24(9):1105–9. https://doi.org/10.1592/phco.24.13.1105.38083.

Evans SJW. An agenda for UK clinical pharmacology pharmacoepidemiology. Br J Clin Pharmacol. 2012;73(6):973–8. https://doi.org/10.1111/j.1365-2125.2012.04248.x.

Farrington CP. Re: "Risk analysis of aseptic meningitis after measles-mumps-rubella vaccination in Korean children by using a case-crossover design". Am J Epidemiol. 2004;159(7):717–8. https://doi.org/10.1093/aje/kwh093.

Farrington P, Pugh S, Colville A, et al. A new method for active surveillance of adverse events from diphtheria/tetanus/pertussis and measles/mumps/rubella vaccines. Lancet. 1995;345(8949):567–9.

Fischer MA, Stedman MR, Lii J, et al. Primary medication non-adherence: analysis of 195,930 electronic prescriptions. J Gen Intern Med. 2010;25(4):284–90. https://doi.org/10.1007/s11606-010-1253-9.

Glynn R, Knight E, Levin R, Avorn J. Paradoxical relations of drug treatment with mortality in older persons. Epidemiology. 2001;12(6):682–9.

Goldacre M. The role of cohort studies in medical research. Pharmacoepidemiol Drug Saf. 2001;10(1):5–11. https://doi.org/10.1002/pds.562.

Gram LF, Hallas J, Andersen M. Pharmacovigilance based on prescription databases. Pharmacol Toxicol. 2000;86(s1):13–5. https://doi.org/10.1034/j.1600-0773.2000.d01-4.x.

Greenland S. An introduction to instrumental variables for epidemiologists. Int J Epidemiol. 2018;47(1):358. https://doi.org/10.1093/ije/dyx275.

Gurwitz JH, Sykora K, Mamdani M, et al. Reader's guide to critical appraisal of cohort studies: 1. Role and design. BMJ. 2005;330(7496):895–7.

Hernán M, Brumback B, Robins J. Marginal structural models to estimate the causal effect of zidovudine on the survival of HIV-positive men. Epidemiology. 2000;11(5):561–70.

Ho PM, Bryson CL, Rumsfeld JS. Medication adherence: its importance in cardiovascular outcomes. Circulation. 2009;119(23):3028–35. https://doi.org/10.1161/CIRCULATIONAHA.108.768986.

Hubbard R, Farrington P, Smith C, Smeeth L, Tattersfield A. Exposure to tricyclic and selective serotonin reuptake inhibitor antidepressants and the risk of hip fracture. Am J Epidemiol. 2003;158(1):77–84. https://doi.org/10.1093/aje/kwg114.

International Declaration on Human Genetic Data: UNESCO. http://portal.unesco.org/en/ev.php-URL_ID=17720&URL_DO=DO_TOPIC&URL_SECTION=201.html. Accessed 15 Oct 2019.

Introduction to Drug Utilization Research. https://apps.who.int/medicinedocs/en/d/Js4876e/. Accessed 15 Oct 15 2019.

Johnson ES, Bartman BA, Briesacher BA, et al. The incident user design in comparative effectiveness research. Pharmacoepidemiol Drug Saf. 2013;22(1):1–6. https://doi.org/10.1002/pds.3334.

Kelly E, Lu CY, Albertini S, Vitry A. Longitudinal trends in utilization of endocrine therapies for breast cancer: an international comparison. J Clin Pharm Ther. 2015;40(1):76–82. https://doi.org/10.1111/jcpt.12227.

Kush RD, Helton E, Rockhold FW, Hardison CD. Electronic health records, medical research, and the tower of babel. N Engl J Med. 2008;358(16):1738–40. https://doi.org/10.1056/NEJMsb0800209.

Li X, Cole SR, Westreich D, Brookhart MA. Primary non-adherence and the new-user design. Pharmacoepidemiol Drug Saf. 2018;27(4):361–4. https://doi.org/10.1002/pds.4403.

Li X, Stürmer T, Brookhart MA. Evidence of sample use among new users of statins: implications for pharmacoepidemiology. Med Care. 2014;52(9):773–80. https://doi.org/10.1097/MLR.0000000000000174.

Li X, Young JG, Toh S. Estimating effects of dynamic treatment strategies in pharmacoepidemiologic studies with time-varying confounding: a primer. Curr Epidemiol Rep. 2017;4(4):288–97. https://doi.org/10.1007/s40471-017-0124-x.

Lu CY. Pharmacoepidemiologic research in Australia: challenges and opportunities for monitoring patients with rheumatic diseases. Clin Rheumatol. 2009;28(4):371–7. https://doi.org/10.1007/s10067-009-1102-6.

Lu CY, Law MR, Soumerai SB, et al. Impact of prior authorization on the use and costs of lipid-lowering medications among Michigan and Indiana dual enrollees in Medicaid and Medicare: results of a longitudinal, population-based study. Clin Ther. 2011;33(1):135–44. https://doi.org/10.1016/j.clinthera.2011.01.012.

Lu CY, Soumerai SB, Ross-Degnan D, Zhang F, Adams AS. Unintended impacts of a medicaid prior authorization policy on access to medications for bipolar illness. Med Care. 2010;48(1):4–9. https://doi.org/10.1097/MLR.0b013e3181bd4c10.

Lu CY, Srasuebkul P, Drew AK, Ward RL, Pearson S-A. Positive spillover effects of prescribing requirements: increased cardiac testing in patients treated with trastuzumab for HER2+ metastatic breast cancer. Intern Med J. 2012;42(11):1229–35. https://doi.org/10.1111/j.1445-5994.2011.02604.x.

Lu CY, Williams KM, Day RO. Has the use of disease-modifying anti-rheumatic drugs changed as a consequence of controlled access to high-cost biological agents through the Pharmaceutical Benefits Scheme? Intern Med J. 2007a;37(9):601–6. https://doi.org/10.1111/j.1445-5994.2007.01396.x.

Lu CY, Williams KM, Day RO. The funding and use of high-cost medicines in Australia: the example of anti-rheumatic biological medicines. Aust New Zealand Health Policy. 2007b;4(1):2. https://doi.org/10.1186/1743-8462-4-2.

Lu CY, Zhang F, Lakoma MD, et al. Changes in antidepressant use by young people and suicidal behavior after FDA warnings and media coverage: quasi-experimental study. BMJ. 2014;348:g3596. https://doi.org/10.1136/bmj.g3596.

Maclure M. The case-crossover design: a method for studying transient effects on the risk of acute events. Am J Epidemiol. 1991;133(2):144–53. https://doi.org/10.1093/oxfordjournals.aje.a115853.

Maclure M, Fireman B, Nelson JC, et al. When should case-only designs be used for safety monitoring of medical products? Pharmacoepidemiol Drug Saf. 2012;21(S1):50–61. https://doi.org/10.1002/pds.2330.

Mamdani M, Sykora K, Li P, et al. Reader's guide to critical appraisal of cohort studies: 2. Assessing potential for confounding. BMJ. 2005;330(7497):960–2. https://doi.org/10.1136/bmj.330.7497.960.

Mantel N, Haenszel W. Statistical aspects of the analysis of data from retrospective studies of disease. J Natl Cancer Inst. 1959;22(4):719–48. https://doi.org/10.1093/jnci/22.4.719.

McKnight J, Scott A, Menzies D, Bourbeau J, Blais L, Lemière C. A cohort study showed that health insurance databases were accurate to distinguish chronic obstructive pulmonary disease from asthma and classify disease severity. J Clin Epidemiol. 2005;58(2):206–8. https://doi.org/10.1016/j.jclinepi.2004.08.006.

McWilliams JM, Meara E, Zaslavsky AM, Ayanian JZ. Use of health services by previously uninsured Medicare beneficiaries. N Engl J Med. 2007;357(2):143–53. https://doi.org/10.1056/NEJMsa067712.

Morgenstern H. Ecologic studies in epidemiology: concepts, principles, and methods. Annu Rev Public Health. 1995;16(1):61–81. https://doi.org/10.1146/annurev.pu.16.050195.000425.

Motheral BR, Fairman KA. The use of claims databases for outcomes research: rationale, challenges, and strategies. Clin Ther. 1997;19(2):346–66. https://doi.org/10.1016/S0149-2918(97)80122-1.

National Cancer Institute Division of Cancer Control & Population Sciences. SEER-medicare linked database. https://healthcaredelivery.cancer.gov/seermedicare/. Published 3 Oct 2019. Accessed 15 Oct 2019.

Normand S-LT, Sykora K, Li P, Mamdani M, Rochon PA, Anderson GM. Readers guide to critical appraisal of cohort studies: 3. Analytical strategies to reduce confounding. BMJ. 2005;330(7498):1021–3. https://doi.org/10.1136/bmj.330.7498.1021.

OECD Guidelines for Quality Assurance in Genetic Testing—OECD. http://www.oecd.org/sti/emerging-tech/oecdguidelinesforqualityassuranceingenetictesting.htm. Accessed 16 Oct 2019.

OptumLabs Health Care Collaboration & Innovation. https://www.optumlabs.com/. Accessed 15 Oct 2019.

Paniz VMV, Fassa AG, Maia M de FS, Domingues MR, Bertoldi AD. Measuring access to medicines: a review of quantitative methods used in household surveys. BMC Health Serv Res. 2010;10:146. https://doi.org/10.1186/1472-6963-10-146.

PDUFA VI: Fiscal years 2018–2022. FDA. June 2019. http://www.fda.gov/industry/prescription-drug-user-fee-amendments/pdufa-vi-fiscal-years-2018-2022. Accessed 15 Oct 2019.

Perrio M, Waller PC, Shakir SAW. An analysis of the exclusion criteria used in observational pharmacoepidemiological studies. Pharmacoepidemiol Drug Saf. 2007;16(3):329–36. https://doi.org/10.1002/pds.1262.

Petersen I, Douglas I, Whitaker H. Self controlled case series methods: an alternative to standard epidemiological study designs. BMJ. 2016;354:i4515. https://doi.org/10.1136/bmj.i4515.

Psaty BM, Koepsell TD, Lin D, et al. Assessment and control for confounding by indication in observational studies. J Am Geriatr Soc. 1999;47(6):749–54. https://doi.org/10.1111/j.1532-5415.1999.tb01603.x.

Ray WA. Evaluating medication effects outside of clinical trials: new-user designs. Am J Epidemiol. 2003;158(9):915–20. https://doi.org/10.1093/aje/kwg231.

Redelmeier DA, Tan SH, Booth GL. The treatment of unrelated disorders in patients with chronic medical diseases. N Engl J Med. 1998;338:1516–20.

Robins J. A new approach to causal inference in mortality studies with a sustained exposure period–application to control of the healthy worker survivor effect. Math Model. 1986;7(9–12):1395–512.

Robins JM, Finkelstein DM. Correcting for noncompliance and dependent censoring in an AIDS clinical trial with inverse probability of censoring weighted (IPCW) log-rank tests. Biometrics. 2000;56(3):779–88. https://doi.org/10.1111/j.0006-341X.2000.00779.x.

Robins JM, Hernan MA, Brumback B. Marginal structural models and causal inference in epidemiology. [Editorial]. Epidemiology. 2000;11(5):550–60.

Rosenbaum PR, Rubin DB. Reducing bias in observational studies using subclassification on the propensity score. J Am Stat Assoc. 1984;79(387):516–24. https://doi.org/10.2307/2288398.

Schneeweiss S. Sensitivity analysis and external adjustment for unmeasured confounders in epidemiologic database studies of therapeutics. Pharmacoepidemiol Drug Saf. 2006;15(5):291–303. https://doi.org/10.1002/pds.1200.

Schneeweiss S. Developments in post-marketing comparative effectiveness research. Clin Pharmacol Ther. 2007;82(2):143–56. https://doi.org/10.1038/sj.clpt.6100249.

Schneeweiss S, Avorn J. A review of uses of health care utilization databases for epidemiologic research on therapeutics. J Clin Epidemiol. 2005;58(4):323–37. https://doi.org/10.1016/j.jclinepi.2004.10.012.

Schneeweiss S, Patrick AR, Stürmer T, et al. Increasing levels of restriction in pharmacoepidemiologic database studies of elderly and comparison with randomized trial results. Med Care. 2007;45(10 Suppl):S131–42. https://doi.org/10.1097/MLR.0b013e318070c08e.

Schneeweiss S, Stürmer T, Maclure M. Case-crossover and case-time-control designs as alternatives in pharmacoepidemiologic research. Pharmacoepidemiol Drug Saf. 1997;6(Suppl 3):S51–9. https://doi.org/10.1002/(SICI)1099-1557(199710)6:3+<S51::AID-PDS301>3.0.CO;2-S.

Schuemie MJ, Ryan PB, Man KKC, Wong ICK, Suchard MA, Hripcsak G. A plea to stop using the case-control design in retrospective database studies. Stat Med. 2019;38(22):4199–208. https://doi.org/10.1002/sim.8215.

Sentinel Initiative. https://www.sentinelinitiative.org/. Accessed 16 Oct 2019.

Strom BL, Carson JL, Halpern AC, et al. Using a claims database to investigate drug-induced Stevens-Johnson syndrome. Stat Med. 1991;10(4):565–76. https://doi.org/10.1002/sim.4780100408.

Strom BL, Kimmel SE, Hennessy S. Pharmacoepidemiology. 5th ed. Chichester: John Wiley & Sons Ltd; 2012.

Suissa S. The case-time-control design. Epidemiology. 1995;6(3):248–53. https://doi.org/10.1097/00001648-199505000-00010.

Suissa S. Effectiveness of inhaled corticosteroids in chronic obstructive pulmonary disease: immortal time bias in observational studies. Am J Respir Crit Care Med. 2003;168(1):49–53. https://doi.org/10.1164/rccm.200210-1231OC.

Suissa S. Immortal time bias in pharmacoepidemiology. Am J Epidemiol. 2008;167(4):492–9. https://doi.org/10.1093/aje/kwm324.

Vaccine Safety Datalink (VSD) I VSD I Monitoring I Ensuring Safety I Vaccine Safety I CDC. https://www.cdc.gov/vaccinesafety/ensuringsafety/monitoring/vsd/index.html. Published 17 June 2019. Accessed 16 Oct 2019.

Vandenbroucke JP, von Elm E, Altman DG, et al. Strengthening the reporting of observational studies in epidemiology (STROBE): explanation and elaboration. Ann Intern Med. 2007;147(8):W-163–94.

Vitry AI, Thai LP, Lu CY. Time and geographical variations in utilization of endocrine therapy for breast cancer in Australia. Intern Med J. 2011;41(2):162–6. https://doi.org/10.1111/j.1445-5994.2010.02304.x.

Wagner AK, Soumerai SB, Zhang F, Ross-Degnan D. Segmented regression analysis of interrupted time series studies in medication use research. J Clin Pharm Ther. 2002;27(4):299–309. https://doi.org/10.1046/j.1365-2710.2002.00430.x.

Walker AM. Confounding by indication. Epidemiology. 1996;7(4):335–6.

Wettermark B. The intriguing future of pharmacoepidemiology. Eur J Clin Pharmacol. 2013;69(1):43–51. https://doi.org/10.1007/s00228-013-1496-6.

Whitaker HJ, Farrington CP, Spiessens B, Musonda P. Tutorial in biostatistics: the self-controlled case series method. Stat Med. 2006;25(10):1768–97. https://doi.org/10.1002/sim.2302.

WHO. How to investigate drug use in health facilities: selected drug use indicators—EDM Research Series No. 007. https://apps.who.int/medicinedocs/en/d/Js2289e/. Published 29 Oct 2018. Accessed 15 Oct 2019.

WHOCC. Definition and general considerations. https://www.whocc.no/ddd/definition_and_general_considera/. Accessed 15 October 2019.

Wilchesky M, Tamblyn RM, Huang A. Validation of diagnostic codes within medical services claims. J Clin Epidemiol. 2004;57(2):131–41. https://doi.org/10.1016/S0895-4356(03)00246-4.

Chapter 10
Randomised Controlled Trials and Pharmacy Practice Research

Louise E. Curley and Joanne C. Lin

Abstract Randomised controlled trials (RCTs) are regarded as the gold standard method for evaluating an intervention and its outcome and have the ability to evaluate the cost-effectiveness of an intervention. This form of research is known to be the most rigorous study design in order to determine a cause-effect relationship. This chapter summarises the randomised controlled trial design methodology, what key features should be present and its advantages and limitations. The place of cluster randomised controlled trials within health services research and in particular pharmacy practice research (PPR) will also be discussed.

PPR has been described extensively in the literature and within other chapters within this book. PPR has evolved through the years, and the number of RCTs within PPR has increased significantly since 2000. This chapter also details examples of recent RCTs within PPR and makes recommendations for future research within this field.

10.1 Introduction

It is important within every avenue of healthcare that the intervention—whether this is the treatment or a service—be evaluated, to ensure that the patient is receiving evidence-based care. Whilst this research has traditionally been focussed on the medication and/or treatment, similar evaluation of services is becoming increasingly common.

Recently, due to pressures on the primary care system, there is an increasing demand worldwide on healthcare services, for a multitude of reasons, including an ageing population (World Health Organization 2016a). Therefore, in some regions, health systems have evolved, and conditions that were once managed by doctors are now being delivered by other healthcare professionals, including pharmacists. The clinical role of the pharmacist was described by Hepler and Strand in the 1990s,

L. E. Curley (✉) · J. C. Lin
School of Pharmacy, University of Auckland, Auckland, New Zealand
e-mail: l.curley@auckland.ac.nz

© Springer Nature Singapore Pte Ltd. 2020
Z. Babar (ed.), *Pharmacy Practice Research Methods*,
https://doi.org/10.1007/978-981-15-2993-1_10

who were the first to discuss the term pharmaceutical care (Hepler and Strand 1990). The role of the pharmacist has been evolving for decades, changing from the 'compounder and dispensing chemist' to 'drug therapy manager' and now encompassing a wide variety of other patient-focussed clinical services (Thamby and Subramani 2014). In an evidence-based health service, it is vital to show evidence of benefit to support these changing roles and perceptions of the pharmacist (Bond 2006; Jorgenson et al. 2011). Due to the increasingly integrated nature of pharmacy within the healthcare profession (Babar and Vitry 2014), 'practicing pharmacists need to actively participate in research in order to reflect on the relevancy of the services they deliver, to help discover new areas that may require research, and to firmly establish the necessity of the profession' (Scahill et al. 2018).

Within health services research, a sub-speciality has developed, known as pharmacy practice research (PPR) (Bond 2015). Its aim is to 'support evidence-based policy and practice decisions where pharmacists are employed, or medicines are prescribed or used' (Bond 2015). In essence, PPR tries to understand the clinical, humanistic and economic impact from the perspectives of the pharmacist, the patient and other healthcare professionals (Bond 2015). There appears to be no globally accepted definition of exactly what PPR is, which has been discussed by other authors (Awaisu et al. 2015; Koshman and Blais 2011).

As PPR has developed over the decades, there has been a call for quality research to be conducted, using rigorous methodologies, and to be delivered by multidisciplinary groups (Bond 2015). Especially, given the evolving nature of the pharmacist's role, this PPR should be collated and evaluated by using a systematic review of literature (Bond 2015). This has the potential to provide evidence for healthcare practice and influence policy (Bond 2015).

This chapter will discuss randomised controlled trials (RCTs) and their place within PPR, as well as provide examples of types of RCTs that have been conducted and recently conducted RCTs in different healthcare settings.

10.2   Hierarchy of Evidence

All evidence is not created equal. Whilst the number of research studies in PPR has increased exponentially over the past six decades, the quality of research prior to 2000 was held in question (Bond 2015). In order to be able to critically evaluate the evidence that is presented, we must have a clear and accurate understanding of the design of research methods and understand the place that each type of design fits within the hierarchy of evidence. When we discuss hierarchy of evidence, this is in relation to assessing the effectiveness of an intervention. It is well established that some research designs are more 'powerful' than others in being able to evaluate the evidence. A hierarchy of evidence has been established and discussed at length amongst the literature (Akobeng 2005). RCTs are amongst the most rigorous and robust methods and are regarded as the gold standard method for evaluating an intervention and its outcome (Sibbald and Roland 1998); they have the ability to evaluate the cost-effectiveness of an intervention and, more than any other methodology, can have a powerful and immediate impact on patient care (Begg et al. 1996). The importance of the intervention studies for the advancement of healthcare has also been highlighted by the Medical Research Council (MRC) of the UK. They have documented and provided guidance on the development, implementation and evaluation of such studies; this guidance was first issued in 2000 and updated in 2008 (MRC AJMRC 2000). However, as with any research, the quality of research is founded on ensuring that the research is designed well. We must, therefore, understand the RCT design and what factors need consideration at each stage. Furthermore, like all designs, RCTs come with their own limitations; understanding the limitations of research is integral to understanding and interpreting results that ensue.

10.3   Randomised Controlled Trials: Purpose, Structure and Limitations

RCTs are usually used to assess an intervention or treatment for efficacy or effectiveness, in terms of 'superiority' (the intervention is better than placebo or standard treatment), 'non-inferiority' (the intervention is no worse than placebo or standard treatment) or 'equivalence' (analogous to non-inferiority but determines whether a novel intervention is just as good as a placebo or standard treatment) (Guerrera et al. 2017).

Bias, confounders and random error can have important impacts on the interpretation and generalisability of the results of a research project; however, a well-designed RCT can effectively reduce or eliminate these errors. The important features and appropriate design strategies of robust RCTs will be discussed, as well as some limitations.

10.3.1 Hypothesis

A trial is an experiment that aims to confirm or refute a particular hypothesis. The study hypothesis needs to specify an anticipated association between predictor and outcome variables so that statistical tests can be carried out (Cummings and Hulley 1988). Good hypotheses are specific, precise and formulated before the study commences (a priori). The subsequent study design will need to be designed to enable a true evaluation of the hypothesis being tested.

10.3.2 Study Population

The study sample must be representative of the target population for the study results to be generalisable. It is important to set inclusion and exclusion criteria to define the population/s that are appropriate to the hypothesis. 'Experimental' trial designs may use extremely stringent eligibility criteria to determine the best possible outcome in highly selected patients, whereas 'pragmatic' trial designs will result in much broader eligibility to better reflect the whole population. It is important to find a balance between very strict and precise criteria (resulting in a 'standardised' patient population) and more heterogeneous conditions, which increase the external validity of the results.

10.3.3 Sample Size

Once the appropriate study population has been determined, it is necessary to estimate the size of the study sample in order to detect a clinically important outcome. The sample size needed to achieve power is inversely proportional to the treatment effect squared (Rosner 2015); an estimate of effect size can be based on previous experience, e.g. from the literature or from a pilot study. An appropriate sample size calculation will determine the required sample size to detect the predetermined statistically significant difference to a certain degree of power.

10.3.4 Randomisation

Randomisation is the cornerstone of the RCT, and all eligible participants should have an equal chance of being allocated to the intervention. Randomisation should also equally distribute any confounding variables between groups (Altman 1991), although it is important to recognise that differences in confounding variables may occur by chance.

It is essential that intervention allocations are concealed from investigators so that bias cannot be introduced at the stage of assigning participants to their groups (Schulz et al. 1995).

The randomisation process should be determined in advance of the start of the study. The method (e.g. coin toss, random number generator and computer-based sets), personnel involved, timing and randomisation register must be reported, following the CONSORT guidelines (Begg et al. 1996). Depending on the size and design of a study, different types of randomisations can be implemented (Schulz et al. 2010):

- Simple randomisation—this is pure randomisation based on a single allocation ratio (1:1).
- Blocked randomisation—blocking is used to ensure that groups will be generated according to a predetermined ratio and can ensure close balance of numbers in each group at any time. For example, randomisation for a block of eight participants would proceed normally until four assignments had been made to one group and the remaining assignments would be to the other group (Altman and

Bland 1999); however, improved balance can come at the cost of reducing unpredictability of the sequence.
- Stratified randomisation—a technique for ensuring that an important baseline characteristic (potential confounder) is more evenly distributed between groups, e.g. age or stage of disease. Stratified randomisation is achieved by performing separate randomisations within subsets of participants, but stratification requires some form of restriction, e.g. blocking within strata, without which stratification is ineffective (Schulz et al. 2010).

10.3.5 Blinding

Blinding is used to withhold information about group allocation from people in the trial who may be influenced by this knowledge as it prevents potential bias. Where practicable, trials should blind five groups of individuals: participants, investigators, data collectors, outcome assessors and data analysts (Karanicolas et al. 2010).

If participants are not blinded, their behaviour in the trial and responses to subjective outcomes may be affected by their knowledge of group allocation. For example, a participant who is aware they are not receiving active treatment may be more likely to seek additional treatment outside the trial and/or leave the trial. Moreover, those aware that they are receiving or not receiving therapy are more likely to provide biased assessments of the effectiveness than blinded participants. Similarly, blinded investigators are much less likely to transfer their attitudes to participants or to provide differential treatment to different groups (Schulz and Grimes 2002).

Blinding of personnel involved in data collection and outcome assessment is vital to ensure unbiased evaluation of outcomes. Subjective outcomes are most at risk of ascertainment bias; however, seemingly objective outcomes often require some degree of subjective assessment and are, therefore, at risk of bias too (Karanicolas et al. 2010).

At the analysis stage of a study, selective use and reporting of statistical tests may also introduce bias. This may be subconscious and unintended, prompted by investigators eager to see a positive result; therefore, the best method to avoid this potential bias is blinding of data analyst/s until all analysis has been completed (Karanicolas et al. 2010).

10.3.6 Limitations

Although RCTs are one of the most robust methods for evaluating effects of treatment on specific populations, they do have limitations that are inherent in their design (Hannan 2008), and there is justifiable concern that the way trials are conducted results in limited external validity and clinical salience (Mulder et al. 2018).

Where observational studies usually apply to a much broader population, RCTs have specific inclusion and exclusion criteria that are often quite restrictive, and there is evidence that RCT populations do not mirror the age, sex and race distribution of the target population (Hannan 2008). In general, they tend to be less sick, younger, better educated and of higher socioeconomic status; this may mean participants are more likely to be adherent, which may lead to overstatement of the treatment effect.

As discussed previously, power analyses are used to determine the sample size necessary to identify meaningful clinical differences between treatments. However, because of time, cost and effort associated with running RCTs, compromises are often made to increase statistical power, e.g. using combined outcomes. However, composite end points can combine outcomes with different levels of severity, subjectivity or incidence (Hannan 2008); therefore, it is important to remember that, when using composite end points, 'the individual components must be appropriately chosen, objectively measured in an unbiased manner, and individually reported' (Lauer and Topol 2003).

## 10.4	Cluster Randomised Controlled Trials, How These Differ and Their Place in Health Services Research

In clinical trials, the randomisation usually occurs at the patient/subject level. One of the major limitations in PPR is how to ensure blinding (Sibbald and Roland 1998; Charrois et al. 2009). If an intervention requires the pharmacy/pharmacist to have patients in both arms of a study, i.e. intervention and control, it is impossible to have a behavioural intervention that is double blinded. Without double blinding, there can easily be contamination of the intervention in the control arm, as the intervention naturally will change the behaviour of the pharmacy/pharmacist (Charrois et al. 2009; Carter 2010; Carter and Foppe van Mil 2010).

A specific type of RCT is the cluster RCT (cRCT) or sometimes referred to as the group randomised trial design (Vetter 2017); the cRCT is now considered by some to be the gold standard of health services research trials, including pharmacy-based intervention trials (Gums et al. 2016). The cRCT is not new; it has been used for many years outside of health services research, including studies that have assessed behaviour and looked at epidemiology and those that have evaluated educational interventions (Vetter 2017; Gums et al. 2016).

In a cRCT, instead of the randomisation being at the patient/subject level, it is undertaken at a group level, or cluster level (Vetter 2017; Tsuyuki 2014). Each of the clusters will be randomised to either intervention or control. In PPR, the cluster of randomisation can be the community pharmacy and the medical practice, or it could be a whole community of people, depending on the intervention and the design of the study (Vetter 2017). In terms of the intervention, this could be a behavioural intervention, for example, a change in practice guidelines and an educational intervention, or the intervention could be of a therapeutic nature (Vetter 2017).

Despite now being recognised by some as the as the gold standard, there are still limitations with cRCTs; cRCTs tend to be complex, have high costs associated, are large in scale and have more complex statistics (Vetter 2017; Gums et al. 2016; Tsuyuki 2014).

According to Gums et al. (2016), a well-designed cRCT must consider the following attributes: sample size, stratification and selection bias. Sample size calculations in cRCTs are more complex than standard RCTs (Gums et al. 2016; Hemming et al. 2017). A minimum of ten clusters are recommended for a two arm cRCT, but calculation of the intra-class correlation coefficient (ICC) will provide a better estimate of number of clusters required (Gums et al. 2016). The ICC is the 'correlation among participants recruited from the same cluster' (Gums et al. 2016). The ICC will allow for the differences between clinics and pharmacies to be taken into account; this may be at the clinic level, i.e. differences in practices (Carter and Foppe van Mil 2010), or could be at the patient level, i.e. differences in patient populations (Carter and Foppe van Mil 2010). You may wonder why this is important. Generally speaking, as the cluster size increases, the precision and power do not increase to the same degree; that is, there reaches a point in cRCTs where adding numbers to the clusters does not yield a return on power and precision (Hemming et al. 2017). Therefore, the ICC is important to calculate. Hemming et al. (2017) have published a practical guide to making these calculations to design an efficient cRCT. The authors state that the number and size of the clusters are a decision that should be made together, not separately (Hemming et al. 2017).

Stratification within the randomisation procedure must be considered in cRCTs; failing to do so may lead to bias in the results of the intervention or control arm outcomes (Gums et al. 2016).

Bias needs to be considered in cRCTs. There are many ways to potentially minimise bias, examples are: have a small intervention as control, such as an educational intervention or a weaker version of the actual intervention or follow-up with an intervention after the study. Another way is to offer the intervention to the cluster after the trial is completed (Gums et al. 2016).

10.5   Randomised Controlled Trials in Pharmacy Practice

There has been an increase in research in PPR in the past three decades (Rotta et al. 2017). The purpose of this chapter is not to synthesise the RCT data on PPR, but to highlight the range of research undertaken.

The DEPICT (Descriptive Elements of Pharmacist Intervention Characterization Tool) project database was established in 2013 (Correr et al. 2013); it was developed to provide a standardised description of the components of pharmacist health interventions and to consider which of these components were the most meaningful for patient outcomes. The project retrospectively applied this to RCTs assessing clinical pharmacy services (Rotta et al. 2017; Correr et al. 2013).

Using the DEPICT database, Rotta et al. (2017) provide an analysis of RCTs in PPR; the authors report that there has been a notable increase in the number of RCTs published in PPR after the year 2000. Despite this increase, the analysis sheds light on the ongoing issue relating to sample size (Rotta et al. 2017); despite the sample size post-2000 increasing to a median of 87, this is still lacking for adequately powered studies (Rotta et al. 2017). This finding is not unique to PPR; issues with sample size have been seen in other health research areas (Freedman et al. 2001) and were reported three decades ago (Moher et al. 1994). Sample size calculations must be conducted carefully to ensure that there is enough power to detect small changes (Altman et al. 2001). Furthermore, researchers need to detail how these sample size calculations were conducted and if there were any deviations from the target sample size in the actual collection of data.

10.5.1 Evaluation of Non-dispensing Services

Studies that use RCT design in PPR span a range of conditions, outcomes and settings. Many RCTs (Rotta et al. 2017) and systematic reviews of RCTs are categorised in this manner (Rotta et al. 2017; Chisholm-Burns et al. 2010; Salgado et al. 2011; de Barra et al. 2018; Nkansah et al. 2010). Evidence from a recent Cochrane review indicates that there was some evidence for pharmacist interventions in certain areas; blood pressure outside the target range and physical functioning both showed improvements with a low certainty of evidence (de Barra et al. 2018). Other RCTs that were included in the analysis evaluated the percentage outside glycated haemoglobin range, hospital attendance/admission, adverse drug effects and mortality, none of which showed significant differences in this meta-analysis (de Barra et al. 2018). This Cochrane review contained 116 reports of 111 trials, but the authors recommend caution with interpretation of these results, as there was a high degree of heterogeneity in the analyses and a variation of risk of bias in the included studies (de Barra et al. 2018).

Possibly the most obvious and frequently reported setting for outpatient pharmacist services is the community pharmacy (Rotta et al. 2017); other localities and multidisciplinary teams can be employed. These will be discussed below.

10.5.2 Home-Based Interventions

Home-based interventions are common in PPR and represented a third of all RCTs in the analysis by Rotta et al. (2017). Most RCTs in the home setting focus on medication reviews or medication management (MacKeigan and Nissen 2008); these home-based services have been established in a number of countries, for example, the home medication review in Australia (Healthdirect Australia n.d.). Despite these services being established, the data surrounding the effectiveness of home-based interventions are conflicting (MacKeigan and Nissen 2008; Flanagan and Barns 2018). The HOMER RCT is one example of such research; patients over the age of 80 were recruited after an emergency admission (if they were returning home and were taking two or more medications) (Holland et al. 2005). The study showed that the pharmacist intervention (home-based medication review) when compared to a control arm (usual care) was associated with a higher rate of hospitalisations, and did not affect patient quality of life or mortality (Holland et al. 2005).

More recently, there are a number of *other* home-based pharmacist services that have been studied (MacKeigan and Nissen 2008). Examples of these services include blood pressure monitoring and compliance (Green et al. 2008; Margolis et al. 2013); a home-based intervention by a nurse and pharmacist post-discharge for patients with congestive heart failure (Stewart et al. 1999, 1998) and a collaborative team care (that included a pharmacist) improved quality of care for patients deemed at high risk, when compared to usual care in a study by Hogg et al. (2009).

A review of home-based interventions that had pharmacist input was published by Flanagan and Barns in 2018. The review identified a wide range of studies that had evaluated pharmacists' services in a home setting, including nine RCTs (Flanagan and Barns 2018). Of these RCTs the majority was conducted in older adults over 60 years of age (Flanagan and Barns 2018), and the outcomes measured varied between studies.

10.5.3 A Service in Rest Home/Similar Facilities

Older people in general have more complex health management requirements; these patients are more likely to have a higher number of long-term conditions, be prescribed more medications and have age-related pharmacokinetic and pharmacodynamic changes (Turnheim 2004). There are a number of challenges in this population including polypharmacy and inappropriate prescribing (Wallerstedt et al. 2014). RCTs within this setting have included medication reviews, education of staff and meetings with multidisciplinary team members (Loganathan et al. 2011).

The evidence for medication reviews in rest home facilities is not clear; a recent meta-analysis of RCTs showed no effect on hospitalisations or on mortality (Wallerstedt et al. 2014). The studies included all involved a pharmacist either alone or as part of a multidisciplinary team, except for two studies that included a physician only or a combination of a geriatricians and geriatric nurses (Wallerstedt et al. 2014).

Pharmacist involvement in educational interventions appears to have mostly positive effects, but there, again, has been mixed results (Loganathan et al. 2011). Outcomes measured in these RCTs largely report the number of medication changes or reductions in inappropriate prescribing (Avorn et al. 1992; Crotty et al. 2004).

A small number of RCTs of multidisciplinary team meetings in rest homes have been conducted; examples include a study by Schmidt et al. (1998) and Crotty et al. (2004), which both showed significant decreases in rates of psychotropic drug use.

10.5.4 Other Settings: Pharmacist Services via Telepharmacy

Pharmacist services for non-hospitalised patients can also occur via other means of communication. Recent published RCTs have used telepharmacy as an example of such a service. Teleservices in the literature have been used when patients may not be able to access pharmacy services or are being trialled as novel services to improve patient outcomes, for example, adherence to medications. A cRCT by Margolis et al. (2013) used tele-monitoring to evaluate blood pressure control. Eight clinics were randomised to pharmacist tele-monitoring and eight to standard care, finding that the intervention resulted significantly better blood pressure control. The *Study of a Telepharmacy Intervention for Chronic Diseases to Improve Treatment Adherence* (STIC2IT) cRCT evaluated the impact of a remotely delivered multi-component intervention on improving adherence to medications for hyperlipidaemia, hypertension and diabetes in comparison to usual care (Choudhry et al. 2018). This cRCT found that this pharmacist intervention led to a statistically significant improvement in medication adherence but not in clinical outcomes (Choudhry et al. 2018). These examples show promise for remotely delivered interventions in healthcare, but more research is needed to elucidate the types of interventions and patients that would benefit.

10.5.5 Multidisciplinary Research, i.e. Physician/Pharmacist Interventions

The World Health Organisation (WHO) Global Strategy on Human Resources for Health projects that 40 million new health and social care jobs will be created by 2030 (World Health Organization 2016b), and there needs to be an additional 18 million health workers in order to attain high and effective coverage of the broad range of health services necessary to ensure healthy lives. The report affects all health workers, from community to specialist levels, and recognises that diversity in the health workforce 'is an opportunity to be harnessed through strengthened collaborative approaches to social accountability, inter-professional education and practice, and closer integration of the health and social services workforces to improve long-term care for ageing populations' (World Health Organization 2016b).

After almost 50 years of enquiry, the WHO states that effective inter-professional education enables effective collaborative practice and that 'collaborative practice strengthens health systems and improves health outcomes' (Gilbert et al. 2010). Therefore, high-quality research is essential to understand the roles and value of health workers in order to build more flexible health workforces to improve the effectiveness of healthcare.

Systematic reviews have been carried out to explore the impact of pharmacist-involved collaborative care in diverse patient groups, disease states and healthcare settings, such as primary care (Riordan et al. 2016), acute care (Hickman et al.

2015), home-based care (Flanagan and Barns 2018) and general practice (Tan et al. 2014). Many RCTs report positive effects on outcomes including improvement in the management of chronic conditions such as cardiovascular disease and diabetes, evidenced by improved blood pressure, HbA1c, cholesterol levels and attainment of health goals (Tan et al. 2014). Pharmacist-involved interventions may also improve prescribing appropriateness and have an impact on hospital readmission rates and mortality (Hickman et al. 2015).

The evidence highlights the benefits of inter-professional communication and collaboration; however, it also suggests a number of factors that can influence the success of interventions. Studies have reported healthcare professional feedback and acceptance rates varying from 18% to 95% (Flanagan and Barns 2018), and another study found it can be challenging to modify behaviour, despite full support and advocacy of an intervention (Raebel et al. 2007). The extent and type of collaboration communication can influence the likelihood of improved outcomes. Tan et al. (2014) found that, across 38 different RCTs of clinical services delivered by pharmacists co-located in general practice clinics, positive effects were seen most often when interventions were multifaceted and involved inter-professional collaboration combined with face-to-face verbal communication. Positive effects were less likely to be observed in interventions with written or no communication. Studies that incorporated additional pharmacist interventions such as assessment of adherence, health and lifestyle information, medication initiation or adjustment and monitoring combined with verbal (telephone or face-to-face) communication with the physician were also more likely to show positive outcomes (Tan et al. 2014).

Several reviews have highlighted a lack of rigour in methodological quality of some studies and difficulty comparing studies due to heterogeneity (Chisholm-Burns et al. 2010; Nkansah et al. 2010; Riordan et al. 2016; Tan et al. 2014; Fish et al. 2002). Common sources of bias included inadequate sample size, performance bias (unclear or inappropriate methods for blinding of participants and/or personnel) and detection bias (inadequate blinding of outcome assessment). Adequately powered multicentre studies that use cluster randomisation with sufficient follow-up are needed to enhance the validity of data, and explicit reporting of quality criteria is necessary to ensure studies produce reliable and high-quality data.

10.6 Economics and RCTs

Robust evidence is needed to quantify the value offered by pharmacists' provision of targeted professional services; however, few RCTs in PPR have evaluated the costs associated with pharmacist-led interventions. The majority of studies has measured the cost-effectiveness of an intervention using a dollar value for an outcome, e.g. $ per day of glycaemic episode avoided (Hendrie et al. 2014), mean € per emergency department visit (Jodar-Sanchez et al. 2015), mean cost per hospital admission (Jodar-Sanchez et al. 2015; Malet-Larrea et al. 2016) or cost savings between intervention and usual care (Manfrin et al. 2017). Across the different outcome measures, all studies showed expanded pharmacy practice to be both effective and cost-effective. However, further costs associated with provision of services are inevitable and pose a significant barrier, particularly in terms of expense related to additional training, cost of service establishment, remuneration and time (Winslade et al. 2016).

Due to the relative paucity of studies including measures of economic viability and cost-effectiveness, larger-scale replication studies are warranted. Future research should focus on using objective measures and strong methodologies to evaluate the effectiveness of services that have a meaningful impact on health outcomes.

10.7 Recommendations

- The evolving role of pharmacists in future healthcare is evident in the literature and in practice worldwide. In order to ensure evidence-based practice research, these services must take place.
- RCTs, in particular cRCTs where appropriate, should be utilised in future PPR where evaluation of pharmacy services is being undertaken.
- Planning the RCT or cRCT is of utmost importance and should be encouraged, for example, by funding bodies.
- Engaging with experts in the development of RCTs/cRCTs should be encouraged to all researchers.
- Health research statisticians should be consulted to calculate sample size, especially in the instance of cRCTs where more complex statistical calculations are required, including the ICC.
- Publication bias is suspected in some research areas, identified in meta-analyses of RCTs. Encourage researchers to seek publication when non-statistically significant differences are found.
- Collaborative care models are encouraged by the WHO and other governance bodies worldwide, and evidence has long shown the positive effect on patient outcomes. The future research in PPR should not be in isolation; it must include multidisciplinary teams.
- Economic evaluation using RCTs is limited but vitally required.
- A systematic review of RCTs spanning across clinical, patient and economic outcomes is needed to holistically synthesise the effect of pharmacist non-dispensing services.

10.8 Conclusion

This chapter focussed on RCTs and cRCTs, both regarded as the gold standard method for evaluating an intervention and its outcome. This form of research is known to be the most rigorous study design in order to determine a cause-effect relationship. PPR is vital for the future of evidence-based healthcare for new and emerging non-dispensing roles for pharmacists. However, quality research is needed in pharmacy practice, and this requires careful planning and engagement with a multidisciplinary team, with statistical and research expertise. The collaborative care model is important for the future provision of healthcare, and research should follow suit; PPR of the future needs to embrace this and not act in isolation. Expansion of the traditional view of where PPR can be based is emerging, creating and evaluating services that are not just based on community pharmacy settings but also in the patient's home, in rest home facilities and remotely via telepharmacy means.

References

Akobeng A. Understanding randomised controlled trials. Arch Dis Child. 2005;90(8):840–4.

Altman DG. Randomisation. BMJ. 1991;302(6791):1481–2.

Altman DG, Bland JM. How to randomise. BMJ (Clinical Research Ed). 1999;319(7211):703–4.

Altman DG, Schulz KF, Moher D, Egger M, Davidoff F, Elbourne D, et al. The revised CONSORT statement for reporting randomized trials: explanation and elaboration. Ann Intern Med. 2001;134(8):663–94.

Avorn J, Soumerai SB, Everitt DE, Ross-Degnan D, Beers MH, Sherman D, et al. A randomized trial of a program to reduce the use of psychoactive drugs in nursing homes. N Engl J Med. 1992;327(3):168–73.

Awaisu A, Alsalimy N, Pharmacy A. Pharmacists' involvement in and attitudes toward pharmacy practice research: a systematic review of the literature. Res Social Adm Pharm. 2015;11(6):725–48.

Babar Z, Vitry A. Differences in Australian and New Zealand medicines funding policies. Aust Prescr. 2014;37:150–1.

Begg C, Cho M, Eastwood S, Horton R, Moher D, Olkin I, et al. Improving the quality of reporting of randomized controlled trials. The CONSORT statement. JAMA. 1996;276(8):637–9.

Bond C. The need for pharmacy practice research. Int J Pharm Pract. 2006;14:1–2.

Bond C. Pharmacy practice research: evidence and impact. In: Pharmacy practice research methods. New York: Springer; 2015. p. 1–24.

Carter BL. Designing quality health services research: why comparative effectiveness studies are needed and why pharmacists should be involved. Pharmacotherapy. 2010;30(8):751–7.

Carter BL, Foppe van Mil JW. Comparative effectiveness research: evaluating pharmacist interventions and strategies to improve medication adherence. Am J Hypertens. 2010;23(9): 949–55.

Charrois TL, Durec T, Tsuyuki RT. Systematic reviews of pharmacy practice research: methodologic issues in searching, evaluating, interpreting, and disseminating results. Ann Pharmacother. 2009;43(1):118–22.

Chisholm-Burns MA, Lee JK, Spivey CA, Slack M, Herrier RN, Hall-Lipsy E, et al. US pharmacists' effect as team members on patient care: systematic review and meta-analyses. Med Care. 2010;48:923–33.

Choudhry NK, Isaac T, Lauffenburger JC, Gopalakrishnan C, Lee M, Vachon A, et al. Effect of a remotely delivered tailored multicomponent approach to enhance medication taking for patients with hyperlipidemia, hypertension, and diabetes: the STIC2IT cluster randomized clinical trial. JAMA Intern Med. 2018;178(9):1182–9.

Correr CJ, Melchiors AC, de Souza TT, Rotta I, Salgado TM, Fernandez-Llimos F. A tool to characterize the components of pharmacist interventions in clinical pharmacy services: the DEPICT project. Ann Pharmacother. 2013;47(7–8):946–52.

Crotty M, Halbert J, Rowett D, Giles L, Birks R, Williams H, et al. An outreach geriatric medication advisory service in residential aged care: a randomised controlled trial of case conferencing. Age Ageing. 2004;33(6):612–7.

Crotty M, Whitehead C, Rowett D, Halbert J, Weller D, Finucane P, et al. An outreach intervention to implement evidence based practice in residential care: a randomized controlled trial [ISRCTN67855475]. BMC Health Serv Res. 2004;4(1):6.

Cummings SR, Hulley SB. Designing clinical research: an epidemiologic approach. Philadelphia: Williams & Wilkins; 1988.

de Barra M, Scott CL, Scott NW, Johnston M, de Bruin M, Nkansah N, et al. Pharmacist services for non-hospitalised patients. Cochrane Database Syst Rev. 2018;(9):CD013102.

Fish A, Watson MC, Bond CM. Practice-based pharmaceutical services: a systematic review. Int J Pharm Pract. 2002;10(4):225–33.

Flanagan PS, Barns A. Current perspectives on pharmacist home visits: do we keep reinventing the wheel? Integr Pharm Res Pract. 2018;7:141.

Freedman K, Back S, Bernstein J. Sample size and statistical power of randomised, controlled trials in orthopaedics. J Bone Joint Surg Br. 2001;83(3):397–402.

Gilbert JH, Yan J, Hoffman SJ. A WHO report: framework for action on Interprofessional education and collaborative practice. J Allied Health. 2010;39(3):196–7.

Green BB, Cook AJ, Ralston JD, Fishman PA, Catz SL, Carlson J, et al. Effectiveness of home blood pressure monitoring, Web communication, and pharmacist care on hypertension control: a randomized controlled trial. JAMA. 2008;299(24):2857–67.

Guerrera F, Renaud S, Tabbò F, Filosso PL. How to design a randomized clinical trial: tips and tricks for conduct a successful study in thoracic disease domain. J Thorac Dis. 2017;9(8):2692–6.

Gums T, Carter B, Foster E. Cluster randomized trials for pharmacy practice research. Int J Clin Pharm. 2016;38(3):607–14.

Hannan EL. Randomized clinical trials and observational studies: guidelines for assessing respective strengths and limitations. JACC Cardiovasc Interv. 2008;1(3):211–7.

Healthdirect Australia. Home medicines review. Available from: https://www.healthdirect.gov.au/home-medicines-review

Hemming K, Eldridge S, Forbes G, Weijer C, Taljaard M. How to design efficient cluster randomised trials. BMJ. 2017;358:j3064.

Hendrie D, Miller TR, Woodman RJ, Hoti K, Hughes J. Cost-effectiveness of reducing glycaemic episodes through community pharmacy management of patients with type 2 diabetes mellitus. J Prim Prev. 2014;35(6):439–49.

Hepler CD, Strand LM. Opportunities and responsibilities in pharmaceutical care. Am J Hosp Pharm. 1990;47(3):533–43.

Hickman LD, Phillips JL, Newton PJ, Halcomb EJ, Al Abed N, Davidson PM. Multidisciplinary team interventions to optimise health outcomes for older people in acute care settings: a systematic review. Arch Gerontol Geriatr. 2015;61(3):322–9.

Hogg W, Lemelin J, Dahrouge S, Liddy C, Armstrong CD, Legault F, et al. Randomized controlled trial of anticipatory and preventive multidisciplinary team care: for complex patients in a community-based primary care setting. Can Fam Physician. 2009;55(12):e76–85.

Holland R, Lenaghan E, Harvey I, Smith R, Shepstone L, Lipp A, et al. Does home based medication review keep older people out of hospital? The HOMER randomised controlled trial. BMJ. 2005;330(7486):293.

Jodar-Sanchez F, Malet-Larrea A, Martin JJ, Garcia-Mochon L, Lopez Del Amo MP, Martinez-Martinez F, et al. Cost-utility analysis of a medication review with follow-up service for older adults with polypharmacy in community pharmacies in Spain: the conSIGUE program. PharmacoEconomics. 2015;33(6):599–610.

Jorgenson D, Lamb D, MacKinnon N. Practice change challenges and priorities: a national survey of practising pharmacists. Can Pharm J. 2011;144(3):125–31.

Karanicolas PJ, Farrokhyar F, Bhandari M. Practical tips for surgical research: blinding: who, what, when, why, how? Can J Surg. 2010;53(5):345–8.

Koshman SL, Blais J. What is pharmacy research? Can J Hosp Pharm. 2011;64(2):154.

Lauer MS, Topol EJ. Clinical trials—multiple treatments, multiple end points, and multiple lessons. JAMA. 2003;289(19):2575–7.

Loganathan M, Singh S, Franklin BD, Bottle A, Majeed A. Interventions to optimise prescribing in care homes: systematic review. Age Ageing. 2011;40(2):150–62.

MacKeigan LD, Nissen LM. Clinical pharmacy services in the home. Dis Manag Health Out. 2008;16(4):227–44.

Malet-Larrea A, Goyenechea E, Garcia-Cardenas V, Calvo B, Arteche JM, Aranegui P, et al. The impact of a medication review with follow-up service on hospital admissions in aged polypharmacy patients. Br J Clin Pharmacol. 2016;82(3):831–8.

Manfrin A, Tinelli M, Thomas T, Krska J. A cluster randomised control trial to evaluate the effectiveness and cost-effectiveness of the Italian medicines use review (I-MUR) for asthma patients. BMC Health Serv Res. 2017;17(1):300.

Margolis KL, Asche SE, Bergdall AR, Dehmer SP, Groen SE, Kadrmas HM, et al. Effect of home blood pressure telemonitoring and pharmacist management on blood pressure control: a cluster randomized clinical trial. JAMA. 2013;310(1):46–56.

Moher D, Dulberg CS, Wells GAJJ. Statistical power, sample size, and their reporting in randomized controlled trials. JAMA. 1994;272(2):122–4.

MRC AJMRC. Framework for the development and evaluation of RCTs for complex interventions to improve health. 2000.

Mulder R, Singh AB, Hamilton A, Das P, Outhred T, Morris G, et al. The limitations of using randomised controlled trials as a basis for developing treatment guidelines. Evid Based Ment Health. 2018;21(1):4–6.

Nkansah N, Mostovetsky O, Yu C, Chheng T, Beney J, Bond CM, et al. Effect of outpatient pharmacists' non-dispensing roles on patient outcomes and prescribing patterns. Cochrane Database Syst Rev. 2010;(7):CD000336.

Raebel MA, Charles J, Dugan J, Carroll NM, Korner EJ, Brand DW, et al. Randomized trial to improve prescribing safety in ambulatory elderly patients. J Am Geriatr Soc. 2007;55(7):977–85.

Riordan DO, Walsh KA, Galvin R, Sinnott C, Kearney PM, Byrne S. The effect of pharmacist-led interventions in optimising prescribing in older adults in primary care: a systematic review. SAGE Open Med. 2016;4:2050312116652568.

Rosner B. Fundamentals of biostatistics. Canada: Nelson Education; 2015.

Rotta I, Souza TT, Salgado TM, Correr CJ, Fernandez-Llimos F, Pharmacy A. Characterization of published randomized controlled trials assessing clinical pharmacy services around the world. Res Social Adm Pharm. 2017;13(1):201–8.

Salgado TM, Moles R, Benrimoj SI, Fernandez-Llimos F. Pharmacists' interventions in the management of patients with chronic kidney disease: a systematic review. Nephrol Dial Transplant. 2011;27(1):276–92.

Scahill S, Nagaria RA, Curley LE. The future of pharmacy practice research–Perspectives of academics and practitioners from Australia, NZ, United Kingdom, Canada and USA. Res Social Adm Pharm. 2018;14(12):1163–71.

Schmidt I, Claesson CB, Westerholm B, Nilsson LG, Svarstad BL. The impact of regular multidisciplinary team interventions on psychotropic prescribing in Swedish nursing homes. J Am Geriatr Soc. 1998;46(1):77–82.

Schulz KF, Altman DG, Moher D. CONSORT 2010 Statement: updated guidelines for reporting parallel group randomised trials. BMJ. 2010;340:c332.

Schulz KF, Chalmers I, Hayes RJ, Altman DG. Empirical evidence of bias. Dimensions of methodological quality associated with estimates of treatment effects in controlled trials. JAMA. 1995;273(5):408–12.

Schulz KF, Grimes DA. Blinding in randomised trials: hiding who got what. Lancet (London, England). 2002;359(9307):696–700.

Sibbald B, Roland M. Understanding controlled trials: Why are randomised controlled trials important? BMJ. 1998;316(7126):201.

Stewart S, Marley JE, Horowitz JD. Effects of a multidisciplinary, home-based intervention on planned readmissions and survival among patients with chronic congestive heart failure: a randomised controlled study. Lancet. 1999;354(9184):1077–83.

Stewart S, Pearson S, Horowitz JD. Effects of a home-based intervention among patients with congestive heart failure discharged from acute hospital care. Arch Intern Med. 1998;158(10):1067–72.

Tan ECK, Stewart K, Elliott RA, George J. Pharmacist services provided in general practice clinics: a systematic review and meta-analysis. Res Soc Adm Pharm. 2014;10(4):608–22.

Thamby SA, Subramani PJ. Seven-star pharmacist concept of WHO. J Young Pharm. 2014;6(2):1.

Tsuyuki RT. Designing pharmacy practice research trials. Can J Hosp Pharm. 2014;67(3):226.

Turnheim K. Drug therapy in the elderly. Exp Gerontol. 2004;39(11–12):1731–8.

Vetter TR. Magic mirror, on the wall—which is the right study design of them all?—Part I. Anesth Analg. 2017;124(6):2068–73.

Wallerstedt SM, Kindblom JM, Nylén K, Samuelsson O, Strandell A. Medication reviews for nursing home residents to reduce mortality and hospitalization: systematic review and meta-analysis. Br J Clin Pharmacol. 2014;78(3):488–97.

Winslade N, Eguale T, Tamblyn R. Optimising the changing role of the community pharmacist: a randomised trial of the impact of audit and feedback. BMJ Open. 2016;6(5):e010865.

World Health Organization. Working for health and growth: investing in the health workforce. 2016a.

World Health Organization. Global strategy on human resources for health: Workforce 2030. 2016b.

Chapter 11
Information Sources for Pharmacy Practice Researchers

Fernanda S. Tonin, Helena H. Borba, Antonio M. Mendes, Astrid Wiens, Roberto Pontarolo, and Fernando Fernandez-Llimos

Abstract The access to relevant and updated information is important to researchers and healthcare professionals to acquire knowledge and to inform, underpin, or shape scientific research. Information is available in different forms, being usually classified accordingly to their format, originality of data, and periodicity of publication (i.e., primary, secondary, and tertiary sources). Given the heterogeneity of pharmacy practice, a stepwise approach moving through tertiary, then secondary, and finally primary literature is useful to find information. After retrieving information, pharmacy practice researchers should have the ability to critically evaluate and use evidence with responsibility. This includes knowing the main tools developed to evaluate the methodological quality and report of evidence. Researchers should be able to properly select a journal for publication and understand the publication process. Thus, the aim of this chapter is to provide a broader overview of information resources in pharmacy practice research.

11.1 Introduction

Almost every scientific discipline uses the concept of "information" within its own different context. In the healthcare, "information" may be defined as the provision of unbiased, evidence-based, and critically evaluated data and experiences (Mononen et al. 2018; Bernknopf et al. 2009). The access to relevant, updated, user-specific, and objective information is required to acquire knowledge and make appropriate clinical decisions (e.g., prescription, dispensing, and use of therapeutic options) and to inform, underpin, or shape scientific research (Sharp et al. 2008). Formal information sources are available in different formats, both printed and electronic, and

F. S. Tonin · H. H. Borba · A. M. Mendes · A. Wiens · R. Pontarolo
Department of Pharmacy, Federal University of Parana, Curitiba, Brazil

F. Fernandez-Llimos (✉)
Laboratory of Pharmacology, Department of Drug Sciences, Faculty of Pharmacy,
University of Porto, Porto, Portugal
e-mail: fllimos@ff.up.pt

© Springer Nature Singapore Pte Ltd. 2020
Z. Babar (ed.), *Pharmacy Practice Research Methods*,
https://doi.org/10.1007/978-981-15-2993-1_11

they vary according to the needs of end users. For researchers, articles published in scientific journals are one of the most valuable sources of information.

The oldest continuously published medical journal was introduced in 1812 by the Massachusetts Medical Society, called *The New England Journal of Medicine and Surgery and the Collateral Branches of Science*, which became in 1828 *The Boston Medical and Surgical Journal*, and later renamed *The New England Journal of Medicine*. Since that time, many other medical associations and journals started to emerge, producing a wide range of intellectual work written about health (Porter 1999; Jakovljevic and Ogura 2016). The more recent advances in communication technology and internet access allowed a faster and broader dissemination of information. Although figures are controversial, much more than 1,000,000 biomedical journal articles are published annually, most of them with online access (Berland et al. 2001; Iwanowicz et al. 2006).

Because healthcare professionals and researchers are daily faced with this extensive amount of information, it is impossible to keep up-to-date to the most reliable, complete, and recent evidence in clinical care (Alper et al. 2004; Davies and Harrison 2007; Eysenbach et al. 2002). The "paradox of the information" reflects the apparent contradiction that the more information we have access to, the more difficulty we have to access and use the required information. This is particularly worrying in the pharmacy area, given the heterogeneity of this field, which encompasses very different categories of basic and applied research (e.g., chemistry, biology, statistics, chemometrics, physics, epidemiology), resulting in a large publication scattering (Minguet et al. 2017; Skau 2007; Mendes et al. 2016, 2019). In addition to this, the lack of a globally agreed definition of pharmacy practice worsens the situation. In 1969, the World Health Organization (WHO) described the mission of pharmacy practice as "to provide medications and other healthcare products and services and to help people and society to make the best use of them" (World Health Organization (WHO) 1996). Modern references include under the scope of pharmacy practice not only patient care activities but also disciplines like pharmacovigilance, pharmacoepidemiology, pharmacy services, and social pharmacy (Wiedenmayer et al. 2006; Almarsdottir and Granas 2016).

In this complex context, pharmacy practice researchers should understand how to retrieve, select, evaluate, and disseminate the most clinically relevant, updated, and objective evidence for each scenario. Thus, the aim of this chapter is to provide a broader overview of information resources and publications of use in pharmacy practice research, including a stepwise approach on how to find information, the main concepts of evidence-based research, how to select a journal for publication, the editorial process, and journals' metrics.

11.2   Information Literacy

A range of models and terminology has been developed by both academics and librarians, to articulate the definition of the term "information literacy." According to the American Library Association (ALA), information literacy is the ability to recognize when information is needed, then to locate and evaluate the appropriate information, and finally to use it effectively and responsibly (ALA Presidential Committee on Information Literacy 1989).

Because information now comes in many different formats and its quality varies enormously, researchers need to develop the cognitive and transferable skills to be able to work efficiently with information. The skills involved in this definition require an understanding of among others the resources available, how to find information, the need to evaluate results, how to work with or exploit results, ethical and responsible use, and how to communicate or share findings (ALA Presidential Committee on Information Literacy 1989; Eisenberg 2008; Hersh et al. 2014).

11.3 Information Sources

11.3.1 Primary, Secondary, and Tertiary Sources

Traditionally, information resources were classified accordingly to their physical format. Primary sources were those providing original data, usually published in printed articles/reports and journals. Secondary sources were those used to guide the review of primary literature, such as abstract compilations, microfiches, and databases. Tertiary sources were those printed "processed information," such as book (Sharp et al. 2008; American Pharmacists Association 2007).

However, with the development of information technologies and the global access to prompt online information, sources can no longer be classified only based on their format. In fact, through internet one can access to primary, secondary, and tertiary sources. In this context, two main aspects are relevant to guide sources' classification: the originality of the information and the periodicity of the publication. The periodicity of publication refers not only to standardized periods of publication of the material (e.g., weekly, annually) but also to the content characteristics. To be periodical, an information source needs to provide different contents in each new edition when compared to the previous one, different to the update of a non-periodical source which includes some new content together with the old one.

Primary sources are periodical publications that provide original data. This material typically consists of journal articles or reports (e.g., original research, clinical trials, case studies, pharmacological research, or opinions). The highest-quality primary sources should undergo a peer-review process to assess scientific soundness and merit (Miranda et al. 2004; Ghaibi et al. 2015) The most positive aspect of this type of sources is that they usually provide the most up-to-date information and they are quickly published. On the other hand, this information can be immature, and, despite the peer-review process, it may not be sufficiently contrasted. Primary sources are useful for research, education, and current awareness.

The definition of secondary sources is controversial. Something agreed upon in these sources is that they contain non-original content, this is to say, compilations of other types of sources. What is not consensual is if their content has to be literally copied from the original sources, like the indexes and modern bibliographic databases, or can be extracted and abstracted from other types of sources, like the narrative reviews or the old abstract books. The first, bibliographic databases, represents a crucial tool to overcome the paradox of information, because they have user-friendly search engines and other features that enable literature searches with high specificity. However, proper training is required for efficient use of these systems, and some of them are costly and require a library or institutional budget (Kier and Goldwire 2018; Stansfield et al. 2014; Clauson et al. 2007).

Tertiary sources are original sources of information that compile and contrast the information contained mainly in primary sources. Different to primary sources, tertiary sources are not periodically published, although they can be periodically updated. Tertiary sources include textbooks, compendia, reference books, formal reports, and other electronic databases (e.g., Micromedex, UpToDate, Dynamed). Their publication process may delay their availability, which may represent their weakest aspect. However, this calm publication process is also their greatest strength making these sources the recommended starting point to obtain information (American Pharmacists Association 2007; Malone et al. 2014).

11.3.2 Official and Nonofficial Information Sources

Information sources can also be classified according to who produces their content. A source is classified as official when it is either produced or approved by an official regulatory body, like the medicines regulatory agencies, or by independent scientific societies or academic groups. Examples of these sources include the European summaries of product characteristics (SmPCs), package leaflet, and European public assessment report (EPAR). On the other hand, sources are classified as nonofficial, which in many cases are also called commercial, if they are produced by for-profit companies (e.g., pharma industry, publishing corporations).

11.4   Searching the Literature

To find information, researchers should perform a literature search, which can be defined as a systematic and comprehensive search of data, using any available information source. Generally, the best method to search for information includes a stepwise approach, moving first through tertiary (e.g., textbooks, full-text databases, review articles), then using secondary (e.g., indexing or abstracting services), to finally identify the relevant primary sources (e.g., original research studies).

11.4.1 Bibliographic Databases and Search Engines

A bibliographic database is the modern version of library bibliographic record drawers with a huge difference: the use of a search engine. Search engines are computerized applications (stand-alone or web applications) that allow searching in a database by means of search terms. This configuration introduces two elements that may contribute to obtaining different results when using different engines: the content of the database and the characteristics of the search engine.

One of the best known secondary sources in healthcare is MEDLINE. The history of this database starts with the monthly catalog of literature that the US National Library of Medicine (NLM) published since 1879 called *Index Medicus*. In 1964, the NLM created the MedLARS (Medical Literature Analysis and Retrieval System), the first large-scale computerized biomedical bibliographic retrieval system that became MEDLINE (MedLARS online) in 1971. With the internet dissemination, in 1996, MEDLINE was included in a free public interface called PubMed. This database contains more than 26 million records covering biomedicine and health from 1950 to the present (Dee 2007; Lindberg 2000; Cummings 1967). Although commonly confused names, MEDLINE is only one of the databases included in PubMed, together with PubMed Central and NCBI Bookshelf. Understanding this difference is crucial to avoid common errors of the systematic searches used to identify the literature for systematic reviews.

Scopus is another bibliographic database of interest in pharmacy practice research. Scopus was created in 2004 absorbing the records of EMBASE that had been created in 1947. As strength, Scopus indexes about 25,000 journals (from many disciplinary fields) and contains more than 70,000 records. However, different to PubMed, access to Scopus requires a costly subscription.

Among other bibliographic databases, the Web of Science comprises the Science Citation Index and the Social Sciences Citation databases. Although the coverage of this database starts from 1900, it only indexes 12.000 journals from all scientific disciplines, which is an important limitation for biomedical searches, especially for pharmacy practice researchers (Mendes et al. 2019).

Some other free-access bibliographic databases can be used to search for literature. Directory of Open Access Journals (DOAJ) provides free access to open-access literature with a poor search engine with limited search functionalities. Other databases index literature from limited geographical regions (e.g., SciELO), which makes them limited in comprehensiveness but more complete for that regions' literature.

11.4.2 Search Strategies

The different origin of bibliographic databases, together with the different functionalities of their search engines, makes searching in more than one database a basic requirement to perform a systematic search. A first difference among search engines is the use of two different systems to build the search query: single bar (used in DOAJ and SciELO), where all the query is placed in search bar, and multiple bar (used in Scopus or WoS) where bars can be combined with Boolean operators. PubMed allows selecting one of the two systems.

Different to a typical Google search, where the searcher grants the engine with a certain level of freedom and the engine displays the results by order of relevance (using a secret algorithm), systematic searches try to balance sensitivity and specificity to produce a completely controlled search. Similarly to the epidemiological concepts, sensitivity is the ability to obtain all the relevant records, although irrelevant records are also retrieved. Specificity is the ability to retrieve only relevant records, although some relevant records can be missed. Thus, a search query is a series of search terms joined with Boolean operators, using brackets, quotation marks, and field descriptors, to increase specificity without losing sensitivity.

Common Boolean operators, also called logic operators, comprise AND, OR, and NOT. AND operator retrieves records that contain the two search terms separated by the operator. OR operator retrieves records that contain any of the two search terms separated by the operator (or both of them). And NOT operator retrieves records that contain none of the two search terms separated by the operator.

To combine Boolean operators in a search bar, the use of parentheses is crucial. Similarly to what happens with Boolean algebra, parentheses explain to the engine what analysis should be first done. A query like ≪(pharmacists OR physicians) AND education≫ will retrieve more records than the query ≪pharmacists OR (physicians AND education)≫. With the first query, the search engine will start elucidating what is inside the parenthesis and first identify records containing the terms pharmacists or the term physicians, but in a second stage, it will select among these records those containing also the term education. This means that the first query will only retrieve records about education, both from pharmacists or physicians. However, in the second query, the engine will start elucidating the parenthesis and retrieve records containing both the term physicians and the term education and then will add to that list all the records containing the term pharmacists. With this, the second query will retrieve records about physicians' education, plus any record about pharmacists (whether about education or not).

In search queries, quotation marks are used to join more than one word in a search string; this means a unique piece of text that searches as a whole. Some search engines, like PubMed, use the Boolean operator AND as default. Searching for ≪pharmacy practice≫ in PubMed is identical than searching for ≪pharmacy AND practice≫, so it will retrieve records containing both terms, but these two terms do not necessarily are together in the text. If one wants to search for records containing the name of the scientific discipline, pharmacy practice, the query ≪"pharmacy practice"≫ should be used to convert the two words joined by a blank space as one chain.

PubMed, and other databases like Scopus, allows searching for the terms allocated in specific fields of the records. A bibliographic record contains a set of metadata, among others: title, abstract, authors, affiliation, etc. If one searches for diabetes, with no specific indication of the field to search that term, the engine will retrieve any record containing that term in any field. For instance, an article written by an author member of the Diabetes Research Group will be indexed with that affiliation, and that record will always be retrieved with the term ≪diabetes≫ if no field descriptor is used to limit where the engine should search for. Each engine has its own set of field descriptors. Among the most commonly used field descriptors in PubMed may be [TI] for tile, [TIAB] for either title or abstract, [LA] for language, and [DP] for publication date.

Keywords are a very special component of bibliographic records. Keywords existed in old paper-based records and allowed storing several identical records in different drawers ordered by subject. Regardless of the term used by the authors in their article to describe diabetes, librarians created a record for that article containing the keyword diabetes mellitus and placed it in the D drawer. To be effective, librarians had to create a controlled vocabulary to consistently use the same words for a type of article. This idea persists in the internet era, and NLM developed the most complete controlled vocabulary from any field, the MeSH thesaurus. MeSH stands for Medical Subject Headings, which are precisely what librarians used many years before. MeSH is placed in a specific field of MEDLINE indexed records and can be searched with the [MH] field descriptor. MeSH terms are organized within MeSH database in a "tree structure." this hierarchal system allows for either broad topic searches (e.g., pharmaceutical services) or more specific searches (e.g., community pharmacy services) (National Library of Medicine 2019). Using the MeSH database to define the subject of interest is a useful way to improve the quality of the search. However, familiarity with these terms is necessary for an efficient and effective search (Kier and Goldwire 2018; Chapman 2009)

An efficient searcher is able to combine all those elements to perform a systematic search, but also must be aware of the limitations of the indexing process. Searching using MeSH enhances the quality of the query since it retrieves more records where authors used inaccurate terms. However searching using only MeSH is incorrect because of three reasons: MeSH may have been incorrectly assigned by NLM cataloguers omitting relevant MeSH for a given article (Minguet et al. 2015); MeSH is never assigned to non-MEDLINE records in PubMed this is to say those indexed in PubMed Central exclusively; and MeSH assignment has a delay different for different journals which can go to several months which means that a search made only with MeSH in these initial months may ignore records of a MEDLINE-journal not yet catalogued

MEDLINE can be searched using other search engines provided by vendors with cost (e.g., Ovid). These search engines can have additional characteristics, like adjacency operators, that retrieve records containing two words separated by a specific number of words (e.g., pharmacists adj3 education will retrieve records with the words pharmacists and education separated by no more than three words). Again, it is important to know if the vendor's search engine uses only MEDLINE database, which may result in ignoring all the literature indexed only in PubMed Central.

11.4.3 Critical Evaluation of the Literature

After retrieving information, researchers should have the ability to critically evaluate the evidence and then use it properly and with responsibility. This process of "evidence-based practice" requires combining literature evaluation skills with the knowledge of practice and clinical experience (Sackett 1995).

Studies of any design should be evaluated using strict and consistent criteria. Some well-recognized international research groups such as the Cochrane Collaboration, the Joanna Briggs Institute, and the EQUATOR Network (*Enhancing the QUAlity and Transparency Of health Research*) provide recommendations, guidelines, and tools for researchers to conduct and report their studies, as well as to evaluate other studies. The Cochrane Collaboration developed the most commonly used instruments to evaluate the risk of bias in different study designs: RoB (risk of bias in randomized trials assessment tool), ROBINS (risk of bias in non-randomized studies of interventions assessment tool), and ROBIS (risk of bias in systematic reviews) (Higgins et al. 2011; Schunemann et al. 2019; Sterne et al. 2016; Whiting et al. 2016). The use of these instruments requires specific training, which should probably be part of the undergraduate pharmacy education curricula but definitely should be part of the postgraduate training for pharmacy practice researchers.

The EQUATOR Network is an organization that brings together researchers, medical journal editors, peer reviewers, developers of reporting guidelines, funding bodies, and other collaborators, aiming to improve the reliability and value of published health research literature by promoting transparent and accurate reporting. A reporting guideline is a structured tool to help healthcare researchers, while performing and writing their research. A reporting guideline provides a list of the minimum information needed to ensure that a manuscript can be understood by a reader, replicated by another researcher, used by a healthcare professional to make clinical decisions, and included in a systematic review or practice guideline (EQUATOR Network 2019). Examples of reporting guidelines include (Schulz et al. 2010; von Elm et al. 2007; Moher et al. 2009; Rotta et al. 2015):

- CONSORT (Consolidated Standards Of Reporting Trials), an initiative for reporting interventional studies. The last updated guidelines for reporting parallel group randomized trials were published in 2010.
- STROBE (Strengthening the Reporting of OBservational studies in Epidemiology) Statement, which is a guideline developed for reporting observational studies.
- PRISMA (Preferred Reporting Items for Systematic Reviews and Meta-Analyses) Statement and its extension for network meta-analysis (PRISMA-NMA), which represent important checklist for conduct and report of secondary studies.
- DEPICT (Descriptive Elements of Pharmacist Interventions Characterization Tool), a guideline to ensure the consistent reporting of clinical pharmacy services to enhance reproducibility in practice.

11.5 Scientific Publishing

Scientific articles in scholarly publications are the most common means of disseminating the knowledge that results from research activities. Selecting the most appropriate journal to submit a paper may be a complex task, especially in multidisciplinary fields like pharmacy (Gagnon 2011; Börner et al. 2003; Touchette et al. 2008). The pressure to publish, rooted in the "publish or perish" culture, stems directly from the perception that progress can only be made by contributing to, sharing, and competing with the knowledge of peers. The rapid growth of published literature (van Assen et al. 2014; Rawat and Meena 2014) obliges researchers to consider several elements for journal selection, such as the length and quality of the journal's editorial process (Cornelius 2012; Wallach et al. 2018), time to indexing (Irwin and Rackham 2017; Rodriguez 2014, 2015), journal metrics (Fernandez-Llimos 2018a), or journal category (Minguet et al. 2017). That means, the ability of researchers to efficiently perform and progress in their career is closely associated with their skills and knowledge about the publishing world.

Researchers should continuously recall that, apart from the progression in academic careers, scholarly publications should serve for more altruistic purposes like sharing new knowledge and reinforce a discipline. Selecting the journal to submit a publication based on journal metrics may not be the best option. In pharmacy practice field, the selection of a journal strictly based on the highest impact factor possible frequently leads to scatter publications outside of the pharmacy practice area, which may weaken the area itself (Rotta et al. 2017). Journals in pharmacy practice use pharmacy practice researchers as peer reviewers, which may avoid some of the problems identified as limitations in pharmacy practice research: duplication of studies, use of inconsistent terminology, lack of standard procedures, lack of core outcome sets, etc. (Pintor-Marmol et al. 2012; Almarsdottir et al. 2014). Similarly, publishing in international journals may increase a study visibility for foreign researcher but may decrease the visibility in the country where the research can be of special relevance. For these reasons, journal's scope and editorial policy should be the two main aspects to consider when selecting a journal to submit a manuscript.

11.5.1 Editorial Process

The scholarly publication process starts when a group of researchers submit a manuscript to a journal. Editorial process can be divided in two phases: manuscript selection and article production.

A journal's editorial board is usually constituted by an editor-in-chief and several associate editors. The editor-in-chief is the highest responsible of the editorial process and the final responsible for manuscript acceptance or rejection.

Associate editors are usually specialized in the sub-areas covered by the scope of the journal.

When a researcher submits the manuscript through the online submission system, trained administrative staff checks the compliance of the instructions for authors that the journal established. If the manuscript does not attend these norms, the corresponding author is warned and requested to modify the submitted files accordingly. Once the manuscript complies the norms, the editor-in-chief can assume the responsibility of the manuscript or select an associate editor to be responsible for it. The editor in charge of the manuscript screens the manuscript to evaluate several aspects: fits under the scope of the journal, presents an original and relevant study, methods look appropriate for the objective, and is correctly written. When a manuscript is negatively evaluated in any of these aspects, a desk rejection (rejection before external evaluation) usually happens. If positively evaluated by the editor in charge, external peer reviewers are selected. Peer reviewers are one of the most important elements in the editorial process because they contribute to the final product by commenting on the manuscript with the aim to improve it (Fernandez-Llimos 2018b). A peer reviewer should produce a two-page report commenting general aspects of the manuscript (e.g., relevance and originality, appropriateness of the study design, quality of the writing) and then enter into a more detailed analysis of the different sections of the manuscript: Does the introduction frame the need of the study? Is the objective clearly stated? Are the methods sufficiently described to ensure the study replicability? Are the results presented clearly and sufficiently detailed? Does the discussion analyze the results comparing with existing literature and provide their implications into practice? Are the conclusions objectively extracted from the results and do they respond to the objectives declared? It is important to remember that peer reviewers are not responsible for manuscript acceptance of the rejection but responsible for producing a report that will help the authors to improve their manuscript. Once the editor in charge of the article receives the reports from all the peer reviewers selected, a decision should be made: accepting (rarely at this stage), rejecting (usually when reviewers' comments give the idea of a poor manuscript), or requesting the authors for modifications according to reviewers' comments. Authors should submit a new version of the manuscript, including the required modification, and should also write a reply to reviewers answering one by one all the reviewers' comments. When the new version is submitted, the editor in charge of the manuscript can send for a second round of external review, with a similar procedure as the first one. This process can be repeated several times (usually no more than three) until the editor in charge presents the results to the editorial board and the editor-in-chief makes the final decision (acceptance or rejection).

Once the paper is accepted, the production phase starts. This process is usually run by a different staff than the editorial board members, and it includes the steps of copy editing, typesetting, inclusion in a specific issue of a journal, and then printing and online publishing (Liesegang et al. 2003; Janke et al. 2017).

11.5.2 Types of Journals

The first two scientific journals were published in 1665 by two scientific societies. That was the common pattern with many other societies creating journals. These societies used publishing companies to print and distribute the journals. Members of the scientific societies had to run with the printing and distribution costs. Then, those for-profit companies started creating their own journals, sometimes affiliated to scientific societies, but not always. Since 1665, internet represented the most important change in scholarly publication. Before internet, journals had to be printed and mailed to libraries, and researchers should move to these libraries to access the articles. After the internet, journals do not need to be printed, and they are available in electronic files accessible from researchers' computers. As a first consequence of this innovation, the two greatest publishing costs disappeared: printing and distributing. By eliminating these two costs, scientific societies could make available through internet their scientific journals at no cost for the readers. However, for-profit companies made also available through the internet their journals with a subscription fee. At that time two types of journals existed: free-access journals and subscription journals. In both types of journals, researchers could publish articles at no cost, but in subscription journals, they had to pay a fee to read other researchers' articles.

In 2002, a group of 15 individuals representing 11 institutions made public the Budapest Open Access Initiative (Budapest Open Access Initiative 2002). This declaration started with the sentence: "An old tradition and a new technology have converged to make possible an unprecedented public good," and described this public good as "The public good they make possible is the world-wide electronic distribution of the peer-reviewed journal literature and completely free and unrestricted access to it by all scientists, scholars, teachers, students, and other curious minds." No one can be against this public good. This declaration coins a new term in scholarly publishing, the open-access journals, referring to those journals that could be accessed with no subscription fee, in opposition to subscription journals. What is not so clear in the Budapest Open Access Initiative is the business model of for-profit companies publishing open-access journals. Thus, another new concept emerged, the article processing charges (APCs). APCs are fees that researchers should pay to journals after having an article accepted to have the article published and with free access to readers.

Many questions and issues arouse from the implementation of this new publishing model, being the ethical concern of "paying to be published" one of the most important. New companies were created to run these new open-access journals that only have revenue if an article is accepted for publication. Several of the signatories of the Budapest Open Access Initiative were staff of some of these companies, although the declaration has no conflict of interest disclaimer. As a consequence of this "paying to be published" together with the "publish or perish" system, unethical companies started the predatory publishing system, reducing the quality of the editorial process. Differentiating ethical open-access publishers from predatory publishers is not easy, with many well-known publishers in the limit of the two practices.

The commercial interests of the two publishing models created a confusing terminology associated to open-access. Gold open-access journals are those where researchers have to pay to have their articles published. Green open-access journals are those that allow depositing the text of the published article in public repositories after an embargo period. Hybrid journals are those subscription journals that open the access of a given article for a fee. However, this confusing terminology unintentionally or intentionally ignores the traditional journals, supported by scientific societies, free and available on the internet, and do not charge APCs to publish. Some authors call these journals as platinum open-access, but this terminology is not always accepted (Fernandez-Llimos 2015).

	Authors pay	Readers pay
Subscription journals	No	Yes
Gold open-access journals	Yes	No
Platinum open-access journals	No	No

11.5.3 Journal Metrics

Bibliometrics can be defined as a set of statistical methods used to measure the different characteristics of publications. As in any metric, it is crucial understanding what the metric measures. Researchers are interested in measuring different aspects of publications, from the quality of the editorial process to some impact indicators. The misuse of bibliometrics is very common that it negatively influences in publishing and researcher performance evaluation. To measure the quality of the editorial process, specific metrics can be used, like duration of the editorial process or the number of external reviewers per manuscript. But funding bodies and researchers want to have an easy to use overall measure of journal quality, which erroneously led to impact indicators.

A first discussion about impact indicators starts with the definition of impact and the implication this definition has on the selection of metrics. Impact is the strong effect produced by something on something else. So, to evaluate the impact of articles published in a journal (as a surrogate of the impact of the journal), one should define on what is impacted: other articles, mass media, regulatory bodies, etc. To consider the impact of one article (or scientific journal) in other articles (or scientific journals), traditional citation metrics are useful. However, to measure the impact of one article (or scientific journal) on social/mass media, alternative metrics are preferred.

Several impact metrics, based on counting the bibliographic references of articles, are available. The impact factor was created in the 1950s and used the journals indexed in Science Citation Index and Social Sciences Citation Index as source of bibliographic references. Impact factor is the quotient between the number of citations made in 1 year to articles published the 2 previous years and the number of articles published in these 2 previous years. In other words, impact factor is the average number of citations originated in 1 year to each article published in the 2 previous years. A massive amount of literature criticizes the impact factor based on limitations both in the numerator and the denominator, but the most important limitation of the impact factor in the pharmacy practice area is based on the scarce coverage of pharmacy practice journals in the bibliographic databases used for the calculations (less than 15%) (Mendes et al. 2019).

CiteScore is an alternative metric to impact factor calculated using the Scopus bibliographic database. Few differences make this metric more useful for pharmacy practice researchers. CiteScore uses 3 years in the calculation, which is more appropriate for this area of citation half-life, and more importantly, it is based on Scopus, which has 91% coverage of pharmacy practice journals (Mendes et al. 2019).

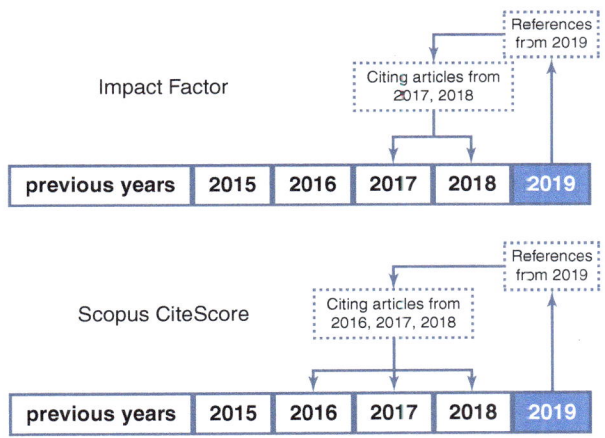

Impact metrics should be carefully used. Metrics are not comparable among different scientific areas, mainly due to their different citation patterns. But the most common misuse of impact metrics is the wrong equivalence between the impact of a journal and the impact of each article of the journal, or even the quality of each article published in that journal. In 2012, a group of researchers and editors created the San Francisco Declaration on Research Assessment, commonly known as DORA, which states as a general recommendation: "Do not use journal-based metrics as a surrogate measure of the quality of individual research articles, to assess an individual scientist's contributions, or in hiring, promotion, or funding decisions." Unfortunately, many funding bodies and researchers still ignore such an important error.

Specific metrics exist to evaluate researchers' impact on science. Among the most commonly accepted is the h-index. This metric combines the number of articles published by a researcher, with the number of citations received by that researcher's articles. Although the h-index has also some limitations, it is a more rational metric to assess individuals' scientific performance than all other journal-based metrics.

11.6   Ethics in Publishing

As in many other areas, scientific publishing is not free of potential misconducts. When the Vancouver group first met in 1979, the document they released was mainly focused on formatting aspects of the submission. Nowadays, the International Committee of Medical Journal Editors (icmje.org) devotes much more efforts to prevent the several aspects of scientific misconduct than to the formatting aspects. From defining who should be listed as authors of an article and the different forms of contributorship to how competing interests should be declared, ICMJE created a series of recommendations that should be attended by journal editors and authors.

Plagiarism is another potential scientific misconduct. Plagiarism is defined as the intentional or unintentional act of appropriation or copying a work (e.g., ideas, expressions, text) as your own, either in part or in whole, without specifying the source or authorship of the original. There are several potential causes for plagiarism including intentional copying, misbelief (i.e., researchers think copying is always accepted as long they include the reference), immature writing skills, and poor time management. To avoid plagiarism, authors should use paraphrasing, quotes, and citations. References of original work must always be listed in full bibliography (Masic 2012, 2014). Journal editors use new technologies (e.g., Similarity Check) to identify plagiarized texts.

The Committee on Publication Ethics (COPE) is an international collaboration that develops guidelines on publication ethics. COPE created a series of flowcharts to be used in the different cases of suspected scientific misconduct (publicationethics.org). Authors should be aware that some of these guidelines recommend "contacting author's institution" or even other authorities and expect institutional investigations to identify benefits resulting from the fraudulent articles.

11.6.1 Data Sharing

Methodology researchers are increasingly criticizing the lack of replicability of articles published as a major symptom of low-quality research. Inappropriate statistical methods and the need of sub-analyses or subgroup analyses are two reasons why sharing original data sets would benefit the science as a whole.

Some research funding policies now encourage investigators to share their raw research data with other researchers. Journals started requiring data sharing as a condition for publication. Several nonprofit organizations are working toward responsible data sharing, by developing public and free databases such as Open Science Framework (OSF, https://osf.io/), which provide a centralized place for many data types.

References

ALA Presidential Committee on Information Literacy. Final report: American Library Association. 1989.

Almarsdottir A, Granas A. Social pharmacy and clinical pharmacy – joining forces. Pharmacy. 2016;4(1):1.

Almarsdottir AB, Kaae S, Traulsen JM. Opportunities and challenges in social pharmacy and pharmacy practice research. Res Social Adm Pharm. 2014;10(1):252–5. https://doi.org/10.1016/j.sapharm.2013.04.002. S1551-7411(13)00053-3 [pii].

Alper BS, Hand JA, Elliott SG, Kinkade S, Hauan MJ, Onion DK, Sklar BM. How much effort is needed to keep up with the literature relevant for primary care? J Med Libr Assoc. 2004;92(4):429–37.

American Pharmacists Association. Drug information handbook. 15th ed. USA: Lexi-Comp Inc; 2007. ISBN: 1591952034.

Berland GK, Elliott MN, Morales LS, Algazy JI, Kravitz RL, Broder MS, Kanouse DE, Munoz JA, Puyol JA, Lara M, Watkins KE, Yang H, McGlynn EA. Health information on the internet: accessibility, quality, and readability in English and Spanish. JAMA. 2001;285(20):2612–21.

Bernknopf AC, Karpinski JP, McKeever AL, Peak AS, Smith KM, Smith WD, Timpe EM, Ward KE. Drug information: from education to practice. Pharmacotherapy. 2009;29(3):331–46. https://doi.org/10.1592/phco.29.3.331.

Börner K, Chen C, Boyack K. In Annual Review of Information Science & Technology, editor. Visualizing knowledge domains. Medfor, NJ: Information Today, Inc./American society for Information Science and Technology; 2003.

Budapest Open Access Initiative. 2002. Available from: http://www.budapestopenaccessinitiative.org/read. Accessed.

Chapman D. Advanced search features of PubMed. J Can Acad Child Adolesc Psychiatry. 2009;18(1):58–9.

Clauson KA, Marsh WA, Polen HH, Seamon MJ, Ortiz BI. Clinical decision support tools: analysis of online drug information databases. BMC Med Inform Decis Mak. 2007;7:7. https://doi.org/10.1186/1472-6947-7-7.

Cornelius JL. Reviewing the review process: identifying sources of delay. Australas Med J. 2012;5(1):26–9. https://doi.org/10.4066/AMJ.2012.1165.

Cummings M. The role of the National Library of Medicine in the national biomedical library network. Ann N Y Acad Sci. 1967;142(2):503–12.

Davies K, Harrison J. The information-seeking behaviour of doctors: a review of the evidence. Health Inf Libr J. 2007;24(2):78–94. https://doi.org/10.1111/j.1471-1842.2007.00713.x.

Dee C. The development of the medical literature analysis and retrieval system (MEDLARS). J Med Libr Assoc. 2007;95(4):416–25.

Eisenberg M. Information literacy: essential skills for the information age. DJLIT. 2008;28(2):39–47.

EQUATOR Network. Enhancing the QUAlity and Transparency Of health Research. 2019. http://www.equator-networkorg/.

Eysenbach G, Powell J, Kuss O, Sa ER. Empirical studies assessing the quality of health information for consumers on the world wide web: a systematic review. JAMA. 2002;287(20):2691–700.

Fernandez-Llimos F. Collaborative publishing: the difference between 'gratis journals' and 'open access journals'. Pharm Pract. 2015;13(1):593. https://doi.org/10.18549/pharmpract.2015.01.593.

Fernandez-Llimos F. Differences and similarities between journal Impact Factor and CiteScore. Pharm Pract. 2018a;16(2):1282. https://doi.org/10.18549/PharmPract.2018.02.1282.

Fernandez-Llimos F. Pharmacy practice 2017 peer reviewers. scholarly publishing depends on peer reviewers. Pharm Pract. 2018b;16(1):1236. https://doi.org/10.18549/PharmPract.2018.01.1236.

Gagnon ML. Moving knowledge to action through dissemination and exchange. J Clin Epidemiol. 2011;64(1):25–31. https://doi.org/10.1016/j.jclinepi.2009.08.013.

Ghaibi S, Ipema H, Gabay M. ASHP guidelines on the pharmacist's role in providing drug information. Am J Health Syst Pharm. 2015;72:573–7.

Hersh WR, Gorman PN, Biagioli FE, Mohan V, Gold JA, Mejicano GC. Beyond information retrieval and electronic health record use: competencies in clinical informatics for medical education. Adv Med Educ Pract. 2014;5:205–12. https://doi.org/10.2147/AMEP.S63903.

Higgins JP, Altman DG, Gotzsche PC, Juni P, Moher D, Oxman AD, Savovic J, Schulz KF, Weeks L, Sterne JA. Cochrane bias methods G, Cochrane statistical methods G. The Cochrane collaboration's tool for assessing risk of bias in randomised trials. BMJ. 2011;343:d5928. https://doi.org/10.1136/bmj.d5928.

Irwin AN, Rackham D. Comparison of the time-to-indexing in PubMed between biomedical journals according to impact factor, discipline, and focus. Res Social Adm Pharm. 2017;13(2):389–93. https://doi.org/10.1016/j.sapharm.2016.04.006.

Iwanowicz SL, Marciniak MW, Zeolla MM. Obtaining and providing health information in the community pharmacy setting. Am J Pharm Educ. 2006;70(3):57.

Jakovljevic M, Ogura S. Health economics at the crossroads of centuries – from the past to the future. Front Public Health. 2016;4:115.

Janke KK, Bzowyckyj AS, Traynor AP. Perspectives on enhancing manuscript quality and editorial decisions through peer review and reviewer development. Am J Pharm Educ. 2017;81(4):73. https://doi.org/10.5688/ajpe81473.

Kier K, Goldwire M. Drug information resources and literature retrieval, 7th edn. ACCP's pharmacotherapy self-assessment program. 2018.

Liesegang TJ, Albert DM, Schachat AP, Minckler DS. The editorial process for medical journals: I. Introduction of a series and discussion of the responsibilities of editors, authors, and reviewers. Am J Ophthalmol. 2003;136(1):109–13. https://doi.org/10.1016/s0002-9394(02)02272-9.

Lindberg D. Internet access to the National Library of medicine. Eff Clin Pract. 2000;3(5):256–60.

Malone P, Kier K, Stanovich JE, Malone MJ. Drug information: a guide for pharmacists. 5th ed. USA: McGraw-Hill Education; 2014. ISBN: 978-0-07-180434-9.

Masic I. Plagiarism in scientific publishing. Acta Inform Med. 2012;20(4):208–13. https://doi.org/10.5455/aim.2012.20.208-213.

Masic I. Plagiarism in scientific research and publications and how to prevent it. Mater Sociomed. 2014;26(2):141–6. https://doi.org/10.5455/msm.2014.26.141-146.

Mendes AM, Tonin FS, Buzzi MF, Pontarolo R, Fernandez-Llimos F. Mapping pharmacy journals: a lexicographic analysis. Res Social Adm Pharm. 2019;15:1464. https://doi.org/10.1016/j.sapharm.2019.01.011.

Mendes AE, Tonin FS, Fernandez-Llimos F. Analysis of ten years of publishing in pharmacy practice. Pharm Pract. 2016;14(4):847. https://doi.org/10.18549/PharmPract.2016.04.847.

Minguet F, Salgado TM, Santopadre C, Fernandez-Llimos F. Redefining the pharmacology and pharmacy subject category in the journal citation reports using medical subject headings (MeSH). Int J Clin Pharm. 2017;39(5):989–97. https://doi.org/10.1007/s11096-017-0527-2.

Minguet F, Salgado TM, van den Boogerd L, Fernandez-Llimos F. Quality of pharmacy-specific medical subject headings (MeSH) assignment in pharmacy journals indexed in MEDLINE. Res Social Adm Pharm. 2015;11(5):686–95. https://doi.org/10.1016/j.sapharm.2014.11.004. S1551-7411(14)00392-1 [pii].

Miranda GF, Vercellesi L, Bruno F. Information sources in biomedical science and medical journalism: methodological approaches and assessment. Pharmacol Res. 2004;50(3):267–72. https://doi.org/10.1016/j.phrs.2003.12.021.

Moher D, Liberati A, Tetzlaff J, Altman DG, Group P. Preferred reporting items for systematic reviews and meta-analyses: the PRISMA statement. Ann Intern Med. 2009;151(4):264–9., W64. https://doi.org/10.7326/0003-4819-151-4-200908180-00135.

Mononen N, Jarvinen R, Hameen-Anttila K, Airaksinen M, Bonhomme C, Kleme J, Pohjanoksa-Mantyla M. A national approach to medicines information research: a systematic review. Res Social Adm Pharm. 2018;14:1106. https://doi.org/10.1016/j.sapharm.2018.01.011.

National Library of Medicine. MeSH (Medical Subject Headings). 2019. https://www.ncbi.nlm.nih.gov/mesh.

Pintor-Marmol A, Baena MI, Fajardo PC, Sabater-Hernandez D, Saez-Benito L, Garcia-Cardenas MV, Fikri-Benbrahim N, Azpilicueta I, Faus MJ. Terms used in patient safety related to medication: a literature review. Pharmacoepidemiol Drug Saf. 2012;21(8):799–809. https://doi.org/10.1002/pds.3296.

Porter D. The history of public health: current themes and approaches. Hygiea Int. 1999;1(1):9–21.

Rawat S, Meena S. Publish or perish: where are we heading? J Res Med Sci. 2014;19(2):87–9.

Rodriguez RW. Delay in indexing articles published in major pharmacy practice journals. Am J Health Syst Pharm. 2014;71(4):321–4. https://doi.org/10.2146/ajhp130421.

Rodriguez RW. Comparison of indexing times among articles from medical, nursing, and pharmacy journals. Am J Health Syst Pharm. 2016;73(8):569–75. https://doi.org/10.2146/ajhp150319.

Rotta I, Salgado TM, Felix DC, Souza TT, Correr CJ, Fernandez-Llimos F. Ensuring consistent reporting of clinical pharmacy services to enhance reproducibility in practice: an improved version of DEPICT. J Eval Clin Pract. 2015;21(4):584–90. https://doi.org/10.1111/jep.12339.

Rotta I, Souza TT, Salgado TM, Correr CJ, Fernandez-Llimos F. Characterization of published randomized controlled trials assessing clinical pharmacy services around the world. Res Social Adm Pharm. 2017;13(1):201–8. https://doi.org/10.1016/j.sapharm.2016.01.003.

Sackett D. Evidence-based medicine. Lancet. 1995;346(8983):1171.

Schulz KF, Altman DG, Moher D, Group C. CONSORT 2010 statement: updated guidelines for reporting parallel group randomized trials. Ann Intern Med. 2010;152(11):726–32. https://doi.org/10.7326/0003-4819-152-11-201006010-00232.

Schunemann HJ, Cuello C, Akl EA, Mustafa RA, Meerpohl JJ, Thayer K, Morgan RL, Gartlehner G, Kunz R, Katikireddi SV, Sterne J, Higgins JP, Guyatt G, Group GW. GRADE guidelines: 18. How ROBINS-I and other tools to assess risk of bias in nonrandomized studies should be used to rate the certainty of a body of evidence. J Clin Epidemiol. 2019;111:105–14. https://doi.org/10.1016/j.jclinepi.2018.01.012.

Sharp M, Bodenreider O, Wacholder N. A framework for characterizing drug information sources. AMIA Annu Symp Proc. 2008;2008:662–6.

Skau K. Pharmacy is a science-based profession. Am J Pharm Educ. 2007;71(1):11.

Stansfield C, Brunton G, Rees R. Search wide, dig deep: literature searching for qualitative research. An analysis of the publication formats and information sources used for four systematic reviews in public health. Res Synth Methods. 2014;5(2):142–51. https://doi.org/10.1002/jrsm.1100.

Sterne JA, Hernan MA, Reeves BC, Savovic J, Berkman ND, Viswanathan M, Henry D, Altman DG, Ansari MT, Boutron I, Carpenter JR, Chan AW, Churchill R, Deeks JJ, Hrobjartsson A, Kirkham J, Juni P, Loke YK, Pigott TD, Ramsay CR, Regidor D, Rothstein HR, Sandhu L, Santaguida PL, Schunemann HJ, Shea B, Shrier I, Tugwell P, Turner L, Valentine JC, Waddington H, Waters E, Wells GA, Whiting PF, Higgins JP. ROBINS-I: a tool for assessing risk of bias in non-randomised studies of interventions. BMJ. 2016;355:i4919. https://doi.org/10.1136/bmj.i4919.

Touchette DR, Bearden DT, Ottum SA. Research publication by pharmacist authors in major medical journals: changes over a 10-year interval. Pharmacotherapy. 2008 28(5):584–90. https://doi.org/10.1592/phco.28.5.584.

van Assen MA, van Aert RC, Nuijten MB, Wicherts JM. Why publishing everything is more effective than selective publishing of statistically significant results. PLoS One. 2014;9(1):e84896. https://doi.org/10.1371/journal.pone.0084896.

von Elm E, Altman DG, Egger M, Pocock SJ, Gotzsche PC, Vandenbroucke JP, Initiative S. The strengthening the reporting of observational studies in epidemiology (STROBE) statement: guidelines for reporting observational studies. Ann Intern Med. 2007;147(8):573–7. https://doi.org/10.7326/0003-4819-147-8-200710160-00010.

Wallach JD, Egilman AC, Gopal AD, Swami N, Krumholz HM, Ross JS. Biomedical journal speed and efficiency: a cross-sectional pilot survey of author experiences. Res Integr Peer Rev. 2018;3:1. https://doi.org/10.1186/s41073-017-0045-8.

Whiting P, Savovic J, Higgins JP, Caldwell DM, Reeves BC, Shea B, Davies P, Kleijnen J, Churchill R, Group R. ROBIS: a new tool to assess risk of bias in systematic reviews was developed. J Clin Epidemiol. 2016;69:225–34. https://doi.org/10.1015/j.jclinepi.2015.06.005.

Wiedenmayer K, Summers R, Mackie C, Gous A, Everard M. Developing pharmacy practice: a focus on patient care. Geneva: WHO; 2006.

World Health Organization (WHO). Good pharmacy practice (GPP) in community and hospital pharmacy settings [WHO/PHARM/DAP/96.1]. Geneva: WHO; 1996.

Chapter 12
Systematic Reviews and Meta-Analysis in Pharmacy Practice

Syed Shahzad Hasan, Therese Kairuz, Kaeshaelya Thiruchelvam, and Zaheer-Ud-Din Babar

Abstract A systematic review is a process of synthesizing research evidence by collecting and summarizing all empirical evidence that meets predefined inclusion and exclusion criteria. Systematic reviews are performed by using systematic methods and often include a meta-analysis component which involves statistical techniques to conduct quantitative synthesis. Pharmacists from different regions of the world and practices—such as academia, hospital, and community—are increasingly using this approach to produce evidence about their new services and interventions, comparing them with services provided by other healthcare professionals or with control groups. This chapter covers the inception of a systematic approach to reviews and their use in pharmacy practice. The quality associated with systematic reviews and meta-analyses are discussed. A quick guide outlines the important steps in conducting a systematic review, and some of the models used in the reporting of meta-analyses—such as direct and indirect evidence models and pooling effect sizes—are introduced.

Abbreviations

CINAHL	Cumulative Index to Nursing and Allied Health Literature
EBP	Evidence-based practice
EMBASE	Excerpta Medica Database
GRADE	Grading of Recommendations, Assessment, Development and Evaluations
IPA	International Pharmaceutical Abstracts

S. S. Hasan · Z. Babar (✉)
Department of Pharmacy, University of Huddersfield, Huddersfield, West Yorkshire, UK
e-mail: z.babar@hud.ac.uk

T. Kairuz · K. Thiruchelvam
School of Biomedical Sciences & Pharmacy, University of Newcastle,
Callaghan, NSW, Australia

© Springer Nature Singapore Pte Ltd. 2020
Z. Babar (ed.), *Pharmacy Practice Research Methods*,
https://doi.org/10.1007/978-981-15-2993-1_12

237

MA   Meta-analysis
NICE   National Institute for Health and Care Excellence
OR   Odds ratio
PICO   Patient, intervention, comparison, outcome
PRISMA   Preferred Reporting Items for Systematic Reviews and
            Meta-Analyses
QUAROM   Quality of Reporting of Meta-analyses
RCT   Randomized controlled trial
RR   [Relative] Risk ratio
SIGN   Scottish Intercollegiate Guidelines Network
SR   Systematic review

12.1 The Importance of Evidence-Based Practice

In the early 1990s, the need for a comprehensive summary of "all" the evidence within a particular domain arose, over and above evidence from primary studies; this was to facilitate the informed decision-making process of clinicians (Grant and Booth 2009). However, these review articles within the field of medicine and prior to the evidence-based practice (EBP) era were largely unsystematic in their approach; furthermore, they were sometimes statistically inaccurate in determining effect sizes of treatment which led to the incorrect and biased conclusions (Mulrow 1987). Reputable British epidemiologist Archie Cochrane initiated the worldwide Cochrane Collaboration in 1992 to provide a platform for updateable systematic reviews of randomized controlled trials (RCT) pertaining to medicine and the field of healthcare (Mulrow 1987). This was the dawn of good-quality systematic reviews which are the mainstay for keeping abreast of scientific knowledge.

12.2 The Many Forms of Reviews

The Collins Dictionary has various definitions of "review" when used as a verb, and the following are relevant to our context: "to look at or examine again" and "to read through or go over in order to correct." When used as a noun, the following definitions are applicable: "a second consideration; re-examination" and "a critical assessment of a book, film, play, concert etc. especially one printed in a newspaper or periodical" (Collins Dictionary 2019). These definitions could also be applicable to scholarly reviews.

A distinguishing feature between reviews is the difference in the degree of rigor and the process; these differences are apparent in the structure and methodology of reviews (Grant and Booth 2009). In their review of a typology of reviews, Grant and Booth (2009) characterized the main review types using an approach termed SALSA (search, appraisal, synthesis, analysis) and described 14 different types of reviews: critical review, literature review/narrative review, mapping review/systematic map, meta-analysis, mixed studies review/mixed methods review, overview, qualitative systematic review/qualitative evidence synthesis, rapid review, scoping review, state-of-the-art review, systematic review, systematic search and review, systematized review, and umbrella review. The authors provide descriptions, perceived strengths and weakness, and examples of each review type (Grant and Booth 2009).

Narrative reviews are perceived to be synonymous with systematic reviews when in fact they are not (Grant and Booth 2009; Uman 2011). A notable difference between them is that systematic reviews involve a systematic search of the literature focusing on a subset of studies related to the topic of the study whereas narrative reviews are mainly descriptive and do not include a systematic search process (Uman 2011). In this chapter, we will focus on systematic reviews and meta-analyses.

12.3 Inception of Systematic Approach to Reviews

James Lind was a Scottish naval surgeon who is well-known for instigating the first RCT; what is less well-known is that he introduced the systematic review method (Chalmers 2003). Lind discarded the "rubbish" and summarized what remained which is regarded as the quintessence of a systematic review (Chalmers 2003). The Cochrane Consumer Network defines a systematic review as summarizing "the results of the available carefully designed healthcare studies (controlled trials), which provide a high level of evidence on the effectiveness of healthcare interventions" (Cochrane Consumer Network 2019).

Systematic reviews involve a comprehensive and detailed plan and search strategy developed a priori aimed at reducing bias by identifying, appraising, and synthesizing relevant research studies on a particular topic (Uman 2011). Systematic reviews have an evolving component referred to as a meta-analysis; this approach uses statistical methods to synthesize data from several studies (quantitative synthesis)—often obtained from a systematic review—into a single quantitative estimate, or a pooled estimate, of the treatment effect size (Petticrew and Roberts 2006). Results of a meta-analysis are often regarded as the highest level of evidence because the summary effect size depicts the strength of the association between two variables; this is a prerequisite to determining causation, which is often the aim of a meta-analysis. The type of effect size to be determined depends on the study designs, the intervention types, the quality of the studies included in the systematic review, and most importantly, the outcomes available from published studies such as RCTs. The most common effect sizes determined in meta-analysis include odds ratio (OR) and [relative] risk ratios (RR). It is equally important to state confidence intervals of the effect sizes as they provide a measure of the precision of the effect size estimate. It is also important to understand the term "uncertainty interval" that is used in systematic reviews/analysis (Naghavi 2019). Uncertainty intervals are a range of values that are likely to include the correct estimate of health loss for a given cause (The Institute for Health Metrics and Evaluation (IHME) 2019).

Since 1999, multiple authors have produced guidelines for reporting systematic reviews and meta-analyses, and it is essential that authors adhere to the most recent guidelines. These include the Quality of Reporting of Meta-analyses (QUORUM) statement (Moher et al. 1999), followed by the use of registers such as the Cochrane Library's Methodology Register. In 2009, the PRISMA (Preferred Reporting Items for Systematic Reviews and Meta-Analyses) statement was published which contains evidence-based requirements—or minimum set of items—that have to be reported in systematic reviews and meta-analyses involving RCTs. PRISMA guidelines may also be used as a basis for reporting reviews of other research such as evaluating interventions (Moher et al. 2009). The advent of the PRISMA guidelines led to standardization and improvement in the quality of systematic reviews and meta-analyses (Willis and Quigley 2011).

12.4 Systematics Reviews and Meta-Analysis in Pharmacy Practice

Systematic reviews in practice have been conducted since the 1990s evaluating the impact of pharmaceutical practices on economic, clinical, and humanistic outcomes. The aim is to gather robust evidence to develop clinical guidelines and to inform policy change in practice (Melchiors et al. 2012). However, as pharmacy practice was evolving, early efforts resulted in only a handful of published systematic reviews that were critically analyzed to provide recommendations aimed at improving pharmacy practice.

Most systematic reviews that discussed pharmacist health interventions with a view to improving pharmaceutical care seemed to lack quality in terms of research question(s) and research design. The use of similar search periods, methodology, and target populations in reviews results in considerable differences in the number of total original studies included in the reviews. The systematic reviews also had shortcomings in the description of intervention(s), test(s), exposure of interest, comparison of interventions, and the outcome(s) of interest (Melchiors et al. 2012).

12.5 Quality of Systematic Reviews and Meta-Analysis in Pharmacy Practice

As part of this chapter, we systematically searched the systematic reviews and meta-analyses published by pharmacy academics, practitioners, or researchers, which were aimed at introducing interventions or improving service or practice of pharmacists or inter-professional teams that included pharmacist(s). The PubMed Central (US National Library of Medicine, Bethesda, MD, USA), CINAHL, EMBASE,

EMCARE, International Pharmaceutical Abstracts (IPA), MEDLINE, and Scopus databases were searched between 1 January 2000 and 19 April 2019. Two authors screened abstracts of reviews published in English against the following criteria: (a) pharmacists' interventions or role; (b) interventions, service, or practice performed by pharmacists or inter-professional team including pharmacist; and (c) outcome measures and impact of interventions on cost savings (medications). Search terms include pharmacological agents, efficacy, harm, and cost of medicines. Original research, narrative, or realist reviews were excluded, as only systematic reviews, with or without meta-analysis, were included.

A total of 156 systematic reviews and meta-analyses were included in the current review. There was a significant increase in recent years: we identified 10 studies in the 5-year period from 2000 to 2005 compared with 70 studies in the period 2016 to 2019 (Fig. 12.1). Melchiors et al. (2012) also commented on the increasing number of systematic reviews; at that time approximately 70.0% of the reviews were published between January 2005 and June 2009 (Melchiors et al. 2012).

In most instances, systematic reviews are reported without a quantitative synthesis (or meta-analysis). This is largely due to heterogeneity of the interventions and outcomes in original studies which makes it inappropriate to conduct a meta-analysis. We found that the majority of systematic reviews was published without a meta-analysis; of the 156 reviews included in the current study, only 42 reviews were reported with a meta-analysis (Table 12.1).

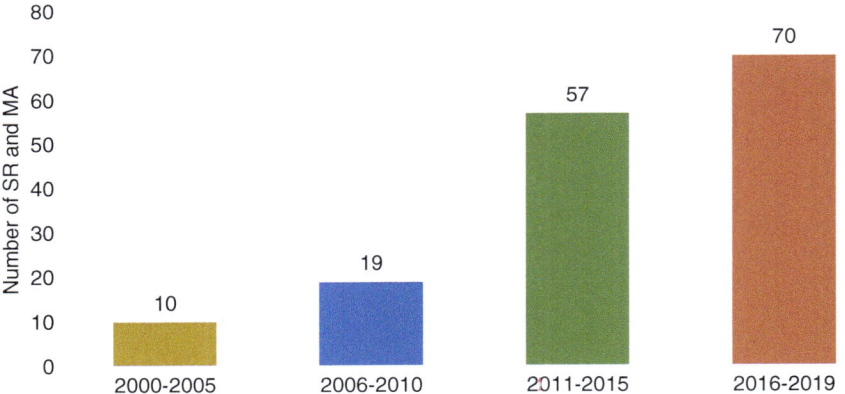

Fig. 12.1 Number of systematic reviews and meta-analysis published between 2000 and 2019

Table 12.1 Summary of the number of SRs and MAs in pharmacy practice

Years	No of reviews	SR + MA	SR only
2000–2005	10	1	9
2006–2010	19	6	13
2011–2015	57	14	43
2016–2019	70	21	49
Total	156	42	114

Note: *SR* systematic review, *MA* meta-analysis

The researchers carefully assessed the studies against a checklist of minimum standards, the Preferred Reporting Items for Systematic Reviews and Meta-Analyses (PRISMA). The PRISMA statement is a list of 27 items, and each question is judged with a "yes," "no," or "not applicable response" (it must be noted that items 14, 16, and 23 only apply to a meta-analysis). The total score was obtained by assigning 1 point for each "yes" answer and 0 points for all other answers (range 0–27) (Liberati et al. 2009).

Figure 12.2 shows that the majority of systematic reviews/meta-analyses (66.99%) was related to pharmacist interventions, pharmacy services, or pharmaceutical care, followed by (in)appropriate use or (in)appropriate prescribing (13.59%); medicine reconciliation, medicine adherence, or medicine optimization (10.19%); and medicine management (9.22%).

The overall mean for the PRISMA score was 19.47 out of a possible 27. The PRISMA score steadily increased from 16.80 (between 2000 and 2005) to 20.08 (between 2016 and 2019) as shown in Fig. 12.3.

Fig. 12.2 Four themes identified in systematic reviews/meta-analyses. The same study may have had more than one theme, and therefore the study may have been categorized under more than one theme

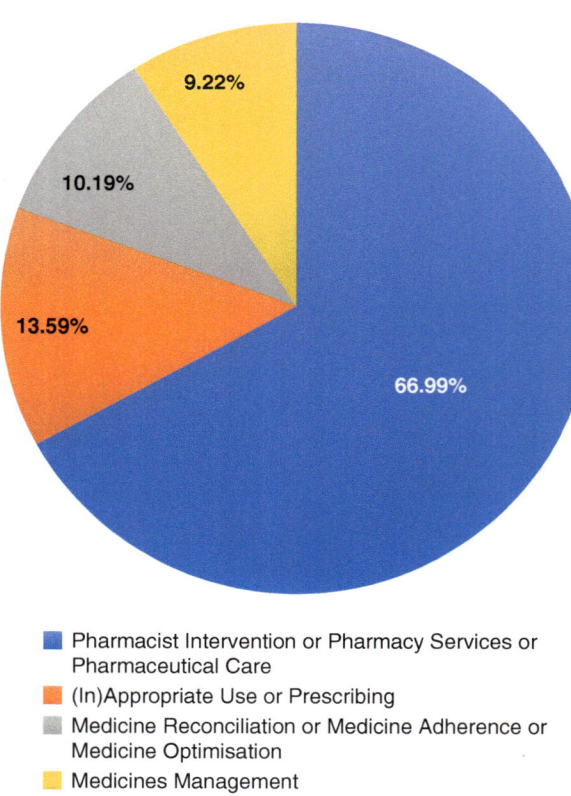

■ Pharmacist Intervention or Pharmacy Services or Pharmaceutical Care
■ (In)Appropriate Use or Prescribing
■ Medicine Reconciliation or Medicine Adherence or Medicine Optimisation
■ Medicines Management

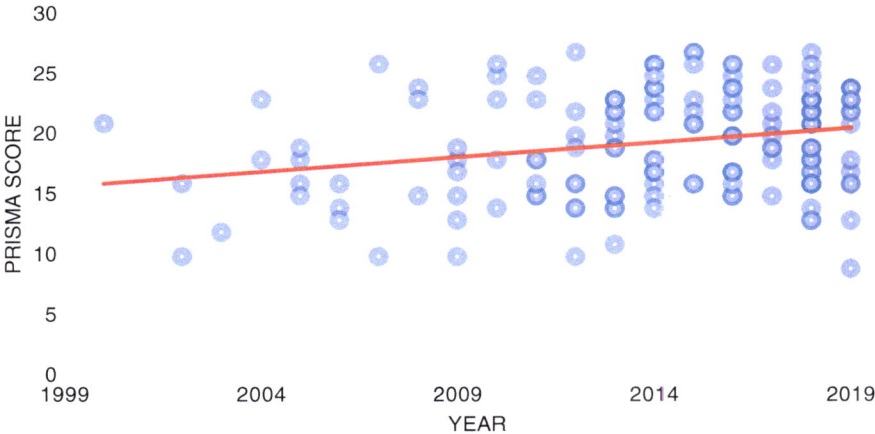

Fig. 12.3 Scattered plot depicting PRISMA score (quality score) for reviews published between 2000 and 2019

12.6   Systematic Review Process: A Quick Guide

Figure 12.4 represents a flow diagram of the process involved in a systematic review. The first step in conducting a systematic review is to formulate a research question which is based on an identified gap in the literature. At this stage, the PICO (patient, comparison, intervention, outcome) model can be helpful in developing a research question and a search strategy (Ahn and Kang 2018). The scope of the review can be determined with the help of clear inclusion and exclusion criteria.

The search strategy is developed with all search terms and synonymous terms, Boolean operators (and, or, not or, and not), as well as truncated words (e.g., chemist/pharm∗ for a systematic search involving pharmacists) and spelling (UK or US). The next step is to determine information sources and databases that will be used to search for eligible studies and the time period/duration of the search. The type of databases that should be searched largely depends on the topic of the systematic review; for example, CINAHL (Cumulative Index in Nursing and Allied Health Literature) would be suitable for data pertaining to nurses, podiatrists, physiotherapists, and other health professionals.

The screening of titles, abstracts, and full texts should be done carefully, and there are online software products (e.g., Covidence) to improve the efficiency of screening and extraction of data processes. Once all articles have been screened, any studies that are deemed ineligible are excluded, and reasons for exclusion should be provided. Two investigators are usually involved in data extraction which is done independently of each other. A third reviewer will be engaged if there are differences in opinion that cannot be resolved between the first two reviewers.

Fig. 12.4 Flowchart illustrating the stages of a systematic review process

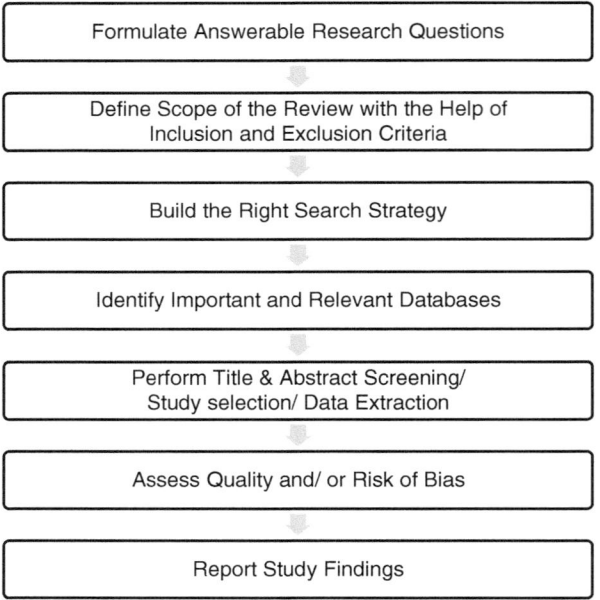

The data extraction/collection process, characteristics of the study, and data items must be described in the report.

The inclusion of studies of low quality and risk of bias will affect the quality of a systematic review and meta-analysis leading to inaccurate results (Guyatt et al. 2008). Even when a review includes RCTs of high quality, it is still essential to determine the quality of the evidence as this will aid in measuring the strength of the recommendations reported in a systematic review or meta-analysis.

There are a number of tools and checklists available to assess quality or risk of bias. Examples include Newcastle-Ottawa scale (developed by the Ottawa Hospital Research Institute) (Kang 2015), GRADE (Grading of Recommendations, Assessment, Development and Evaluations) system (Dijkers 2013; Ahn and Kang 2018), and SIGN (Scottish Intercollegiate Guidelines Network) methodology checklist for observational studies (Scottish Intercollegiate Guidelines Network 2012). Risk of bias in RCTs and non-RCTs can be evaluated by the Cochrane Collaboration's tool (Higgins et al. 2011) and the Effective Practice and Organisation of Care (Effective Practice and Organisation of Care (EPOC) 2019) criteria; the latter is based on ten standard criteria: random sequence generation, allocation concealment, blinding, incomplete outcome data, selective reporting, other risk of bias, similar baseline outcome measurements, similar baseline characteristics, reliable primary outcome measures, and the adequate protection against contamination. Authors should report their judgment of the included studies as to whether they are of low risk, high risk, or "unclear bias." Some of the abovementioned criteria are explained in the paper titled Clinical Research Methodology I: Introduction to Randomized Trials by Kao et al. (2008).

Once the studies have been assessed, those that are of sufficient quality are included in the systematic review. The size and format of each variable may differ; therefore, size and format of outcome variables will also vary. Slight changes will be necessary when the data are combined (Ahn and Kang 2018). This is a crucial stage in determining whether the systematic review can proceed to a meta-analysis. Differences in variables may cause difficulties when data are combined perhaps due to different evaluation instruments of the same outcome variables, evaluations which were done at different time points, differences in the size and direction of the effect, and differences in homogeneity of the studies; in such cases, analysis may be limited to a systematic review.

Presentation or reporting of results includes a summary description of each study that was included in the (systematic) review. In addition to the summary tables, a conclusion will be derived with a pooled estimate in the case of a meta-analysis. There are reporting guidelines to help researchers report the findings in a standardized way. Preferred Reporting Items for Systematic Reviews and Meta-Analyses (PRISMA) is the most widely used checklist to report findings of a systematic review and meta-analysis. Cochrane Handbook provides information on how to conduct and report systematic reviews of interventions, and systematic reviews of diagnostic test accuracy can also be used (Higgins et al. 2019).

12.7 The Meta-Analysis

Unlike a systematic review, the focus of a meta-analysis is on the direction and magnitude of the effects across studies (Doi and Barendregt 2013). Meta-analysis is not a process of simple pooling; it is a method in which combining and comparing are carried out in a specific order (to avoid reversals such as Simpson's paradox) (Doi and Barendregt 2013). Some commonly used effect sizes include standardized mean difference and correlation (measurements are inherently continuous, used with group contrast research, treatment groups, and naturally occurring groups), odds ratio or relative risk (used with group contrast research although measurements are inherently dichotomous), and proportion or diagnostic studies (used in central tendency research, prevalence rates, sensitivity, and specificity). Table 12.2 presents examples of the use of different effect sizes in pharmacy practice-related meta-analyses.

Table 12.2 Use of different effect sizes in pharmacy practice research

Effect size	Example
Standardized mean difference	Babar et al. (2019)
Odds ratio	Carter et al. (2009)
Relative risk	Holland et al. (2007)
Proportion	Hasan et al. (2019)

12.8   Direct and Indirect Evidence Models

There are various approaches to performing a meta-analysis, and the variety of approaches has led to the development of different types of meta-analysis. The meta-analysis techniques synthesize quantitative data to produce more accurate estimate of an effect than an individual study (Doi and Barendregt 2013). Generally, a meta-analysis can provide two types of data: aggregate and individual participant data. Aggregate data are more commonly reported in meta-analyses and represent the summary estimates that we have discussed in this chapter. Aggregate data are derived from direct evidence or indirect evidence. Direct aggregate data or evidence can be directly synthesized within studies that are conceptually similar (e.g., head-to-head comparison of drug A vs drug B in a randomized trial or conventional meta-analysis), whereas indirect aggregate data estimates the effect from multiple direct comparisons that share a common comparator (e.g., trials on drug C vs drug D plus trial on drug A vs drug B, when C and A are the comparison of interest) (Debray et al. 2013; Thomas et al. 2015).

Individual participant data (IPD) are the raw data collected from the study centers, which use one-step clustering or two-step clustering meta-analysis method to synthesize evidence. The one-step clustering method simultaneously models individual participant data from all studies taking into account participant clustering within studies. Clustering refers to the identification of similar groups in multivariate data sets, for example, hierarchical clustering. On the other hand, the two-step clustering model tabulates summary statistics from aggregate data of individual studies and then tabulates overall statistics as a weighted average of study statistics. The use of aggregate data is more robust hence the conversion to aggregate data when individual data are available (Debray et al. 2013; Thomas et al. 2015).

12.9   Pooling Effect Sizes

The type of approach to consider for a meta-analysis is largely dependent on the statistical models used for data aggregation or pooling. Conventional meta-analyses use direct comparisons from randomized controlled trials as standard guidelines from organizations such as guidelines from the National Institute for Health and Care Excellence (NICE) (National Institute for Health and Clinical Excellence (NICE) 2014) and the Cochrane Collaboration (Higgins et al. 2011) which tend to choose direct evidence over indirect evidence. The following are some of the statistical models to present aggregate data.

12.9.1 The Fixed-Effect Model

For aggregate data of direct evidence, there are various models that may be used for pooling effect sizes. The fixed-effect model, also termed the inverse variance method, is one of the standard approaches used to compute average effect size across all studies (Woolf 1955). In this model, larger studies and studies with less random variation are given greater weight than smaller studies (Doi and Barendregt 2013). The fixed-effect model is used when the variability within study results is small and when the studies have similar methodologies and study designs; this model considers the effect of the treatment to be the same and that any variation is due to a random error. The major limitation is that it does not take into account that the innate variability that exists between studies gave rise to the development of random effect model (Doi and Barendregt 2013).

12.9.2 The Random Effects Model

The random effects model is one of the most common techniques used to synthesize heterogeneous research (DerSimonian and Laird 1986). This model is used when size of the treatment effect differs among studies; this model therefore assumes heterogeneity between the studies which are being combined, and this is not random in nature (Ahn and Kang 2018). The "weighted average" is achieved in two steps: (1) inverse variance method and (2) unweighting of inverse variance weighting by applying a random effects variance component (REVC). In the process, variability in effect sizes and unweighting can reach a point when the overall result simply becomes the unweighted average effect size across the studies (Doi and Barendregt 2013). Doi et al. have introduced a model named "inverse variance quasi-likelihood based alternative (IVhet) to the random effects (RE) model." IVhet model coverage remains at the nominal (usually 95%) level for the confidence interval and also maintains the inverse variance weights of individual studies (Doi et al. 2015).

12.9.3 The Quality Effects Model

Another model for direct evidence of aggregate data is one that incorporates additional information, known as the quality effects model (Doi and Thalib 2008). This approach adjusts for inter-study variability by incorporating the variance of a relevant (quality) component. This is in addition to the variance taken into account for random error that is used in a fixed-effect model. One of the advantages of the quality effects meta-analysis is that it allows the researcher to use available methodological evidence over subjective random effects, narrowing the gap between methodology and statistics in clinical research. A synthetic bias variance is tabulated based upon quality information to adjust weights, and the adjusted weights are used in the meta-analysis (Doi and Thalib 2008).

12.9.4 The Network Meta-Analysis

For aggregate data of indirect evidence, network meta-analysis methods are used, for example, when multiple treatments are being assessed in a single process. There are two methodologies that can be used in network meta-analyses. The first is the Bucher method which compares treatments indirectly by preserving the randomization of the originally assigned patient groups (Bucher et al. 1997). This method allows a simple indirect comparison of outcomes, or a comparison across a network of treatments, where different interventions are compared to common comparator (Bucher et al. 1997).

The second method, Bayesian NMA, involves indirect treatment comparisons within more complex networks of treatments with multi-arm trials. This approach combines both direct and indirect evidence of the interventions being compared (Lu and Ades 2004). This method allows standard pairwise meta-analysis, i.e., performing multiple pairwise comparisons across the interventions to produce the relative treatment effects (Lu and Ades 2004).

12.10 Homogeneity Test

A homogeneity test should be done to test if the results of several studies are sufficiently similar to warrant their combination into a pooled estimate. This would make it possible to determine if the effect size estimated from different studies is the same. There are three types of homogeneity tests that can be done: (1) forest plot, (2) Cochrane's Q test (Chi-squared), and (3) Higgin's I^2 statistics (Ahn and Kang 2018).

12.11 Conclusion

This chapter has provided a detailed description of systematic reviews and meta-analyses and their methodological approaches; the evidence-based approach includes a comprehensive list of references. It is interesting to note that both quantity and quality systematic reviews and meta-analyses in pharmacy practice have increased over a period of 20 years. Moving forward, systematic reviews and meta-analyses in pharmacy practice should be performed according to the standards outlined in various checklists. This would increase the quality of evidence as well as acceptability of pharmacy practice evidence.

Acknowledgments We would like to thank Dr. Keivan Ahmadi from Lincoln Medical School (UK) for providing constructed feedback on meta-analysis component.

References

Ahn EJ, Kang H. Introduction to systematic review and meta-analysis. Korean J Anesthesiol. 2018;71(2):103–12.

Babar ZU, Kousar R, Hasan SS, Scahill S, Curley LE. Glycemic control through pharmaceutical care: a meta-analysis of randomized controlled trials. J Pharm Health Serv Res. 2019;10(1):35–44.

Bucher HC, Guyatt GH, Griffith LE, Walter SD. The results of direct and indirect treatment comparisons in meta-analysis of randomized controlled trials. J Clin Epidemiol. 1997;50(6):683–91.

Carter BL, Rogers M, Daly J, Zheng S, James PA. The potency of team-based care interventions for hypertension: a meta-analysis. Arch Intern Med. 2009;169(19):1748–55.

Chalmers I. The James Lind initiative. J R Soc Med. 2003;96(12):575–6

Cochrane Consumer Network. What is a systematic review? 2019. Available from: https://consumers.cochrane.org/what-systematic-review.

Collins Dictionary. Definition of 'review'. 2019. Available from: https //www.collinsdictionary.com/dictionary/english/review.

Debray TP, Moons KG, Abo-Zaid GM, Koffijberg H, Riley RD. Individual participant data meta-analysis for a binary outcome: one-stage or two-stage? PLoS One. 2013;8(4):e60650.

DerSimonian R, Laird N. Meta-analysis in clinical trials. Control Clin Trials. 1986;7:177–88.

Dijkers M. Introducing GRADE: a systematic approach to rating evidence in systematic reviews and to guideline development. Knowl Translat Update. 2013;1:1–9.

Doi SAR, Barendregt JJ. Meta-analysis I: computational methods. In: Doi, Williams, editors. Methods of clinical epidemiology. Berlin, Heidelberg: Springer Publishing; 2013. p. 229–52.

Doi SA, Barendregt JJ, Khan S, Thalib L, Williams GM. Advances in the meta-analysis of heterogeneous clinical trials I: the inverse variance heterogeneity model. Contemp Clin Trials. 2015;45(Pt A):130–8.

Doi SA, Thalib L. A quality-effects model for meta-analysis. Epidemiology. 2008;19(1):94–100.

Effective Practice and Organisation of Care (EPOC). Norwegian Knowledge Centre for the Health Services. Suggested risk of bias criteria for EPOC reviews. 2019. Available from: https://epoc.cochrane.org/sites/epoc.cochrane.org/files/uploads/Suggested%20risk%20of%20bias%20criteria%20for%20EPOC%20reviews.pdf.

Grant MJ, Booth A. A typology of reviews: an analysis of 14 review types and associated methodologies. Health Inf Libr J. 2009;26(2):91–108.

Guyatt GH, Oxman AD, Vist GE, Kunz R, Falck-Ytter Y, Alonso-Coello P, et al. GRADE: an emerging consensus on rating quality of evidence and strength of recommendations. BMJ. 2008;336:924–6.

Hasan SS, Zaidi STR, Nirwan JS, Ghori MU, Javid F, Ahmadi K, Babar ZD. Use of central nervous system (CNS) medicines in aged care homes: a systematic review and meta-analysis. J Clin Med. 2019;8:1292.

Higgins JPT, Altman DG, Sterne JAC. Chapter 8: Assessing risk of bias in included studies. Cochrane statistical methods group and the Cochrane Bias methods group. 2011. Available from: http://handbook.cochrane.org/chapter_8/8_assessing_risk_of_bias_in_included_studies. htm.

Higgins JPT, Thomas J, Chandler J, Cumpston M, Li T, Page MJ, Welch VA, editors. Cochrane handbook for systematic reviews of interventions version 6.0 (updated July 2019). Cochrane. 2019. Available from www.training.cochrane.org/handbook.

Holland R, Desbororough J, Goodyer L, Hall S, Wright D, Loke YK. Does pharmacist-led medication review help to reduce hospital admissions and deaths in older people? A systematic review and meta-analysis. Br J Clin Pharmacol. 2007;65(3):303–16.

Kang H. Statistical considerations in meta-analysis. Hanyang Med Rev. 2015;35:23–32.

Kao LS, Tyson JE, Blakely ML, Lally KP. Clinical research methodology I: introduction to randomized trials. J Am Coll Surg. 2008;206(2):361–9.

Liberati A, Altman DG, Tetzlaff J, et al. The PRISMA statement for reporting systematic reviews and meta-analyses of studies that evaluate healthcare interventions: explanation and elaboration. BMJ. 2009;339:b2700.

Lu G, Ades AE. Combination of direct and indirect evidence in mixed treatment comparisons. Stat Med. 2004;23(20):3105–24.

Melchiors AC, Correr CJ, Venson R, Pontarolo R. An analysis of quality of systematic reviews on pharmacist health interventions. Int J Clin Pharm. 2012;34:32–42.

Moher D, Cook DJ, Eastwood S, Olkin I, Rennie D, Stroup DF. Improving the quality of reports of meta-analyses of randomised controlled trials: the QUOROM statement. Quality of reporting of meta-analyses. Lancet. 1999;354:1896–900.

Moher D, Liberati A, Tetzlaff J, Altman DG, The PRISMA Group. Preferred reporting items for systematic reviews and meta-analyses: the PRISMA statement. BMJ. 2009;339:b2535. https://doi.org/10.1136/bmj.b2535.

Mulrow CD. The medical review article: state of the science. Ann Intern Med. 1987;106:485–8.

Naghavi M. Global, regional, and national burden of suicide mortality 1990 to 2016: systematic analysis for the Global Burden of Disease Study 2016. BMJ. 2019;364:194.

National Institute for Health and Clinical Excellence (NICE). Developing NICE guidelines: the manual. London: National Institute for Health and Clinical Excellence; 2014.

Petticrew M, Roberts H. Systematic reviews in the social sciences: a practical guide. Malden, MA: Blackwell Publishing; 2006.

Scottish Intercollegiate Guidelines Network. Methodology checklist 3: cohort studies. Scottish Intercollegiate Guidelines Network: Scotland, Edinburgh; 2012.

The Institute for Health Metrics and Evaluation (IHME). Available from http://www.healthdata.org/gbd/faq#What%20is%20an%20uncertainty%20interval? Accessed 06 Dec 2019.

Thomas PAD, Moons KGM, van Valkenhoef G, Orestis E, Hummel N, Rolf GHH, Johannes RB, on behalf of the GetReal Methods Review Group. Get real in individual participant data (IPD) meta-analysis: a review of the methodology. Res Synth Methods. 2015;6(4):293–309.

Uman LS. Systematic reviews and meta-analyses. J Can Acad Child Adolesc Psychiatry. 2011;20(1):57–9.

Willis BH, Quigley M. The assessment of the quality of reporting of meta-analyses in diagnostic research: a systematic review. BMC Med Res Methodol. 2011;11:163.

Woolf B. On estimating the relation between blood group and disease. Ann Hum Genet. 1955;19:251–3.

Chapter 13
The Future of Pharmacy Practice Research

Zaheer-Ud-Din Babar and Anna Birna Almarsdóttir

Abstract The chapter starts by outlining the current and future scenario related to pharmacy practice research. This chapter then sets the scene by discussing issues that are pertinent for practice research. These issues are changes in population demographics, changes in technology, the role of the pharmacy as an institution and consumer behaviour as well as changes in the pharmacy profession. It also outlines the major shifts in pharmacy practice research, which include interprofessional collaboration and teamwork with patients, describing and measuring outcomes of interventions as well as patients' cultural diversity. It concludes by drawing attention to methodologies that would be most commonly used in future pharmacy practice research. Some of the future methodological challenges could be the emergence of big and complex datasets, dealing with electronic health records and pharmacy practice researchers' adoption of a myriad of mixed methodologies. The Chapter also includes a conceptual model at the end.

13.1 Introduction

It is estimated that 81% of American adults take at least one medicine per week and one quarter of them take at least five (Slone Epidemiology Center at Boston University, 2005). Medicines continue to be the most common medical treatment offered to patients, and they contribute significantly to the healthcare budget (Babar and Susan, BMJ Open 4:e004415, 2014).

Around the globe, medicine use is changing with changing disease patterns and advances in technology and science (Kaplan et al., World Health Organization,

Z. Babar (✉)
Department of Pharmacy, School of Applied Sciences, University of Huddersfield, Huddersfield, UK
e-mail: z.babar@hud.ac.uk

A. Birna Almarsdóttir
Department of Pharmacy, Faculty of Health and Medical Sciences, University of Copenhagen, Copenhagen, Denmark

© Springer Nature Singapore Pte Ltd. 2020
Z. Babar (ed.), *Pharmacy Practice Research Methods*,
https://doi.org/10.1007/978-981-15-2993-1_13

Geneva, 2013). However, the less than optimal use of medicines commonly results in poor health outcomes and unnecessary cost. The traditional roles of dispensing, distribution and administration fall under the umbrella of pharmacy practice, but so too does the optimal use of medicines and the activity associated with this. This chapter discusses the current state of pharmacy practice and the associated research in this field. In addition, there is a focus on the methods being used, the context and likely content of future practice research and the potential policy implications of such research. The key drivers of change that will influence the field of pharmacy practice research include (1) population demographics, (2) technology (informatics and health/pharmaceutical/device technologies), (3) pharmacy as 'institution' and as 'profession', (4) consumers of healthcare services and (5) new research capabilities building on technological changes. These drivers of change for pharmacy practice research are considered here, and four plausible shifts that are likely to emerge in the coming decades are argued.

13.2   Population Demographics

According to official United Nations (UN) population estimates, the world population of 7.7 billion will increase to 8.5 billion in 2030 and will further increase to 9.7 billion in 2050 and 10.9 billion in the year 2100 (United Nations 2019).

The population increase between now and 2050 is expected to come from developing countries. The increase is projected to take place in high-fertility countries, mainly sub-Saharan African countries. By contrast, the population of the more developed regions is expected to change minimally or even shrink between 2019 and 2050 because of sustained low levels of fertility and, in some places, high rates of emigration. In 2018, for the first time in history, persons aged 65 years or over worldwide outnumbered children under age 5. Projections indicate that by 2050 there will be more than twice as many persons above 65 as children under 5. By 2050, the number of persons aged 65 years or over globally will also surpass the number of adolescents and youth aged 15–24 years (United Nations 2019).

Global demographic change encompasses far more than declining fertility and an ageing population. Social and human capital is far more mobile than it once was. Immigration has resulted in multicultural populations in most developed countries (Kymlicka 2010). For example, in the USA, 321 different languages are spoken. By 2050, current racial and ethnic minorities will constitute 50% of the total population of the USA (US Census Bureau 2014).

Health disparities among these populations are of particular concern (Ling et al. 2008), and it will be important to think about how these demographic changes will affect medicine use, health, disease and public policy. This demographic change will be coupled with technological shifts alongside an ageing population living with long-term conditions. Together, these issues will have considerable influence on pharmacy practice activities and the optimal use of medicines (Babar et al. 2014). As such, a proactive research agenda that focuses on these challenges is warranted.

The process of globalisation has led to an increasingly interconnected world, with both benefits and costs to the health sector. The speed and ease of shared information, advancements to healthcare delivery and health policy and the increased pace of discovery through international research collaborations can all facilitate improvements to population health. At the same time, a significant increase in international travel forges the spread of communicable diseases, for example, the 2003 epidemic of severe acute respiratory syndrome (SARS) and the growth of antibiotic-resistant pneumococcus species. Health priorities, for which the supply and use of medicines is often central, must increasingly be viewed from a global perspective (Murdan et al. 2014).

13.3   Technology

The traditional model of community pharmacy is being challenged, and technology is the largest driver of change in pharmacy practice. The increased use of technology includes automation (robotics), e-prescribing, e-communication, integrated patient records, electronic health monitoring and internet retailing. These technological advances impact on how patients and consumers are accessing and using pharmacy services and medicines (Smith et al. 2013). Robotics and electronic prescribing are reshaping the dispensing of medicines, and this has the potential to release pharmacists to undertake more patient-centred care (Smith et al. 2013). However, the pace of technological development varies among countries. For example, dispensing with robots has become widespread within hospital pharmacy and in community pharmacy in some countries such as the Netherlands when compared with the UK.

There is already increased availability of diagnostics (among these pharmacogenomics tests) and electronic health monitoring devices either as stand-alone or as part of smart phones. This means that consumers are now in a position to be more aware of their health status. Companies like Google and Apple have developed new applications, tools and devices whereby consumers are much more aware of their health status and will be able to store their electronic health record (EHR). This technological development means that consumers are already more aware of disease states and medications, and as a result, pharmacists need to remain current with skill sets and knowledge. This also introduces important data streams that are already tapped into by commercial enterprises, but researchers in pharmacy practice need to be prepared to tap into.

Use of the internet to supply pharmaceuticals is also becoming more common, for example, through established networks such as Amazon. It is even possible that such players may take over the bulk of standardised dosage form medicine distribution. Pharmacogenomic tests are becoming available to patients, which pushes the industry and pharmacists to deliver medicines and services that can take this information into account for each individual patient (The Medical Futurist 2016). There are currently advances being made in printing of medicines (the so-called pharmacoprinting and 3D printing) that tailors specific treatment regimens to each patient's needs and lifestyle (Kaae et al. 2018). It is not certain how this new technology will be handled in the healthcare and community pharmacy sectors, and there are a number of scenarios being proposed; it could be envisioned that pharmacies would receive the 'blueprint' prescription for the personalised medicine for each patient from the doctor and then print the doses for the patient using chemical 'ink' (Kaae et al. 2018; Gayomali 2013). In this manner active components, excipients and dosages can be tailored to the specific needs of the individual (Gayomali 2013). Artificial intelligence (AI) is making inroads into healthcare, and this impacts pharmacy practice in at least three ways: first, medicines will become more tailored to individual needs as AI is able to work on the data being collected about each individual patient to come up with solutions for their medical needs; second, AI may overtake many of the roles of information provision by humans; last, AI will impact the training and education of health professionals, among these pharmacists and pharmacy technicians.

Developments such as these already are changing and are further expected to revolutionise the face of healthcare and pharmacy practice and the research underpinning it. With this in mind, the future research agenda must align with addressing these influences and challenges.

13.4   Role of Pharmacy as 'Institution' and 'Profession'

13.4.1 Community Pharmacy as 'Institution'

With over 40,000 registered pharmacists in England alone, pharmacy is the third largest health profession after medicine and nursing. Internationally, health systems are increasingly recognising the role of pharmaceutical care and community pharmacy (Scottish Government 2013; Pharmaceutical Care 2012). As many health systems are under pressure due to shortages of funding and manpower, community pharmacy has a window of opportunity in many countries where they are the most accessible type of care.

In England community pharmacy is under pressure, as NHS funding for dispensing and other services is constrained, reimbursement of drug costs is diminishing, non-pharmaceutical sales are falling and the oversupply of pharmacies and pharmacists also contributes to this pressure (Health and Social Care Information Centre 2012). Internationally, this will only be reversed if pharmacies are able to create new extended roles based on patient-centred care and persuade funders to purchase services as part of wider programmes of public health, treatment of common ailments, care for people with long-term conditions and so forth (Smith et al. 2013).

However, much has been written about the role of pharmacy as an institution in society and the state of play—'where it is' and 'where it should be going'—community pharmacy seems to be marginalised in the health and social care system at local and national levels. Pharmacy is seen by others as an insular profession, busy with its own concerns and missing out on debates and decisions that other health and social care organisations are engaging with in the wider world of health policy (Smith et al. 2013; Lewis et al. 2014).

It is not clear to healthcare and social professionals, policymakers, patients and the population at large what is meant by the terms 'pharmaceutical care' and 'medicine optimisation'. Even within pharmacy itself, there is an alarming lack of consensus about these concepts and about which pharmacist services fall under them (Blöndal 2017). Consumers also have misconceptions about the role of pharmacists.

A 2008 consumer survey in the UK found that 43% of people would consider consulting a pharmacist for tests related to their long-term condition but that only 6% had actually done so (Which 2008). This raises very important questions about the actual availability and services that pharmacists can provide for patients, in comparison with the assertions often made about the potential of pharmacy to deliver such care (Smith et al. 2013).

The global picture of the 'place' of community pharmacy as an institution is also rather varied. In some parts of the world, pharmacy has been gaining a foothold, as is seen in the USA (Lewis et al. 2014). Conversely, relatively strong professional systems have been dismantled and restructured where pharmacy has moved to a more commercial identity, such as in some Nordic countries (Almarsdóttir and Traulsen 2009; Wisell et al. 2019). The question could be raised as to whether community pharmacies in their current form may disappear if only seen as commercial sellers of medicines and be replaced by mail order, robot technology and automatic delivery of medications. However, this grim picture of the future of community pharmacy may be offset by the fact that community pharmacists in some countries are increasingly being asked by burdened healthcare systems to take on new more patient care-oriented tasks such as vaccinations, adherence counselling and non-medical prescribing. This makes for new opportunities for research within pharmacy practice utilising the enormous data being generated about patient care both at the pharmacy and in other parts of the systems where patients may be treated.

In the coming decades, community pharmacies (as other healthcare institutions) will use more virtual reality and online consulting than ever before, fuelled by demand from new generations of patients who feel more comfortable with this means of communication. Distribution to the customers may be happening mostly by internet retailing, drones or kiosks (The Medical Futurist 2016). New remuneration and incentive systems will have to be proposed and devised for community pharmacies (Nagaria et al. 2019). This change in communication and remuneration opens up a fruitful avenue of pharmacy practice research.

13.4.2 The Pharmacy Profession

In line with the developments of pharmacy as 'institution', earlier research focused on the dual role of the community pharmacist as a business person, which was juxtaposed to that of a healthcare professional (Kronus 1975; Hindle and Cutting 2002). In this focus, their education, job content and satisfaction have been of interest. Deprofessionalisation and loss of autonomy to business have been important topics within this research. Researchers in Canada and Australia have suggested that despite increased efforts and important policy initiatives (Canadian Pharmacists Association 2008; The Fifth Community Pharmacy Agreement 2010), pharmacists themselves are the ultimate barriers to change (Rosenthal et al. 2010; Mak et al. 2011), whilst others believe that there needs to be a bigger emphasis on professional competency, enhanced leadership skills and a push towards organisational change

(Tsuyuki and Schindel 2008; Scahill et al. 2009). Each year, 84% of adults in England visit a pharmacy at least once, 78% of these attendances being for health-related reasons. Whilst medicine use reviews (MUR) and new medicine services for chronic illnesses are now widely available in pharmacies, some pharmacies are still not taking advantage of the opportunities afforded by these programmes to provide screening, diagnosis, advice, medicine support and public health services. There needs to be a significant change in this area, as the low preparedness of pharmacists indicates that research on pharmacists and how the world views them is not the most promising way forward. Instead, the research focus needs to shift to how patients, other healthcare professionals and pharmacists work together, i.e. to where and how clinical services are carried out, the outcomes of these services and how to best integrate pharmacists into the healthcare team through innovative care models. At the same time, the pharmacy profession has to adjust to new technology, such as robotics, AI and virtual modes of communication, and this brings an extra disruptive scenario that is important to study.

Another important dimension is that access differences between rural (and less privileged) areas and urban (more privileged) areas are increasing, so the pharmacists in order to serve remote areas will have to be a broader healthcare provider. The pharmacist—if placed in a remote area—will have a special place in a given community, know his or her 'patients' histories and provide basic care for their illnesses with appropriate medicines (The Medical Futurist 2016), which will make for important rural pharmacy practice research.

13.5   Role and Expectations of Consumers

The lay public is becoming more literate and better educated with more resources at their disposal than was the case 20–30 years ago. The literature dealing with trends in consumerism of healthcare defines the 'new consumer' as having the following characteristics: being information strong, information seeking, non-authoritarian and increasingly demanding (Winkler 1987; Herzlinger 1997; Traulsen and Noerreslet 2004).

One very important phenomenon is the baby boomers coming into retirement age (Barr 2014). As noted above, this demographic shift will put pressure on health-care systems and speed up the requirement for development of new models of care which are cost-effective, integrated and team based. The boomers' political prowess and sheer numbers will force pharmacy to adapt to this through monitoring care-fully what this group wants from pharmacy and the wider healthcare sector and how the cohort might influence the healthcare agenda. Digital health empowers these citizens and makes for a more equal partnership between patients and providers. Polypharmacy patients are a special group of the older generations and polypharmacy is still on the rise. This trend in healthcare has led to research into deprescribing taking off as field of interest within pharmacy practice. There are many viable research avenues related to this focus, such as how rapid technological and societal developments (i.e. patient empowerment and pharmacoprinting) will play with respect to deprescribing.

Another important and impactful phenomenon is the 'digtal natives', who are the younger generations born after the advent of the internet and cheap computing. These young people (as opposed to older generations) feel comfortable with internet-based communication, use their phones for a wide range of needs and do not find face-to-face interaction to be more natural than electronic as mode of communication. The baby boomers are of course also tech savvy and use IT, but they are also interested in physical consultation.

Social media is used by many (especially chronically ill) patients to garner support and empower them in relations to healthcare (Kingod 2018). One way of increasing empowerment is using augmented reality (AR) which gives more real-life and vivid information in order to learn about the patient's drugs, instead of the patient information leaflet that is very hard to understand by patients. In a broad sense, the asymmetry of information between healthcare professionals and patients is decreasing as a result of both technological advances and because the younger generations will find it more natural to be a partner in healthcare.

Medical normality, what is an illness and what should be treated with medicines and medical devices, is becoming ever more fluid (REF). This phenomenon appears in that lifestyle-related problems are being increasingly being treated with medicines. Conversely, some groups of patients are increasingly being treated by non-pharmaceutical means instead of medicines, i.e. for chronic pain.

13.6   New Horizons for Pharmacy Practice Research

As the institution and profession of pharmacy develops within the realm of rapidly changing healthcare technology, healthcare systems and patient populations, it faces future challenges and has to respond to these. This will mean four types of major shifts for research within pharmacy practice. Some of these shifts are well under way in many countries.

13.6.1   From Uniform Pharmacy Practice/Pharmacist Implemented Interventions to Cross-Disciplinary or Interprofessional Collaboration and Team Work with Patients

The opinion has been voiced that pharmacy practice research all too often has been aimed at evaluating narrowly focused pharmacy services and the world view of these (Almarsdottir et al. 2013). In addition, the challenges faced by healthcare systems are forcing providers and professionals to implement more large-scale team-based healthcare services. This is an opportunity for pharmacists to get involved and/or build on models of care that have been generated internationally. Smaller projects started by enthusiastic 'trail blazers' within pharmacy have often shown positive results, since these pioneer pharmacists have high motivation and sound connections within the community they work in. Making their models transferrable to a larger scale and different settings is the challenge facing both practitioners and researchers. Pharmacy practice researchers can play an important role, with their knowledge of pharmaceutical policy analysis and implementation research. As a consequence, increased emphasis has to be put on researchers being well versed in implementation science and action research. Action research and related research approaches inherently involve all pertinent stakeholders in projects and in implementing organisational changes to improve medicines use.

In order to get more recognised as important collaborators in interprofessional collaboration, pharmacy practice researchers will have to prepare to ally with researchers from disciplines outside mainstream health services research, such as anthropology, language psychology, innovation science, philosophy, education and rhetorics. These less 'orthodox' disciplines are becoming more recognised by funders as relevant and important research fields that will help understand and change the healthcare system. Pharmacy practice researchers have often worked without using social science theory and models, but it is of great importance when expanding the alliance to new disciplines to emphasise the theoretical underpinnings of the research. As an example, when working with pharmacist-general practitioner collaborative models, one should review already existing models that can explain how collaborations can be built and tested (Bardet et al. 2015).

13.6.2 From Describing and Measuring Outcomes of Interventions Towards Systematising and Understanding Implementation of Large-Scale Initiatives

Policymakers and administrators commission healthcare services and purchase specific clinical interventions. It will not suffice to plan an intervention without being able to demonstrate its value to purchasers, based on theoretical and empirical merits. Questions that need to be answered include:

- What does the intervention entail?
- Why are individual components of the intervention chosen?
- What is the long-term cost for the organisation?
- Is the intervention cost-effective to the organisation, the healthcare system or society?
- And what impact will interventions have on the way the organisation works?

There has been enough research into effects and outcomes carried out (Smith et al. 2013). What is required is a shift to focus on implementation research and how decision makers can be influenced to incorporate pharmacy in large-scale health services planning. Researchers will also need to follow the trend towards increased team work within healthcare and refrain from studying interventions undertaken by pharmacy in a vacuum.

Placing the patient at the centre of the system has been a weakness of pharmacy practice research which is focused on itself as a subject of study. Future pharmacy practice research will have to shift towards studying collaborative models, identifying problem areas and reaching consensus on systematised approaches. It will be even more important to listen to professions that pharmacists will collaborate with and to social and organisational scientists in order to avoid the programmes' failure due to unobserved negative attitudes. Clinical pharmacology is one of the most important disciplines to ally with in this respect (Burckart 2012). Similarly, healthcare authorities and their administrators may want to impress by implementing new services such as medication reviews but may omit setting up real outcome goals and institute process indicators that will not improve process. For example, an outcome measure of how many interventions the pharmacists suggest to GPs may actually be counterproductive and lead to both lower quality and alienation of doctors from the project. Researching successful collaborative approaches will be one of the most important strands in pharmacy practice in the future (see, for example, Snyder et al. 2010).

13.6.3 Patients Are Increasingly Culturally Diverse and Active Analysers and Decision Makers Who Use IT to Their Advantage

With the baby boomers ageing, there will be a domineering group of people expecting healthy ageing who involve many different approaches to prevention and life enhancement. They are more health literate, critical and information seeking than the generations before them, and they have a stronger voice in healthcare politics (Barr 2014). Younger generations also bring new ways of using healthcare and health information. This will impact all of healthcare research. On the pharmacy practice front, this will go hand in hand with demand for evidence for practising in a certain way. Why pharmacists do as they do will be questioned, just as for other healthcare professionals. This will mean that interventions need to be interpreted and founded not only in professional but in patient rationalities.

The trends reviewed regarding the ageing of the population constituting the baby boomers, coupled with fast-evolving IT decision support systems for patients and healthcare professionals, will mean that they have more (evidence-based) information about health and medicines ready at their fingertips which they are able to use due to their high level of health literacy and will show little or no submissiveness to authority, rather looking at health professionals as partners in their decisions about healthcare and lifestyle. This will make physicians, pharmacists and other healthcare professionals into 'guides/facilitators/advocates' and not all-knowing experts. Another important development is that insulated patient communities are emerging due to social media. These communities build on and amplify their own rationalities and are not open to incorporating healthcare information in their decision-making (Kingod 2018).

Practising pharmacists and their pharmacy researcher colleagues will have to adapt to this new reality by studying how they use the informatics available and how this information/informatics influences citizens. It will become even more imperative for pharmacists to maintain patient-centredness, since the patients of all ages who trust healthcare professions will require pharmacists to have a holistic view of them and be guides in their quest for good health.

Cultural differences—especially within countries with significant immigration—make for a burgeoning field of research within the pharmacy practice sector. This trend will be escalated as the empowered citizens are primarily a phenomenon of the inhabitants of industrialised developed countries. There will also be large minority groups within this part of the world who have recently immigrated and will need a totally different healthcare approach, due to less health and IT literacy.

13.6.4 Blurring of Boundaries Between What Has Been Termed Pharmacy Practice Research and Related Fields

Many researchers who classify themselves pharmacy practice researchers also work in departments that define their work as part of drug utilisation research (DUR), clinical pharmacy, pharmaceutical policy, health services research, health economics or social pharmacy. Some pharmacy practice researchers can even relate to having one or more of these as areas of expertise. As pressure increases to participate in large multidisciplinary research consortia, the relationship between those working in the fields of DUR, pharmacoepidemiology, social science theories and clinical pharmacy research will be expected to intensify and develop a common front towards the public. There is increased interest in the capacities for real-world data collection at pharmacies. This can be sold to interested parties, such as the pharmaceutical industry. This in turn will mean that the boundaries between pharmacy practice research and disciplines such as health economics, outcomes research, DUR and pharmacoepidemiology will be blurred. Other research areas such as pharmacogenetics and drug formulation—which have not traditionally been integrally connected with pharmacy practice research—may also increasingly be invited to 'enter this space' or may be a competence of many who define themselves as pharmacy practice researchers.

13.7 Future Uses of Methods in Pharmacy Practice Research

As demonstrated within previous chapters of this book, there are a wide variety of methods in use within pharmacy practice research. Historically, the research area has been characterised by being more inclusive of qualitative methods than related pharmaceutical subjects such as pharmacoepidemiology and drug utilisation research (DUR). One of the reasons for this has been noted as the inclusion of the patient/user perspective in pharmacy practice research. This is currently more fluid and changing, as being outlined in the chapter on pharmacoepidemiological methods in the book. These related fields are moving towards more breadth in methodological and design choices (Wettermark et al. 2016).

Another important development is the increased availability of 'big data' in many countries around the globe. Big data in healthcare refers to electronic health datasets so large and complex that they are difficult (or impossible) to manage with traditional software and/or hardware nor can they be easily managed with traditional or common data management tools and methods (Raghupathi and Raghupathi 2014). This development will increase the pressure on pharmacy practice researchers to be knowledgeable about the use of extensive datasets in understanding the patient/user perspective and in evaluating pharmacy practice-related healthcare initiatives. More breadth will be required of researchers within the field, although those involved in qualitative methodologies may also have to become savvier in using big secondary qualitative data.

Pharmacy practice researchers will increasingly be using new social science methods. Social sciences are increasingly crossing disciplinary boundaries in their use of methods. Examples of this are computer-assisted content analysis, simulating scenarios of how actors may behave, comparative scenario analysis of plausible futures and ever more use of case studies to identify holes in data collection and explaining outlier cases when using larger datasets. Examples of qualitative methods that are not entirely new, but will be used more in the future, are narratives, photovoice, netnography, praxiography, psycholinguistics and rhetorical analysis. Examples of quantitative methods that are not entirely new, but will increasingly be used in the future, are machine learning, data mining and language recognition. Other likely advances in already used methods are using avatars as interviewers and machine learning where there is improved syntax and language processing capabilities for text, audio and visual data. Due to the increased availability of time series and other real-world big datasets, there will be heightened possibilities of using natural experiments (also termed quasi-experiments). Forecasting based on these large datasets will become ever more relevant in order for pharmacy practice to survive in an ever faster changing environment.

Due to the expansion of techniques available and challenges faced, researchers will have to be able to use a larger palette of methods and be ready to use mixed methods. They will have to be even more knowledgeable about various designs and methods when working in teams of researchers who do not have the same educational background. Pharmacy practice researchers need to be clearer about who they are, where they sit on the epistemological spectrum and what special competences they bring to large-scale interdisciplinary projects.

Funders of research have views of what they want to achieve and how this should be evaluated. As key stakeholders, they are likely to require a broad healthcare services focus and be less likely to fund pharmacy-focused research. These projects are then often led and administered by social science-trained persons who make crucial decisions on funding. Therefore, pharmacy practice researchers will have to closely follow developments in methods and theories within the social sciences.

13.8   Futuristic Model of Pharmacy Practice

This model depicts multiple elements, and influencers that are likely to impact on the future of pharmacy practice. As can be seen from Fig. 13.1, there are various layers of this model showing how different factors transcend, interact and the overall impact they have on the future. The central core impacting on future is "medicines", "drugs", and "pharmaceuticals" and it's the core business of pharmacy. But the way medicines are "accessed" and "used" could impact on patient health outcomes. However, the current and future use of medicines largely depend on "workforce", "digital health" and "professional acceptance." These factors are important and they would impact on the future and the way pharmacy is practiced.

The outer layer to this is the "health", to which pharmacy and medicines are a fundamental part of health and a discussion is perhaps difficult about the future without having a broader health context into it. "Public policy", "consumers", "patients" and the "governments" sit on another vital layer outside to it. These are key players which would set the tone for a broader engagement with the future of health and ultimately towards the "future of pharmacy". The last layer outside is the "change". The change is permanent and there could be many external, internal, intrinsic and extrinsic factors continually forcing change.

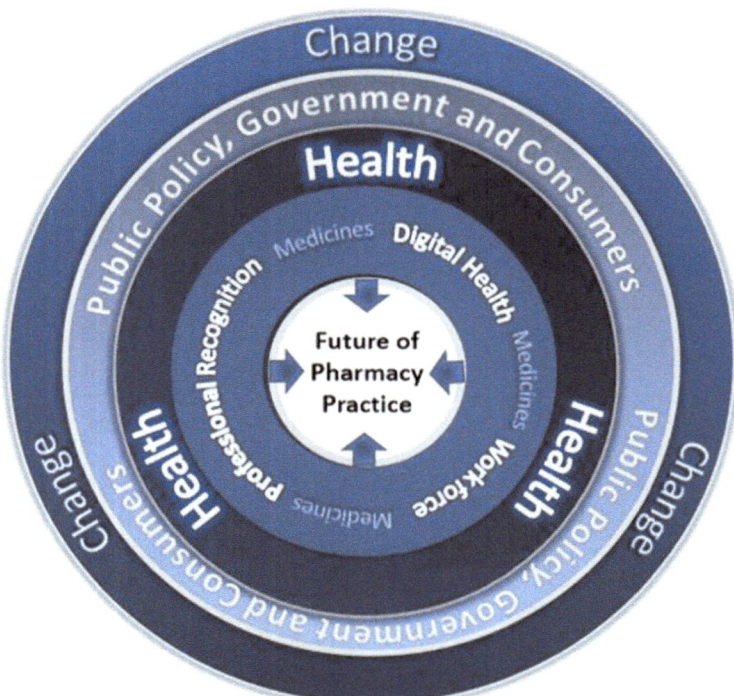

Fig. 13.1 The futuristic model of pharmacy practice

13.9 Summary

The chapter has outlined the changes in pharmacy practice research. The key drivers of change to influence pharmacy practice research are population parameters, changes in technology, consumers of healthcare services and new research capabilities building on technological changes. As the institution and profession of pharmacy develop within the realm of rapidly changing healthcare technology, it faces future challenges and has to respond to these. The growing focus on pharmacy practice research would include interprofessional collaboration and teamwork with patients, describing and measuring the outcomes of interventions as well as cultural diversity of patients. The future methodological development in pharmacy practice research would be the emergence of big data and dealing with large and complex electronic health records. Due to the expansion of techniques available and challenges faced, researchers will have to be able to use a larger palette of methods and be ready to use mixed methods. Also, as most research projects are often led and administered by social science researchers, pharmacy practice researchers will have to closely follow developments in methods and theories within the social sciences.

References

Almarsdottir AB, Kaae S, Traulsen JM. Opportunities and challenges in social pharmacy and pharmacy practice research. Res Social Adm Pharm. 2013;10(1):252–5.

Almarsdóttir AB, Traulsen JM. Multimethod research into policy changes in the pharmacy sector – the Nordic case. Res Social Adm Pharm. 2009;5(1):82–90.

Babar ZU, Gray A, Kiani A, Vogler S, Ballantyne P, Scahill S. The future of medicines use and access research: using the Journal of Pharmaceutical Policy and Practice as a platform for change. J Pharm Policy Pract. 2014;7:8. http://www.joppp.org/content/7/1/8

Babar Z-U-D, Susan F. Identifying priority medicines policy issues for New Zealand. BMJ Open. 2014;4(5):e004415.

Bardet JD, Vo TH, Bedouch P, Allenet B. Physicians and community pharmacists collaboration in primary care: a review of specific models. Res Soc Adm Pharm. 2015;11:602–22.

Barr P. The boomer challenge. Trustee. 2014;67:13–6.

Blöndal AB. Bringing pharmaceutical care to primary care in Iceland. Doctoral dissertation, University of Iceland. 2017.

Burckart GJ. Clinical pharmacology and clinical pharmacy: a marriage of necessity. Eur J Hosp Pharm. 2012;19:19–21.

Canadian Pharmacists Association. Blueprint for pharmacy: designing the future together. Ottawa, ON: Canadian Pharmacists Association; 2008. http://blueprintforpharmacy.ca/docs/pdfs/2011/05/11/BlueprintVision.pdf. Accessed 11 Nov 2014.

Gayomali C. Can you 3D print drugs? The week, 26 June. 2013. http://theweek.com/article/index/246091/can-you-3d-print-drugs.

Health and Social Care Information Centre. General pharmaceutical services in England: 2002–03 to 2011–12. 2012. www.hscic.gov.uk/searchcatalogue?productid¼4973 1&q¼title%3a%22gene ral+pharmaceutical+services%22&sort¼relevance&size¼10&page¼ #top.

Herzlinger RE. Market-driven health care: who wins, who loses in the transformation of America's largest service industry. New York: Addison–Wesley; 1997.

Hindle K, Cutting N. Can applied entrepreneurial education enhance job satisfaction and financial performance? An empirical investigation in the Australian Pharmacy Profession. J Small Bus Manag. 2002;40:162–7.

Kaae S, Lind JLM, Genina N, Kälvemark Sporrong S. Unintended consequences for patients of future personalized pharmacoprinting. Int J Clin Pharm. 2018;40:321–4.

Kaplan W, Wirtz VJ, Mantel-Teeuwisse A, Stolk P, Duthey B, Laing R. Priority medicines for Europe and the World: 2013 update. Geneva: World Health Organization; 2013.

Kingod N. The tinkering m-patient: co-constructing knowledge on how to live with type 1 diabetes through Facebook searching and sharing and offline tinkering with self-care. Health. 2018:1–17. https://doi.org/10.1177/1363459318800140.

Kronus CL. Occupational values, role orientations and work settings: the case of pharmacy. Socio Q. 1975;16:171–83.

Kymlicka W. The current state of multiculturalism in Canada and research themes on Canadian multiculturalism 2008–2010. 2010. http://www.cic.gc.ca/english/pdf/pub/multi-state.pdf.

Lewis NJW, Shimp LA, Rockafellow S, Tingen JM, Choe HM, Marcelino MA. The role of the pharmacist in patient-centered medical home practices: current perspectives. Integr Pharm Res Pract. 2014;3:29–38.

Ling AM, Panno NJ, Shader ME, Sobinsky RM, Whitehead HN, Hale KM. The evolving scope of pharmacy practice: perspectives from future pharmacists. 2008. http://www.pharmacy.ohiostate.edu/forms/outreach/intro-to-pharmacy/Evolving_Scope_of_Pharmacy_Practice.pdf.

Mak VSL, Clark A, Poulsen JH, et al. Pharmacists' awareness of Australia's health care reforms and their beliefs and attitudes about their current and future roles. Int J Pharm Pract. 2011;20(1):33–40.

Murdan S, Blum N, Francis SA, Slater E, Alem N, Munday M, Taylor J, Smith F. The global pharmacist. UCL School of Pharmacy. 2014. http://www.ioe.ac.uk/Global_Pharmacist_-_FINAL.PDF.

Nagaria RA, Hasan SS, Babar ZUD. Pharmacy, pharmaceuticals and public policy: solving the puzzle. Res Soc Adm Pharm. 2019; https://doi.org/10.1016/j.sapharm.2019.07.010.

Pharmaceutical Care. Policies and practices for a safer, more responsible and cost-effective health system. European Directorate for the Quality of Medicines & HealthCare. 2012. https://doi.org/EDQM.www.edqm.eu/en/pharmaceutical-care-1517.html.

Raghupathi W, Raghupathi V. Big data analytics in healthcare: promise and potential. Health Inform Sci Syst. 2014;2:3.

Rosenthal M, Austin Z, Tsuyuki RT. Are pharmacists the ultimate barrier to pharmacy practice change? CPJ. 2010;143(1):37–42.

Scahill SL, Harrison J, Sheridan J. The ABC of New Zealand's ten year vision for pharmacists: awareness, barriers and consultation. Int J Pharm Pract. 2009;17(3):135–42.

Scottish Government. Prescription for excellence: a vision and action plan for the right pharmaceutical care through integrated partnerships and innovation. Edinburgh: Scottish Government; 2013. www.scotland.gov.uk/publications/2013/09/3025.

Slone Epidemiology Center at Boston University. Patterns of medication use in the United States 2005: a report from the Slone Survey. 2005. http://www.bu.edu/slone/SloneSurvey/AnnualRpt/SloneSurveyWeb.Report2005.pdf. Accessed 23 June 2008.

Smith J, Picton C, Dayan M. Now or never: shaping pharmacy for the future, the report of the Commission on future models of care delivered through pharmacy November 2013. London: Royal Pharmaceutical Society of Great Britain; 2013. http://www.rpharms.com/promoting-pharmacy-pdfs/moc-report-full.pdf.

Snyder ME, Zillich AJ, Primack BA, Rice KR, McGivney MAS, Pringle JL, Smith RB. Exploring successful community pharmacist-physician collaborative working relationships using mixed methods. Res Social Adm Pharm. 2010;6(4):307–23.

The Fifth Community Pharmacy Agreement between the Commonwealth of Australia and the Pharmacy Guild of Australia. 2010. http://www.guild.org.au/docs/default-source/public-documents/tab%2D%2D-the-guild/Community-Pharmacy-Agreements/fifth-community-pharmacy-agreement.pdf. Accessed 11 Nov 2014.

The Medical Futurist. The bright future of pharmacies. Downloaded 29. 2016. July 2019 from: https://medicalfuturist.com/the-bright-future-of-pharmacies/.

Traulsen JM, Noerreslet M. The new consumer of medicine – the pharmacy technicians' perspective. Pharm World Sci. 2004;26:203–7.

Tsuyuki RT, Schindel TJ. Changing Pharmacy Practice: The Leadership Challenge. Canadian Pharmacists Journal / Revue Des Pharmaciens Du Canada, 2008;141(3):174–180. https://doi.org/10.3821/1913701X2008141174CPPTLC20CO2.

U.S. Census Bureau. Population projections, U.S. interim projections by age, sex, race, and Hispanic origin: 2000–2050. 2014. http://www.census.gov/ipc/www/usinterimproj/.

United Nations, Department of Economic and Social Affairs, Population Division. World population prospects 2019: highlights (ST/ESA/SER.A/423). 2019.

Wettermark B, Elseviers M, Almarsdottir AB, Andersen M, Benko R, Bennie M, Eriksson I, Godman B, Krska J, Poluzzi E, Taxis K, Vander Stichele R, Vlahovic-Palcevski V. Introduction to drug utilization research. In: Elseviers M, et al., editors. Drug utilization research: methods and applications. Chichester: Wiley-Blackwell; 2016. p. 3–12. ISBN: 978-1-118-94978-8.

Which. A test of your own medicine. Oct 2008. p. 12–15.

Winkler F. Consumerism in health care: beyond the supermarket model. Policy Polit. 1987;15(1):1–8.

Wisell K, Winblad U, Kälvemark Sporrong S. Diversity as salvation? – a comparison of the diversity rationale in the Swedish pharmacy ownership liberalization reform and the primary care choice reform. Health Policy. 2019;123:457. https://doi.org/10.1016/j.healthpol.2019.03.005.